Principles and Practice of Dermatology

Principles and Practice of Dermatology

Edited by **Heidi Mueller**

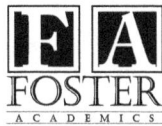

FOSTER ACADEMICS

New Jersey

Published by Foster Academics,
61 Van Reypen Street,
Jersey City, NJ 07306, USA
www.fosteracademics.com

Principles and Practice of Dermatology
Edited by Heidi Mueller

International Standard Book Number: 978-1-63242-456-3 (Hardback)

Printed in the United States of America.

Contents

Preface

Dermatology deals with the diagnosis and treatment of skin disorders. Skin is the largest organ of body and functions as a cover for internal organs. Due to this it is vulnerable to the damaging effects of pollutants, irritants, ultraviolet and infrared rays, pathogens, etc. It plays an important role in regulating the temperature of the body. The diseases treated under this field of medical science are fungal infections, dermatitis, psoriasis, skin cancer, warts, cold sores, ectopic eczema, etc. This book is compiled in such a manner, that it will provide in-depth knowledge about the theory and practice of dermatology. It is a valuable compilation of topics, ranging from the basic to the most complex advancements in the field of dermatology. It is a beneficial source of knowledge offering the readers new and valuable insights into this discipline. This book is an essential guide for dermatologists, academicians and those who wish to pursue this discipline further.

The information shared in this book is based on empirical researches made by veterans in this field of study. The elaborative information provided in this book will help the readers further their scope of knowledge leading to advancements in this field.

Finally, I would like to thank my fellow researchers who gave constructive feedback and my family members who supported me at every step of my research.

Editor

Evaluation of the Quantitative and Qualitative Alterations in the Fatty Acid Contents of the Sebum of Patients with Inflammatory Acne during Treatment with Systemic Lymecycline and/or Oral Fatty Acid Supplementation

Adilson Costa,[1,2] Aline Siqueira Talarico,[1] Carla de Oliveira Parra Duarte,[1]
Caroline Silva Pereira,[1] Ellem Tatiani de Souza Weimann,[1]
Lissa Sabino de Matos,[1] Livia Carolina Della Coletta,[1] Maria Carolina Fidelis,[1]
Thaísa Saddi Tannous,[1] and Cidia Vasconcellos[3]

[1] Service of Dermatology of the Pontifical Catholic University of Campinas, Campinas, SP, Brazil
[2] KOLderma Clinical Trials Institute, Campinas, SP, Brazil
[3] Department of Dermatology of the University of Sao Paulo, Sao Paulo, SP, Brazil

Correspondence should be addressed to Adilson Costa; adilson_costa@hotmail.com

Academic Editor: Lajos Kemeny

Background. Acne is a dermatosis that involves an altered sebum pattern. *Objectives.* (1) To evaluate if a treatment based on antibiotics (lymecycline) can alter fatty acids contents of the sebum of patients with acne; (2) to evaluate if oral supplementation of fatty acids can interfere with fatty acids contents of the sebum of patients with acne; (3) to evaluate if there is any interaction in fatty acids contents of the sebum of patients with acne when they use both antibiotics and oral supplementation of fatty acids. *Methods.* Forty-five male volunteers with inflammatory acne vulgaris were treated with 300 mg of lymecycline per day, with 540 mg of γ-linolenic acid, 1,200 mg of linoleic acid, and 510 mg of oleic acid per day, or with both regimens for 90 days. Every 30 days, a sample of sebum from the forehead was collected for fatty acids' chromatographic analysis. *Results.* Twelve fatty acids studied exhibited some kind of pattern changes during the study: C12:0, C14:0, C15:0, C16:1, C18:0, C18:1n9c+C18:1n9t, C18:2n6t, C18:3n6, C18:3n3, C20:1, C22:0, and C24:0. *Conclusions.* The daily administration of lymecycline and/or specific fatty acids may slightly influence some fatty acids levels present in the sebum of patients with inflammatory acne vulgaris.

1. Introduction

Acne is a chronic dermatosis that affects the pilosebaceous follicles. The physiopathogenesis of this condition involves periglandular dermal inflammation mechanisms, sebum hyperproduction, follicular hyperkeratosis, an increase of colonization of *Propionibacterium acnes* (*P. acnes*), and hormones [1–3]. We have observed that many of these pathogenic mechanisms are governed by a bio-immuno-molecular phenomenon that serves as the basis for research on and the future development of possible individual treatments for this dermatosis [4].

Fatty acids (FAs) constitute an essential part of corporeal lipids, especially FAs with chains composed of 12 to 24 carbons and 0 to 6 double bonds [5]. Essential fatty acids (EFAs) are FAs that the body is not capable of producing, such as linoleic acid (LA, 18:2n-6) and α-linolenic acid (ALA, 18:3n-3), which cannot be produced due to lack of Δ12- and Δ15-desaturases [5]. In the human body, EFAs are primarily found in phospholipids and in the triglycerides (TGs) which participate in sebum (SB) formation [6].

SB of patients with AV is different from those without this condition. One of the main characteristics is the lower concentration of LA, and this low AL concentration facilitates follicular hyperkeratosis [7–9], SB hyperproduction [3, 10, 11], and periglandular dermal inflammation [12]. LA is present in acyl-glycosyl ceramides; hence, it participates in the maintenance of the skin barrier [13]. If LA is absent from the SB, the integrity of the skin barrier is compromised, and the free fatty acids (FFAs) resulting from the hydrolysis of TGs by the lipases of *P. acnes* [14] act on the infundibular epithelium, causing hyperkeratosis and inflammation [3, 10, 11].

Antibiotics can alter the composition of the SB of patients with AV; tetracycline antibiotics are the most effective [15]. Lymecycline (LM; 150 mg–300 mg/day) is a semisynthetic derivative antibiotic of the tetracycline group [16, 17]. There are no reports in the literature about the influence of lymecycline on SB.

An example of the systemic use of EFAs to treat skin diseases is the treatment of atopic dermatitis, a skin condition that results in the disruption of the skin barrier [18, 19]. For individuals with AV, there are reports of clinical benefits with the use of EFAs [20–22], including the possibility of reducing the size of the sebaceous glands (SGs) [10]. There are no reports in the literature about the influence of EFAs on the FA composition of SB, nor is there any indication that EFAs can be used for the treatment of acne [23].

Given that the LM is a modern antibiotic used for the treatment of acne [16, 17], we conducted a study to evaluate the possible clinical improvements of this dermatosis after treatment with this antibiotic and how these improvements are related to the variation of the FA composition of SB. In addition, because SB is rich in FAs [24–26] and because past studies have shown that the levels of some FAs are altered in the SB of patients with AV [7–10, 12], we added a daily supplement composed of FAs present in SB to determine whether these FAs could individually interfere with and/or maximize the possible alterations caused by LM in these patients.

2. Methods

This study was approved by the Ethics Committees on Clinical Research of two universities and complied with all rules laid down by the Declaration of Helsinki. In this single-center, randomized, single-blind, parallel, and phase IV study, forty-five male volunteers with inflammatory AV (either papulopustular or cystic) were recruited from the Service of Dermatology of the Pontifitial Catholic University of Campinas (Campinas/SP, Brazil). Patients were between 12 and 40 years of age and had phototype I to VI (Fitzpatrick phototype scale).

These volunteers were divided (by previous statistical randomization using the method of numerical drawing) into three treatment groups of 15 individuals each and were treated with the following regimens for 90 consecutive days: Group 1: 300 mg/day of LM (Tetralysal, Galderma do Brasil Ltda., Ortolândia/SP, Brazil); Group 2: 540 mg of γ-linolenic acid, 1,200 mg of linoleic acid, and 510 mg of oleic acid per day (Tiliv L, borage seed oil (*Borago officinalis*), Arese Pharma Ltda., Valinhos/SP, Brazil); and Group 3: the combination of the treatments used for Groups 1 and 2. The products were ingested with water at lunchtime. This study was conducted between February and October 2011.

The volunteers analyzed on the first study day (D0) returned for monthly consultations for 90 days (D90) to provide samples of facial SB (for chromatographic analysis), to receive treatment products (except on D90), and to allow us to assess therapeutic adherence and side effects. Over all visits, the volunteers were instructed to refrain from washing their face for 12 hours prior to the clinical evaluation. They also remained in a room with temperature set at 21°C for 30 minutes prior to the collection of SB.

2.1. Obtaining SB Samples.
SB samples were obtained from a $32 \, cm^2$ area of the forehead through multiple swabbings with sterile cotton swabs intended for commercial hygienic use. The cotton balls were removed from the plastic shafts and soaked with 4 drops of n-hexane. These cotton balls were placed in 2 mL vials and stored for transportation at a temperature of 4°C.

2.2. Preparation of SB Samples.
The cotton balls were placed in a sterile Erlenmeyer flask, to which were added 10 mL of methanolic KOH at 0.5 N and 8 glass beads. The flask was placed in a condenser that, after the heating-cooling-ebullition cycles were complete, was washed with 15 mL of sterilizing solution (3.8 g of ammonium chloride 99.5%, 115 mL of methanol, and 6 mL of concentrated sulfuric acid); another heating-ebullition cycle was performed. After 10 minutes, the Erlenmeyer flask was cooled with ice for 10 minutes. This condensed liquid was placed in 10 mL of n-hexane and was then shaken for 90 seconds. Finally, 2 mL was used for the chromatographic analysis.

2.3. Chromatographic Analysis Method.
Gas chromatography was performed with a flame ionization detector (GC 7890 A, Agilent Technologies Brasil Ltda., Barueri/SP, Brazil) (GC-DIC) and an HP-Innowax polyethylene glycol column (length: 30 m; internal diameter: 0.25 mm; depth of stationary phase: 0.25 μm) that was calibrated for analysis using polyethylene glycol at a dilution of 1 : 20. AFA standard was used (47885-U/602-004-00-3, Supelco 37 Component FAME Mix, Sigma-Aldrich Brasil Ltda., Sao Paulo/SP, Brazil), and a separate standard was used for squalene (S3626/111-02-4, Squalene, Sigma-Aldrich Brasil Ltda., Sao Paulo/SP, Brazil). The FAs analyzed and their respective retention times (RT) are presented in Figure 1.

After 45 minutes, the amount of each of the FA was obtained in milli-absorbance units (mAU) (Figure 1), and these values were converted into percentages in the sample. It should be noted that the first peak was for the solvent (n-hexane).

2.4. Statistical Methods.
A significance level of 5% was used. The aim of this study was to evaluate the two different factors used in this study, groups and visits, and the differences were tested by two-way analysis of variance (ANOVA) with repeated measures. The Huynh-Feldt correction was used to determine any differences in the percentages of the various FAs in the SB.

Fatty acids	Retention times (minutes)	Fatty acids	Retention times (minutes)	Fatty acids	Retention times (minutes)	Fatty acids	Retention times (minutes)	Fatty acids	Retention times (minutes)
C4:0	1.75	C14:0	16.07	C17:1	23.58	C20:0	29.22	C20:5n3	33.29
C6:0	2.17	C14:1	16.95	C18:0	25.18	C20:1	29.6	C22:0	33.66
C8:0	3.33	C15:0	18.45	C18:1n9c+ C18:1n9t	25.58	C20:2	30.55	C22:1n9	34.23
C10:0	6.34	C15:1	19.34	C18:2n6c	26.53	C20:3n6	31.13	C22:2	35.73
C11:0	8.59	C16:0	20.81	C18:2n6t	26.63	C21:0	31.21	C23:0	36.71
C12:0	11.06	C16:1	21.37	C18:3n6	27.17	C20:3n3	31.65	C24:0	40.69
C13:0	13.57	C17:0	23.02	C18:3n3	27.86	C20:4n6	32	Squalene $(C_{30}H_{50})$	41.66

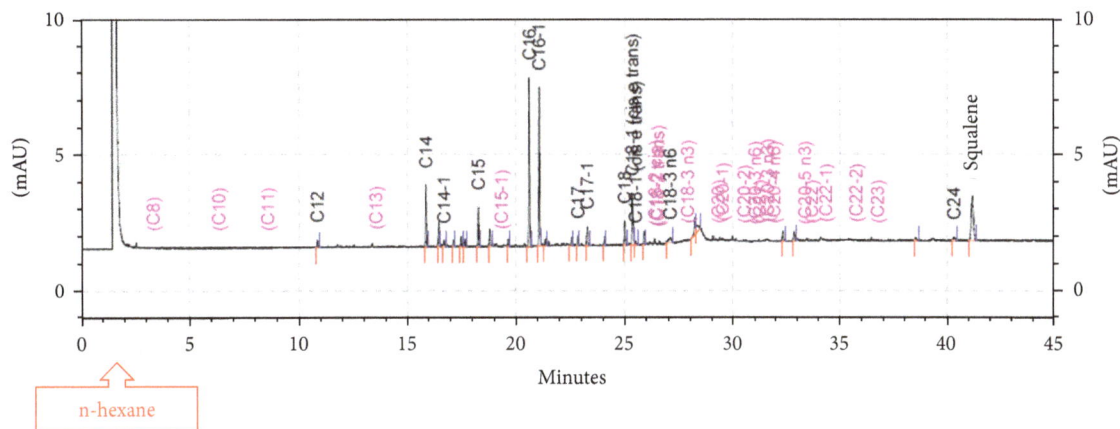

FIGURE 1: Evaluated fatty acids, their respective retention times, and example of chromatographic result graphic.

3. Results

For the differences that were statistically significant, Bonferroni's correction for multiple comparisons was used to identify the circumstance(s) under which such difference(s) occurred. The data were analyzed with STATA version 11.0, SPSS version 17.0, and SAS version 8.0.

Five volunteers (11.1%) did not complete the study for personal reasons. No side effects were observed in any of the groups. The characteristics of the volunteers who completed the study were as follows: average age = 18.3 years; AV grade II = 82.5% ($n = 33$) and III = 17.5% ($n = 7$); phototype I = 22.5% ($n = 9$), II = 27.5% ($n = 11$), and III = 50% ($n = 20$); and the average duration of AV = 5.8 years. For all groups, all volunteers ingested the complete dosage of the products throughout the study. The groups did not differ significantly with respect to age ($P = 0.626$), acne grade ($P = 0.327$), phototype ($P = 0.548$), or duration of the disease ($P = 0.959$).

Only the SB of those volunteers who completed the study ($n = 40$) was evaluated because the five volunteers who did not complete the study did not differ from the others. The content of the SB was analyzed, and 20.54% of the FA peaks obtained were not detected in the commercially used fatty acid standard (their amounts were under than 0.1%). C4:0, C6:0, C8:0, C10:0, C11:0, C20:3n6, and C20:4n6 FAs were not

found at any time during the study in any of the groups. The average FA composition found on D0 is presented in Table 1.

Table 2 contains a summary of changes in the FAs of the study participants determined using GC-DIC. It should be noted that no statistically significant changes were observed in the squalene pattern during the study for any of the groups (Table 3).

After the descriptive analysis, a two-way ANOVA with repeated measures was performed (Tables 4(a) and 4(b)) to compare the two different factors observed in this study: groups and visits.

Twelve of the FAs evaluated in this study showed significant changes in their contents in the SB based either on the groups and/or over the course of the visits (Figure 2). C18:1n9c+C18:1n9t showed differences only among the groups and not over the course of the visits; C14:0, C15:0, C16:1, C18:0, C18:2n6t; C18:3n6, C18:3n3; C20:1, C22:0, and C24:0 showed differences only over the course of the visits (Tables 4(a) and 4(b)). C12:0 showed differences both among the groups and over the course of the visits (Tables 4(a) and 5). This pattern was observed in all three of the groups under evaluation. During the study, C12:0 presented a higher concentration in Group 3 compared with Group 2 ($P = 0.035$), and Group 2 presented a higher concentration of C18:1n9c+C18:1n9t compared with Group 1 ($P = 0.024$) (Table 5).

TABLE 1: Distribution of patients with acne vulgaris according to the outcome of gas chromatography carried out on D0.

Fatty acid	n = 40	
	Average% (standard deviation)	Median% (min.–max.)
C12:0	0.32 (0.44)	0 (0.00–1.39)
C13:0	0.02 (0.08)	0 (0.00–0.45)
C14:0	5.79 (1.85)	5.94 (1.22–10.38)
C14:1	0.33 (0.41)	0 (0.00–1.16)
C15:0	3.77 (1.11)	3.97 (0.88–5.45)
C15:1	0.01 (0.05)	0 (0.00–0.34)
C16:0	17.92 (5.31)	17.66 (4.83–29.25)
C16:1	15.63 (4.86)	16.73 (2.83–24.92)
C17:0	0.69 (0.57)	0.87 (0.00–1.59)
C17:1	2.23 (0.93)	2.36 (0.00–4.82)
C18:0	3.74 (1.27)	3.50 (1.77–6.62)
C18:1n9c+C18:1n9t	9.50 (2.59)	9.83 (3.33–15.30)
C18:2n6c	0.32 (0.51)	0 (0.00–1.80)
C18:2n6t	0.53 (1.26)	0 (0.00–5.45)
C18:2n6c+C18:2n6t	0.85 (1.31)	0 (0.00–5.45)
C18:3n6	0.20 (0.73)	0 (0.00–3.27)
C18:3n3	0.52 (1.29)	0 (0.00–4.44)
C20:0	1.62 (5.09)	0 (0.00–26.83)
C20:1	1.78 (4.71)	0 (0.00–22.09)
C20:2	0.12 (0.79)	0 (0.00–4.99)
C21:0	0.02 (0.10)	0 (0.00–0.66)
C20:5n3	0.12 (0.75)	0 (0.00–4.74)
C22:0	0.52 (1.47)	0 (0.00–6.35)
C22:1n9	0.14 (0.69)	0 (0.00–4.30)
C24:0	0.27 (0.47)	0 (0.00–1.42)
Squalene	13.34 (4.91)	12.88 (2.88–23.15)
Total identified	79.46 (14.42)	84.44 (40.44–100)

Alterations in sebum patterns were observed throughout the treatments for eleven FAs in all three of the groups: C12:0 ($P = 0.014$), C14:0 ($P = 0.031$), C15:0 ($P = 0.025$), C16:1 ($P < 0.001$), C18:0 ($P = 0.041$), C18:2n6t ($P = 0.021$), C18:3n6 ($P = 0.009$), C18:3n3 ($P = 0.011$), C20:1 ($P = 0.023$), C22:0 ($P = 0.032$), and C24:0 ($P = 0.042$).

Some FAs showed an increase in their amounts during specific visits: C12:0, from D0 to D30 and from D0 to D60 ($P = 0.041$ and $P = 0.031$, resp.); C14:0, from D30 to D90 ($P = 0.007$); C15:0, from D30 to D90 ($P = 0.006$); C16:1, from D0, D30, and D60 to D90 ($P = 0.003$, $P < 0.001$ and $P = 0.005$, resp.); C18:3n6, from D0 to D60 ($P = 0.037$); C24:0, from D0 to D30 ($P = 0.026$) (Tables 4(a) and 4(b)). However, a decrease in C18:3n6 was observed for all three of the groups from D60 to D90 ($P = 0.042$) (Tables 4(a)

and 4(b)). Nevertheless, C18:0, C18:2n6t, C18:3n3, C20:1, and C22:0 had statistically significant changes on at least one visit for all three of the groups, but it was not possible to identify when the change occurred (Tables 4(a) and 4(b)).

4. Discussion

FAs form the lipids in SB [24–26]. On the face of an adult with regular skin, the FAs with the highest concentrations in the SB are, in decreasing order, C16:0, C18:1, C16:1+C18:2, C14:0, and C18:0. The C18:1, C18:2, and C16:1 FAs are more commonly found in the T-zone (the space including the forehead, nose, and chin), whereas C18:0 is found in the U-zone (the remainder of the face, surrounding the T-zone) [27].

In this study, neither lymecycline, nor FA supplementation were able to markedly influence FA levels in sebum. They slightly influenced the FAs levels in the patients with AV evaluated.

There are no reports in the published literature on the evaluation of the behavior of FAs in the SB of patients with acne who are being treated with an antibiotic regime based on LM.

A previous study evaluated supplementation with the same daily dose of oral FAs as that studied herein (for the same follow-up period of 90 days) in patients with AV and compared the use of FAs to the use of a placebo [10]. Despite the absence of differences in the level of clinical improvement of acne between the groups, there was a reduction in the volume of FAs at the end of the treatment with these FA, relative to the FA volumes in the placebo group observed in a histological analyses conducted by a Dermatophatologist. These findings suggest that there are possible clinical benefits from the use of these products that can be maximized by adjusting the dosage or treatment duration [10].

On D0, the FAs that were present at higher than average concentrations in our volunteers' SB were C16:0 (17.92%), C16:1 (15.63%), squalene (13.34%), C18:1n9c+C18:1n9t (9.5%), C14:0 (5.79%), C15:0 (3.77%), C18:0 (3.74%), C17 (2.23%), C20:1 (1.78%), and C20:0 (1.62%). We noted that this SB has a composition different from that of regular skin [27] because the squalene, C15:0, C17:0, C20:1, and C20:0 were observed in the SB of these patients with AV, whereas C18:2 was not found.

Squalene is considered the principal lipid that is increased in the SB of patients with AV, and the production of squalene is performed directly by sebocytes [28–30]. The presence of squalene is a marker of the likelihood and severity of AV because this compound enhances the comedogenicity and proliferation of *P. acnes* [24–31].

On D0, the average squalene level was 13.34%, similar to that reported in the literature (10% to 20%); [31, 32] in patients without AV, the average squalene level is 15% [31]. This result does not support the findings of Kotani and Kusu, 2002 [27], who did not find squalene in the SB of their volunteers without AV. During the treatment of the different groups, the squalene concentration did not vary significantly, either between groups or between visits. There are several possible explanations for this result: (1) the synthesis of squalene in the SGs [29] is independent of external agents; (2) this lipid is a constant marker of the likelihood of AV [31], regardless of the

TABLE 2: Descriptive statistic of twelve fatty acids that presented changes during the study, based on group treatment and visits.

Fatty acid	Visit	Group 1 (n = 12)		Group 2 (n = 14)		Group 3 (n = 14)	
		Average (sd)	Median (min.–max.)	Average (sd)	Median (min.–max.)	Average (sd)	Median (min.–max.)
C12:0	D0	0.3 (0.4)	0.0 (0–0.9)	0.3 (0.4)	0.0 (0–1.4)	0.4 (0.5)	0.0 (0–1.2)
	D30	0.5 (0.4)	0.7 (0–0.9)	0.3 (0.4)	0.0 (0–0.9)	0.8 (0.3)	0.8 (0–1.4)
	D60	0.7 (0.4)	0.8 (0–1.1)	0.6 (0.7)	0.3 (0–2.1)	0.6 (0.5)	0.7 (0–1.7)
	D90	0.6 (0.5)	0.7 (0–1.3)	0.3 (0.4)	0.0 (0–1.0)	0.7 (0.4)	0.8 (0–1.1)
C14:0	D0	5.7 (2.2)	6.1 (1.2–9.4)	5.8 (1.8)	5.7 (3.4–10.4)	5.7 (1.7)	6.1 (1.5–7.3)
	D30	5.8 (1.0)	5.4 (4.7–7.8)	5.5 (0.7)	5.3 (4.5–6.8)	5.8 (1.2)	5.8 (3.3–7.9)
	D60	5.9 (1.4)	6.0 (2.9–7.7)	5.8 (1.4)	5.9 (2.6–8.0)	6.3 (1.4)	6.1 (4.5–10.4)
	D90	6.5 (1.0)	6.1 (5.0–8.2)	6.1 (1.3)	6.3 (2.9–8.3)	6.7 (1.3)	6.9 (4.9–8.7)
C15:0	D0	3.7 (1.3)	4.3 (0.9–5.1)	3.9 (1.1)	4.0 (1.9–5.5)	3.6 (1.0)	3.7 (1.0–4.7)
	D30	4.0 (0.6)	3.8 (3.1–5.4)	3.7 (0.6)	3.7 (2.9–5.4)	3.7 (0.7)	3.7 (1.9–4.8)
	D60	3.8 (0.9)	3.8 (2.0–4.8)	3.9 (0.7)	4.1 (2.1–4.8)	4.0 (0.9)	4.1 (2.8–6.3)
	D90	4.2 (0.6)	4.1 (3.4–5.5)	4.3 (0.7)	4.3 (2.2–5.4)	4.3 (0.7)	4.4 (2.8–5.2)
C16:1	D0	14.6 (5.3)	17.2 (2.8–18.3)	16.3 (4.4)	17.2 (8.6–24.9)	15.3 (4.5)	16.1 (3.5–21.1)
	D30	16.2 (3.2)	15.3 (12.5–21.4)	15.2 (1.7)	15.4 (12.4–17.9)	16.3 (3.1)	15.9 (8.9–20.9)
	D60	16.3 (4.2)	17.7 (8.0–21.2)	16.6 (3.9)	17.7 (7.1–21.0)	17.0 (2.5)	16.9 (12.3–22.1)
	D90	18.8 (3.4)	18.7 (13.2–25.1)	19.2 (3.4)	19.6 (12.2–25.1)	18.8 (3.4)	18.7 (13.2–25.1)
C18:0	D0	3.7 (1.4)	3.3 (1.8–6.6)	3.8 (1.3)	3.9 (2.3–6.5)	3.6 (1.1)	3.4 (2.5–6.0)
	D30	2.8 (0.6)	2.8 (1.9–4.2)	3.7 (1.5)	3.1 (2.1–8.0)	3.0 (0.8)	2.8 (2.2–5.2)
	D60	2.7 (0.5)	2.8 (1.9–3.5)	3.4 (1.1)	3.3 (1.9–5.3)	3.3 (1.1)	3.0 (2.2–5.4)
	D90	2.6 (0.8)	2.5 (1.9–5.0)	3.3 (1.5)	2.6 (1.7–6.4)	3.3 (0.9)	3.3 (2.0–5.4)
C18:1n9c+C18:1n9t	D0	8.5 (2.9)	8.8 (3.3–12.9)	10.2 (2.3)	10.7 (6.3–14.1)	9.6 (2.1)	9.8 (3.9–13.4)
	D30	8.2 (2.0)	8.0 (4.0–11.4)	9.7 (2.5)	9.2 (6.5–16.8)	9.2 (1.4)	9.0 (6.6–12.0)
	D60	8.3 (1.7)	8.0 (5.4–11.9)	9.4 (2.5)	9.6 (4.1–13.0)	9.7 (1.7)	9.7 (7.8–13.9)
	D90	8.3 (1.6)	7.9 (6.5–12.2)	9.2 (1.9)	8.9 (5.7–13.0)	9.6 (1.5)	9.5 (7.4–12.1)
C18:2n6t	D0	0.2 (0.3)	0.0 (0–0.8)	0.6 (0.6)	0.4 (0–1.8)	0.3 (0.5)	0.0 (0–1.3)
	D30	0.5 (0.5)	0.6 (0–1.3)	0.5 (0.7)	0.3 (0–2.4)	0.6 (0.3)	0.7 (0–1.1)
	D60	0.4 (0.5)	0.3 (0–1.1)	0.5 (0.5)	0.6 (0–1.4)	0.7 (0.6)	0.8 (0–2.3)
	D90	0.3 (0.4)	0.1 (0–1.2)	0.4 (1.0)	0.0 (0–3.6)	0.4 (0.6)	0.0 (0–1.9)
C18:3n6	D0	0.3 (0.9)	0.0 (0–3.3)	0.2 (0.8)	0.0 (0–3.0)	0.1 (0.4)	0.0 (0–1.7)
	D30	0.6 (1.1)	0.0 (0–3.7)	0.3 (0.6)	0.0 (0–1.8)	0.7 (1.5)	0.0 (0–5.5)
	D60	0.8 (1.8)	0.0 (0–6.2)	1.7 (2.5)	0.0 (0–8.2)	0.7 (0.9)	0.3 (0–2.3)
	D90	0.0 (0.1)	0.0 (0–0.5)	0.3 (0.9)	0.0 (0–3.1)	0.3 (0.7)	0.0 (0–2.1)
C18:3n3	D0	0.3 (1.1)	0.0 (0–3.9)	0.5 (1.3)	0.0 (0–4.5)	1.0 (1.7)	0.0 (0–4.4)
	D30	0.2 (0.7)	0.0 (0–2.6)	0.2 (0.8)	0.0 (0–3.1)	0.3 (1.1)	0.0 (0–3.9)
	D60	0.0 (0.0)	0.0 (0–0)	0.0 (0.0)	0.0 (0–0)	0.0 (0.0)	0.0 (0–0)
	D90	0.0 (0.0)	0.0 (0–0)	0.0 (0.0)	0.0 (0–0)	0.0 (0.1)	0.0 (0–0.4)
C20:1	D0	2.1 (5.6)	0.0 (0–19.4)	0.3 (1.1)	0.0 (0–4.2)	2.9 (5.9)	0.4 (0–22.1)
	D30	0.2 (0.7)	0.0 (0–2.4)	0.2 (0.8)	0.0 (0–3.1)	0.0 (0.0)	0.0 (0–0)
	D60	0.0 (0.1)	0.0 (0–0.5)	0.0 (0.0)	0.0 (0–0)	0.0 (0.0)	0.0 (0–0)
	D90	0.0 (0.0)	0.0 (0–0)	0.0 (0.0)	0.0 (0–0)	0.0 (0.0)	0.0 (0–0)
C22:0	D0	0.9 (1.9)	0.0 (0–6.4)	0.4 (1.2)	0.0 (0–4.5)	0.3 (1.3)	0.0 (0–4.8)
	D30	0.1 (0.3)	0.0 (0–0.9)	0.0 (0.0)	0.0 (0–0)	0.0 (0.2)	0.0 (0–0.6)
	D60	0.0 (0.0)	0.0 (0–0)	0.0 (0.0)	0.0 (0–0)	0.0 (0.1)	0.0 (0–0.4)
	D90	0.0 (0.0)	0.0 (0–0)	0.0 (0.0)	0.0 (0–0)	0.0 (0.0)	0.0 (0–0)
C24:0	D0	0.4 (0.5)	0.0 (0–1.3)	0.3 (0.4)	0.0 (0–1.0)	0.4 (0.6)	0.0 (0–1.4)
	D30	0.6 (0.5)	0.7 (0–1.6)	0.5 (0.4)	0.7 (0–1.0)	0.7 (0.6)	0.7 (0–1.8)
	D60	0.5 (0.6)	0.0 (0–1.4)	0.3 (0.4)	0.0 (0–1.0)	0.5 (0.6)	0.6 (0–1.6)
	D90	0.3 (0.4)	0.0 (0–0.9)	0.6 (0.5)	0.9 (0–1.2)	0.5 (0.5)	0.3 (0–1.7)

TABLE 3: Quantitative squalene variation during the study, based on group treatment and visit.

Fatty acid	Visit	Group 1 ($n = 12$)		Group 2 ($n = 14$)		Group 3 ($n = 14$)	
		Average (sd)	Median (min.–max.)	Average (sd)	Median (min.–max.)	Average (sd)	Median (min.–max.)
Squalene	D0	13.5 (6.0)	13.7 (3.0–23.2)	12.4 (4.1)	12.0 (5.3–20.3)	14.1 (4.9)	14.2 (2.9–20.9)
	D30	15.5 (3.5)	15.5 (9.9–21.1)	13.5 (4.0)	13.3 (4.5–21.9)	13.9 (3.7)	14.6 (6.9–19.0)
	D60	14.2 (4.1)	14.8 (7.6–19.6)	12.8 (2.8)	14.0 (7.9–16.1)	14.3 (4.3)	13.9 (7.3–25.0)
	D90	17.0 (3.2)	16.6 (13.0–24.1)	14.2 (3.2)	13.6 (8.1–19.1)	14.0 (6.0)	14.9 (1.4–23.0)

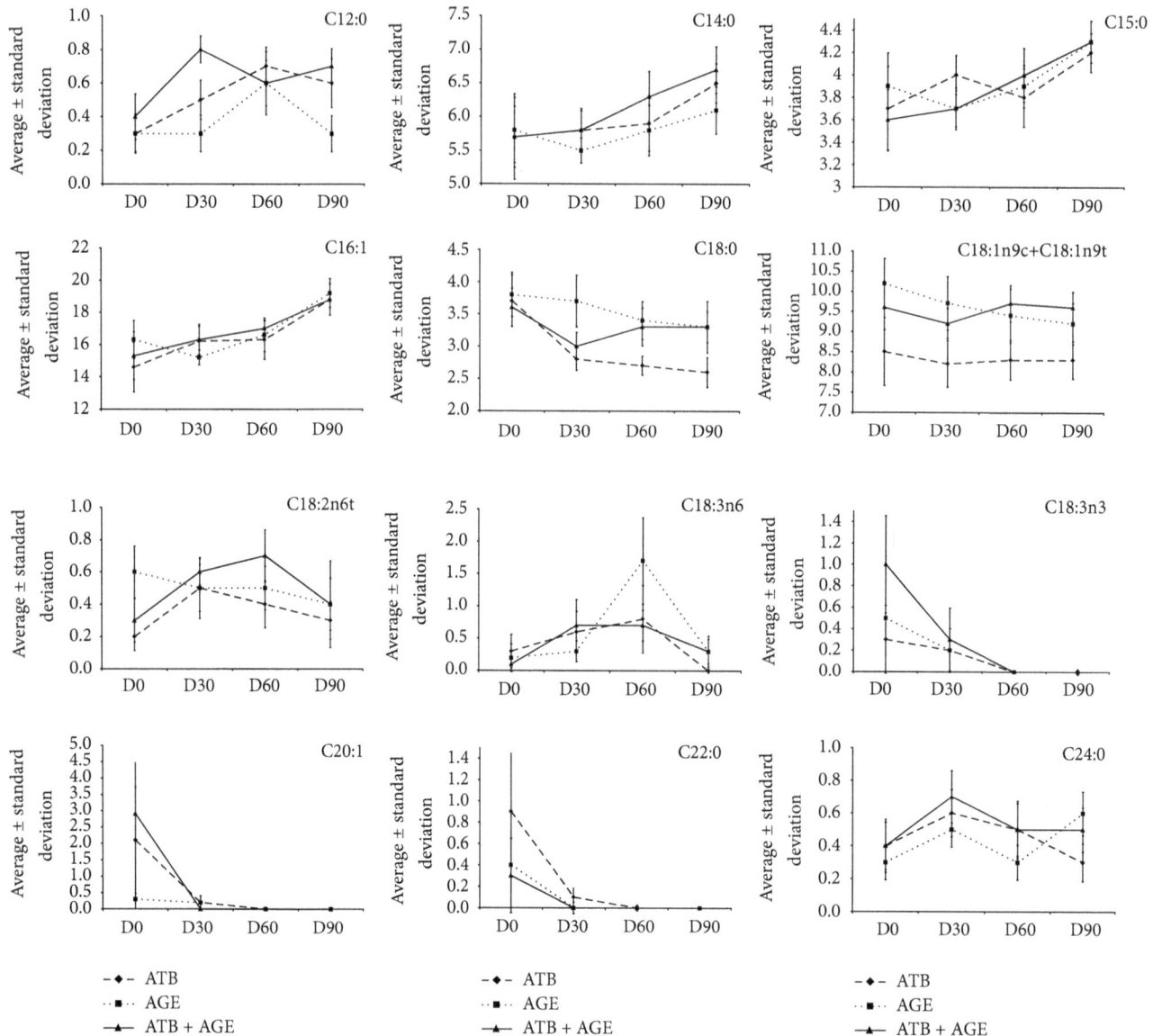

FIGURE 2: Graphic representation of fatty acids which showed differences in chromatographic pattern during the study.

action of antibiotics and EFAs, similar to the results obtained with the use of hormonal antiandrogens [33] but different from the results for treatment with oral isotretinoin, during which squalene disappears from the SB; [34] or (3) the hot climate of this region, which stimulates the hyperproduction of sebum [35, 36] and, consequently, of squalene [29], may have influenced the results. This information conflicts with the theory of Ikaraocha et al., 2004 [37].

The most common profile of irritant FAs consists of saturated FAs between C8 and C12 [38–40]. In our study population, we did not observe FAs smaller than C12. Throughout our study, we observed changes in the profile of the SB for some FAs with chains larger than those with this level of irritation.

C12:0 (lauric acid) is an FA with a medium chain length that has bactericidal activity against several infectious agents

TABLE 4: (a) Results of analysis of variances (ANOVAs) for every fatty acid from C12:0 to C18:2n6c+C18:2n6t, based on group treatment and visit. (b) Results of analysis of variances (ANOVAs) for every fatty acid from C18:3n6 to C24:0 (with squalene and total identified fatty acids), based on group treatment and visit.

(a)

Fatty acid	Factor	Degrees of freedom of numerator	Degrees of freedom of denominator	F-test	P value
C12:0	Group	2	37	3.578	**0.038**
	Visit	3	111	3.688	**0.014**
	Group * Visit	6	111	1.361	0.237
C13:0	Group	2	37	0.524	0.597
	Visit	2	86	0.851	0.445
	Group * Visit	5	86	1.525	0.195
C14:0	Group	2	37	0.422	0.659
	Visit	3	98	3.235	**0.031**
	Group * Visit	5	98	0.358	0.885
C14:1	Group	2	37	0.155	0.857
	Visit	2	86	0.154	0.885
	Group * Visit	5	86	0.745	0.582
C15:0	Group	2	37	0.033	0.967
	Visit	2	91	3.516	**0.025**
	Group * Visit	5	91	0.375	0.862
C15:1	Group	2	37	1.406	0.258
	Visit	1	40	1.161	0.292
	Group * Visit	2	40	1.103	0.345
C16:0	Group	2	37	2.270	0.117
	Visit	3	96	1.947	0.136
	Group * Visit	5	96	0.284	0.926
C16:1	Group	2	37	0.290	0.750
	Visit	3	93	7.596	**<0.001**
	Group * Visit	5	93	0.535	0.749
C17:0	Group	2	37	0.127	0.881
	Visit	3	102	1.599	0.198
	Group * Visit	6	102	0.416	0.853
C17:1	Group	2	37	0.264	0.769
	Visit	3	102	0.634	0.581
	Group * Visit	6	102	1.098	0.371
C18:0	Group	2	37	3.113	0.056
	Visit	3	105	2.905	**0.041**
	Group * Visit	6	105	0.578	0.739
C18:1n9c+C18:1n9t	Group	2	37	4.612	**0.016**
	Visit	3	111	0.439	0.725
	Group * Visit	6	111	0.284	0.944
C18:2n6c	Group	2	37	0.799	0.457
	Visit	3	111	2.004	0.118
	Group * Visit	6	111	0.553	0.767
C18:2n6t	Group	2	37	0.147	0.864
	Visit	1	42	5.401	**0.021**
	Group * Visit	2	42	0.328	0.749
C18:2n6c+C18:2n6t	Group	2	37	0.197	0.822
	Visit	2	70	2.229	0.118
	Group * Visit	4	70	0.569	0.677

(b)

Fatty acid	Factor	Degrees of freedom of numerator	Degrees of freedom of denominator	F-test	P value
C18:3n6	Group	2	37	0.377	0.689
	Visit	2	76	4.945	**0.009**
	Group * Visit	4	76	0.985	0.423
C18:3n3	Group	2	37	0.626	0.541
	Visit	2	67	5.118	**0.011**
	Group * Visit	4	67	0.634	0.625
C20:0	Group	2	37	0.178	0.838
	Visit	2	68	2.121	0.132
	Group * Visit	4	68	0.159	0.949
C20:1	Group	2	37	0.923	0.406
	Visit	1	40	5.392	**0.023**
	Group * Visit	2	40	1.099	0.347
C20:2	Group	2	37	0.925	0.406
	Visit	1	39	0.899	0.354
	Group * Visit	2	39	0.925	0.410
C21:0	Group	2	37	1.299	0.285
	Visit	2	67	0.334	0.697
	Group * Visit	4	67	0.402	0.789
C20:3n3	Group	2	37	0.029	0.971
	Visit	1	43	2.905	0.090
	Group * Visit	2	43	0.1	0.929
C20:5n3	Group	2	37	2.133	0.133
	Visit	1	41	2.168	0.147
	Group * Visit	2	41	2.550	0.085
C22:0	Group	2	37	0.535	0.590
	Visit	1	40	4.796	**0.032**
	Group * Visit	2	40	0.431	0.653
C22:1n9	Group	2	37	1.177	0.319
	Visit	2	79	0.322	0.739
	Group * Visit	4	79	1.145	0.343
C22:2	Group	2	37	1.002	0.377
	Visit	1	39	3.802	0.056
	Group * Visit	2	39	1.002	0.380
C23:0	Group	2	37	1.177	0.319
	Visit	1	39	1.239	0.275
	Group * Visit	2	39	1.177	0.321
C24:0	Group	2	37	0.254	0.777
	Visit	3	111	2.821	**0.042**
	Group * Visit	6	111	1.595	0.155
Squalene	Group	2	37	1.252	0.298
	Visit	3	99	1.761	0.165
	Group * Visit	5	99	0.704	0.631
Total identified	Group	2	37	1.548	0.226
	Visit	3	101	1.087	0.354
	Group * Visit	5	101	0.241	0.953

[41, 42], including *P. acnes, Staphylococcus aureus*, and *Streptococcus epidermidis* [43, 44], but no cytotoxicity to sebocytes [43, 45]. C12:0 is rarely found in the SB of healthy humans, with absolute rates of 1% to 2% [43, 46]. At all times during the treatment, a higher concentration of lauric acid was observed in Group 3 than in Group 2 ($P = 0.035$). Additionally, there were increases in the level of this FA in all groups between D0 and D30 ($P = 0.041$) and between D0 and D60 ($P = 0.031$).

TABLE 5: Multiple comparison method for C12:0 and C18:1n9c+C18:1n9t based on treatments.

Fatty acid	Comparison	Differences (estimated average)	Standard deviation	P value	95% Confidence interval
	Group 1 versus Group 2	0.174	0.109	0.361	(−0.100; 0.447)
C12:0	Group 1 versus Group 3	−0.105	0.109	>0.999	(−0.378; 0.169)
	Group 2 versus Group 3	−0.278	0.105	**0.035**	**(−0.541; −0.015)**
	Group 1 versus Group 2	−1.341	0.479	**0.024**	**(−2.543; −0.139)**
C18:1n9c+C18:1n9t	Group 1 versus Group 3	−1.200	0.479	0.051	(−2.402; 0.002)
	Group 2 versus Group 3	0.141	0.461	>0.999	(−1.014; 1.296)

C14:0 (myristic acid) represents 14% of the FFAs present in SB [27]. This FA has important antimicrobial against several bacteria (both Gram-positive and Gram-negative) and fungi [47]. The level of C14:0 in the SB of patients with AV included in this study was lower, perhaps because (1) it was diluted due to hyperseborrhea [8, 48], (2) it promoted a skin microenvironment prone to infection by *P. acnes* in individuals with AV, and [1–3] (3) the amount of this FA in SB decreases in age groups with higher incidences of AV [24]. We observed an increase in the myristic acid level in all groups from D30 to D90 ($P = 0.007$). This change could represent a bactericidal profile in the SB due to the use of the treatments studied in this clinical trial.

C15:0 (pentadecanoic acid) is an unusual FA found in human SB. The main source of C15:0 in humans is milk ingestion (human beings cannot synthetize C15:0 on their own), and it is stored in fatty tissues. C15:0 is an FA that is characteristically found as a constituent lipid in *P. acnes*. Our findings were different than those of Saino et al. (1976) [49], who suggested that it was possible to predict that an incremental increase in the amount of *P. acnes* could lead to worse acne lesions. Even in Groups 1 and 3 (which were treated with lymecycline), an increase in the C15:0 levels from D30 to D90 ($P = 0.006$) was observed, which could indicate that pentadecanoic acid is not an important constitutional element for this bacteria or that it is, in fact, a marker of unfeasible (devitalized) bacteria.

C16:1 (palmitoleic acid) is primarily observed in SB from the forehead and nose, and the amount of this FA decreases over time [27, 50]. C16:1 has antibacterial activity against nasal (*Pseudomonas aeruginosa*), skin (*Staphylococcus aureus*, *Streptococcus salivarius*, and *Fusobacterium nucleatum*), and oral bacteria (*Streptococcus mutans*, *Candida albicans*, *Aggregatibacter actinomycetemcomitans*, *Fusobacterium nucleatum*, and *Porphyromonas gingivalis*) but not against *P. acnes* [46, 51, 52]. The application of C16:1 to the skin of guinea pig disrupts the skin barrier, enabling the influx of Ca^{2+} into the interior of the keratinocytes, resulting in proliferation and comedogenesis [53, 54].

In healthy males, C16:1, when added by LA, represents 16.4% of the Fas in the SB [27]. In our work, the average concentration of C16:1 was 15.63% of the FAs. At the end of the study, we verified that there was an increase of the level of this FA in the SB of the volunteers of all groups between D0 and D90 ($P = 0.003$). There were also significant increases in the level of this FA between D30 and D90 ($P < 0.001$) and between D60 and D90 ($P = 0.005$).

C18:0 (stearic acid) acts to maintain the skin's pH and the integrity of the skin barrier [55]. It has no anti-inflammatory effect because it does not activate peroxisome proliferator activated receptor-α agonists (PPAR-α) [56]. FAs C18:0, C18:1, and C18:2 are closely linked to a rare skin cytosolic protein, epidermal fatty acid-binding protein (E-FABP), which is related to keratinocytic differentiation; C18:0 also participates in the synthesis of sphingolipids, which maintain the integrity of the epidermal membranes of keratinocytes and assist in the formation of ceramides [57–59]. In our volunteers, we verified that the average concentration of C18:0 was 3.74% which is lower than the 7.8% concentration found by Kotani and Kusu (2002) [27]. We observed that the concentration on at least one visit was statistically significantly different than the concentrations on the other visits in all three of the groups, but we could not identify at which visit this difference occurred.

C18:1n9c (oleic acid) has a concentration of 17% in normal human SB [27]. This FFA has bactericidal activity against methicillin-resistant *Staphylococcus aureus* [60]. It has been hypothesized that this FA may adhere to *P. acnes* in the interior of the pilosebaceous follicles, after action of the bacterial lipase [61]. The anti-*P. acnes* activity of this FA has already been explained by the ability of this FA to increase the β-defensin 2 expression by sebocytes [43, 62]. In addition, this FA decreases the *in vitro* expression of keratinocytic proinflammatory cytokines (TNF-α, I-L-8, and IL-1) and fibroblastic cytokines (IL-8) after UVB exposure [63, 64].

At high topical concentrations, C18:1n9c alters the skin barrier [65–70], which explains why the content of this FA is increased in the type-1 skin ceramides during the winter [71]. C18:1n9c alters the skin barrier because it increases the influx of Ca^{2+} into the keratinocytes [53, 72–74]. Elaidic acid (C18:1n9t) has an important effect on the extracellular matrix because it inhibits metalloproteinase-A (MMP-A) and MMP-B, which, respectively, degrade collagen and elastic fibers. In addition, C18:1n9t activates TGF-beta (a protector of collagen) and inhibits the activation of pro-MMP-3 by plasmin (which triggers the degradation of collagen) [75–77].

The combined detection of C18:1n9c+C18:1n9t occurs because the retention times for these two compounds in the GC-DIC analysis are similar. In our study, Group 2 exhibited a higher level of association of these FAs than Group 1 ($P = 0.024$). In addition, there was a trend of improved findings when FAs were used in combination with LM ($P = 0.051$).

C18:2n6t (LA) is an important EFA found on the skin that decreases with age (it is 40% lower in the elderly) [50].

LA is hyperconcentrated in the SB in AV, which is likely secondary to hyperseborrhea [8, 26, 78–80], leading to a scarcity of these ceramides in comedones [81]. Whenever there is a nutritional deficiency of LA and α-linolenic acid, these fatty acids are replaced with palmitoleic and oleic acids to form eicosatrienoic acids [82]. The proportion of LA in the SB of patients with AV is approximately 0.3% [7]; in our volunteers, however, its concentration was 0.85% when both the *cis* and *trans* forms were added together. In at least one visit, a statistically significant difference was found in the LA concentration in relation to the other visits, but it was not possible to identify when this difference occurred. Indeed, we cannot forget that SB alterations in this FA in SB are not unusual, which led us to suspect the following:

(1) the exogenous administration of supplemental LM and/or LA is not capable of altering the levels of this EFA in the SB because these levels are far lower than what is observed with the use of oral isotretinoin [34] or it association with cyproterone acetate or ethynylestradiol use, [83] which are treatments to reduce sebaceous excretion and to increase the proportion of the excretion that is sebaceous;

(2) the absorption of LA by the SG at the time of oral administration either does not occur or is not sustained over time. There are three potential mechanisms for this possibility: (1) 1,200 mg/day is not sufficient; (2) the LA produced in the SG is completely dependent on sebocytes for the synthesis of joined carbon fragments; or (3) for an effect to be observed, LA must be ingested for a period longer than the 90 days of this study;

(3) exogenous LA has the capacity to increase the synthesis of SB by the sebocytes by stimulating PPAR-δ, PPAR-α and *stearoyl-coenzyme A desaturase* [84–86], which leads to the dilution of the LA itself as well as of other FFAs of the SB [8, 26, 48, 78–80];

(4) the ingestion of high dosages of LA has an effect on the maintenance of the skin barrier, which is clinically expressed as a reduction in xerosis exclusively;

(5) the ingestion of LA causes the deposition of one of its desaturation/elongation subproducts in the skin and/or other organs, which has been observed in animal experiments (joint administration of LA and α-linolenic acid) [87];

(6) exogenously administered LA is directed to the replacement of C16:1n9 and C18:1n9 as needed to replenish them in cases of deficiency [82], thereby decreasing the availability of LA in the SB;

(7) administration of oleic and γ-linolenic acids together with LA may interfere with their absorption by the SG.

γ-linolenic acid (C18:3n6) is the first product of the intracorporeal saturation of LA [18, 19, 88]. There are no data in the scientific literature regarding the level of γ-linolenic acid in the SB of patients with AV. In our laboratory study, this FA was found at an average percentage of 0.2%. In animals, the ingestion of γ-linolenic acid triggers a reduction in epidermal hyperproliferation by stimulating ceramide production [89], thus maintaining the integrity of the skin barrier [90]. Perhaps, for this reason, γ-linolenic acid reduces the epidermal complications of radiotherapy [91]. In humans, the ingestion of γ- and α-linoleic acids reduces skin inflammation because these FAs decrease the production of PGE-2 by blood mononuclear cells and suppress proliferation [92, 93]. For these reasons, the topical use of γ-linolenic acid at 2.2% soothes uremic itching [94]. In our study, for all groups, the level of C18:3n6 in the SB decreased from D0 to D60 ($P = 0.037$) and from D60 to D90 ($P = 0.042$).

C18:3n3 (α-linoleic acid) is rarely found in the adipose tissues of mammals due to its rapid metabolism into docosahexaenoic acid and/or beta-oxidation to acetyl-CoA and CO_2 [95]. C18:3n3 is an EFA; thus, it must be obtained through food [5, 6, 13, 20, 21, 79, 80]. No information is available about its participation in the SB in either normal patients or in patients with AV. In our study population, the C18:3n3 concentration was 0.52%. Oral ingestion of C18:3n3 assists lymphocytic functioning [96], promotes an anti-inflammatory state [93, 97], inhibits coagulase-negative *Staphylococcus aureus* [98], and maintains the integrity of the skin barrier [90, 99, 100]. On at least one visit, a statistically significant difference was found in LA compared with the other visits, but it was not possible to identify when this difference occurred. Perhaps such a difference would occur in any treatment based on the inability of C18:3n3 to resist subsequent metabolic cycles [95].

C20:1 (gadoleic acid) is obtained through the ingestion of seeds (e.g., mustard seeds and hominy) and is likely derived from the action of elongases on oleic acid [101, 102]. Its concentration in human SB has not been described; in our study population, C20:1 was present at a low percentage (1.78%). On at least one visit, a statistically significant difference in LA was found in relation to the other visits, but it was not possible to identify when this difference occurred.

C22:0 (behenic acid) is poorly absorbed from food (only approximately 30%) and has low bioavailability; however, C22:0 is important for the formation of blood cholesterol [103]. It is deposited in brown fat [104] and also participates in the formation of ceramides [105]. The C22:0 concentration in human SB is not known, but in our study population, it was very scarce (approximately 0.5%). On at least one visit, a statistically significant difference was found in the C22:0 pattern in all three of the groups, but it was not possible to identify on which visit this difference occurred.

C24:0 (lignoceric acid) is an FA that is present in several tissues and in the skin. It is highly linked to fatty acid transport protein 4 (FATP4) in the corneum layer [106]. For this reason, it and other long-chain FAs (8 to 24 carbons) are important for the maintenance of the skin barrier [107]. Despite the important of these Fas, C24:0 was the most abundant among them but represented only 0.39% of the total Fas [108]. Therefore, during the winter, when xerosis is more evident, its concentration decreases [109]. In our findings, the C24:0 concentration was 0.27%, less than that reported in the literature [109]. There was no final difference in the concentrations of C24:0 in the SB of all three groups, but we verified that there was an increase in its percentage from D0 to D30 ($P = 0.026$).

5. Conclusions

In this study, we verified that both LM and oral FA supplementation based on linoleic, γ-linolenic, and oleic acids may slightly influence the FAs levels in the SB of individuals with AV. We concluded that (1) LM and oral FA supplementation based on linoleic, γ-linolenic, and oleic acids may alter the profiles of some FA in the SB of patients; (2) the concentration of squalene in the SB did not decrease in any experimental group; (3) the concentrations of C12:0, C14:0, and C16:1 increased in all three groups during the treatment period; (4) LM and/or the ingestion of LA did not increase the level of LA in the SB; and (5) the concentration of γ-linolenic acid increased during the first 60 days of treatment and decreased during the following 30 days of treatment with LM and/or oral FA supplementation. All these FA measurements for the considerable time of 90 days will be an important reference for similar works in the future.

Conflict of Interests

The authors declare that they have no conflict of interests.

Acknowledgments

Galderma do Brasil Ltda., Ortolândia/SP, Brazil, and Arese Pharma Ltda., Valinhos/SP, Brazil, donated Tetralysal and Tiliv L, respectively.

References

[1] M. H. Winston and A. R. Shalita, "Acne vulgaris: pathogenesis and treatment," *Pediatric Clinics of North America*, vol. 38, no. 4, pp. 889–903, 1991.

[2] K. M. Hassun, "Acne: etiopathogenesis," *Anais Brasileiros de Dermatologia*, vol. 75, no. 1, pp. 7–15, 2000.

[3] A. Costa, M. M. A. Alchorne, and M. C. B. Goldschmid, "Fatores etiopatogênicos da acne vulgar," *Anais Brasileiros de Dermatologia*, vol. 83, no. 5, pp. 451–459, 2008.

[4] I. Kurokawa, F. W. Danby, Q. Ju et al., "New developments in our understanding of acne pathogenesis and treatment," *Experimental Dermatology*, vol. 18, no. 10, pp. 821–832, 2009.

[5] E. Tvrzicka, L. S. Kremmyda, B. Stankova, and A. Zak, "Fatty acids as biocompounds: their role in human metabolism, health and disease—a review. Part 1: classification, dietary sources and biological functions," *Biomedical Papers*, vol. 155, no. 2, pp. 117–130, 2011.

[6] C. Prottey, "Essential fatty acids and the skin," *British Journal of Dermatology*, vol. 94, no. 5, pp. 579–587, 1976.

[7] A. M. Morello, D. T. Downing, and J. S. Strauss, "Octadecadienoic acids in the skin surface lipids of acne patients and normal subjects," *Journal of Investigative Dermatology*, vol. 66, no. 5, pp. 319–323, 1976.

[8] D. T. Downing, M. E. Stewart, P. W. Wertz, and J. S. Strauss, "Essential fatty acids and acne," *Journal of the American Academy of Dermatology*, vol. 14, no. 2, pp. 221–225, 1986.

[9] W. J. Cunliffe, D. B. Holland, S. M. Clark, and G. I. Stables, "Comedogenesis: some aetiological, clinical and therapeutic strategies," *Dermatology*, vol. 206, no. 1, pp. 11–16, 2003.

[10] A. Costa, M. Alchorne, N. Michalany, and H. Lima, "Acne vulgar: estudo piloto de avaliação do uso oral de ácidos graxos essenciais por meio de analises clínica, digital e histopatológica," *Anais Brasileiros de Dermatologia*, vol. 82, pp. 129–134, 2007.

[11] A. Costa, D. Lage, and T. A. Moises, "Acne e dieta: verdade ou mito?" *Anais Brasileiros de Dermatologia*, vol. 85, no. 3, pp. 346–353, 2010.

[12] A. H. T. Jeremy, D. B. Holland, S. G. Roberts, K. F. Thomson, and W. J. Cunliffe, "Inflammatory events are involved in acne lesion initiation," *Journal of Investigative Dermatology*, vol. 121, no. 1, pp. 20–27, 2003.

[13] P. Berbis, S. Hesse, and Y. Privat, "Acides gras essentiels et peau," *Allergy and Immunology*, vol. 22, no. 6, pp. 225–231, 1990.

[14] J. H. Cove, K. T. Holland, and W. J. Cunliffe, "An analysis of sebum excretion rate, bacterial population and the production rate of free fatty acids on human skin," *British Journal of Dermatology*, vol. 103, no. 4, pp. 383–386, 1980.

[15] G. M. Pablo and J. E. Fulton Jr., "Sebum: analysis by infrared spectroscopy. II. The suppression of fatty acids by systemically administered antibiotics," *Archives of Dermatology*, vol. 111, no. 6, pp. 734–735, 1975.

[16] H. Gollnick, W. Cunliffe, D. Berson et al., "Management of acne: a report from a global alliance to improve outcomes in acne," *Journal of the American Academy of Dermatology B*, vol. 49, supplement 1, pp. S1–S2, 2003.

[17] M. Ramos-e-Silva, A. Nogueira, C. Reis et al., "Brazilian acne consensus," *Expert Review of Dermatology*, vol. 1, no. 1, pp. 151–186, 2006.

[18] D. F. Horrobin, "Fatty acid metabolism in health and disease: the role of delta-6-desaturase," *American Journal of Clinical Nutrition*, vol. 57, supplement 5, pp. S732–S737, 1993.

[19] M. Andreassi, P. Forleo, A. Di Lorio, S. Masci, G. Abate, and P. Amerio, "Efficacy of γ-linolenic acid in the treatment of patients with atopic dermatitis," *Journal of International Medical Research*, vol. 25, no. 5, pp. 266–274, 1997.

[20] D. T. Downing, "The effect of sebum onepidermal lipid composition," in *Acne and Related Disorders: An International Symposium, Cardiff*, 1988.

[21] M. H. A. Rustin, "Dermatology," *Postgraduate Medical Journal*, vol. 66, no. 781, pp. 894–905, 1990.

[22] M. G. Rubin, K. Kim, and A. C. Logan, "Acne vulgaris, mental health and omega-3 fatty acids: a report of cases," *Lipids in Health and Disease*, vol. 7, article 36, 2008.

[23] D. Thiboutot, H. Gollnick, V. Bettoli et al., "New insights into the management of acne: an update from the Global Alliance to Improve Outcomes in Acne Group," *Journal of the American Academy of Dermatology*, vol. 60, supplement 5, pp. S1–S50, 2009.

[24] N. K. M. Nordstrom and W. C. Noble, "Application of computer taxonomic techniques to the study of cutaneous propionibacteria and skin-surface lipid," *Archives of Dermatological Research*, vol. 278, no. 2, pp. 107–113, 1985.

[25] L. F. U. Uribe, A. M. Cabezas, and M. T. C. Molina, "Glândulas sebáceas y acne," *Derematología*, vol. 2, no. 1, pp. 22–24, 1986.

[26] M. E. Stewart, W. A. Steele, and D. T. Downing, "Changes in the relative amounts of endogenous and exogenous fatty acids in sebaceous lipids during early adolescence," *Journal of Investigative Dermatology*, vol. 92, no. 3, pp. 371–378, 1989.

[27] A. Kotani and F. Kusu, "HPLC with electrochemical detection for determining the distribution of free fatty acids in skin surface lipids from the human face and scalp," *Archives of Dermatological Research*, vol. 294, no. 4, pp. 172–177, 2002.

[28] M. E. Stewart and D. T. Downing, "Chemistry and function of mammalian sebaceous lipids," in *Skin Lipids: Advances in Lipid Research*, P. M. Elias, Ed., vol. 24, pp. 263–302, Academic Press, San Diego, Calif, USA, 1991.

[29] J. A. Cotterill, W. J. Cunliffe, B. Williamson, and L. Bulusu, "Age and sex variation in skin surface lipid composition and sebum excretion rate," *British Journal of Dermatology*, vol. 87, no. 4, pp. 333–340, 1972.

[30] K. Ohsawa, T. Watanabe, and R. Matsukawa, "The possible role of squalene and its peroxide of the sebum in the occurrence of sunburn and protection from damage caused by U.V. irradiation," *Journal of Toxicological Sciences*, vol. 9, no. 2, pp. 151–159, 1984.

[31] A. Pappas, S. Johsen, J. C. Liu, and M. Eisinger, "Sebum analysis of individuals with and without acne," *Dermatoendocrinol*, vol. 1, no. 3, pp. 157–611, 2009.

[32] E. W. Powell and G. W. Beveridge, "Sebum excretion and sebum composition in adolescent men with and without acne vulgaris," *British Journal of Dermatology*, vol. 82, no. 3, pp. 243–249, 1970.

[33] S. Patel and W. C. Noble, "Analysis of human skin surface lipid during treatment with anti-androgens," *British Journal of Dermatology*, vol. 117, no. 6, pp. 735–740, 1987.

[34] J. S. Strauss, M. E. Stewart, and D. T. Downing, "The effect of 13-cis-retinoic acid on sebaceous glands," *Archives of Dermatology*, vol. 123, no. 11, pp. 1538–1541, 1987.

[35] W. J. Cunliffe, J. L. Burton, and S. Shuster, "The effect of local temperature variations on the sebum excretion rate," *British Journal of Dermatology*, vol. 83, no. 6, pp. 650–654, 1970.

[36] M. Williams, W. J. Cunliffe, and B. Williamson, "The effect of local temperature changes on sebum excretion rate and forehead surface lipid composition," *British Journal of Dermatology*, vol. 88, no. 3, pp. 257–262, 1973.

[37] C. I. Ikaraocha, G. O. L. Taylor, J. I. Anetor, and J. A. Onuegbu, "Pattern of skin surface lipids in some Southern-Western Nigerians with acne vulgaris," *West African Journal of Medicine*, vol. 23, no. 1, pp. 65–68, 2004.

[38] R. E. Kellum, "Acne vulgaris. Studies in pathogenesis: relative irritancy of free fatty acids from C_2 to C_{16}," *Archives of Dermatology*, vol. 97, no. 6, pp. 722–726, 1968.

[39] M. A. Stillman, H. I. Maibach, and A. R. Shalita, "Relative irritancy of free fatty acids of different chain length," *Contact Dermatitis*, vol. 1, no. 2, pp. 65–69, 1975.

[40] J. G. Voss, "Acne vulgaris and free fatty acids. A review and criticism," *Archives of Dermatology*, vol. 109, no. 6, pp. 894–898, 1974.

[41] G. Bergsson, J. Arnfinnsson, S. M. Karlsson, Ó. Steingrímsson, and H. Thormar, "In vitro inactivation of Chlamydia trachomatis by fatty acids and monoglycerides," *Antimicrobial Agents and Chemotherapy*, vol. 42, no. 9, pp. 2290–2294, 1998.

[42] C. B. Huang, Y. Alimova, T. M. Myers, and J. L. Ebersole, "Short- and medium-chain fatty acids exhibit antimicrobial activity for oral microorganisms," *Archives of Oral Biology*, vol. 56, no. 7, pp. 650–654, 2011.

[43] T. Nakatsuji, M. C. Kao, L. Zhang, C. C. Zouboulis, R. L. Gallo, and C. M. Huang, "Sebum free fatty acids enhance the innate immune defense of human sebocytes by upregulating β-defensin-2 expression," *Journal of Investigative Dermatology*, vol. 130, no. 4, pp. 985–994, 2010.

[44] A. Ruzin and R. P. Novick, "Equivalence of lauric acid and glycerol monolaurate as inhibitors of signal transduction in *Staphylococcus aureus*," *Journal of Bacteriology*, vol. 182, no. 9, pp. 2668–2671, 2000.

[45] S. M. Puhvel and R. M. Reisner, "Effect of fatty acids on the growth of Corynebacterium acnes in vitro," *Journal of Investigative Dermatology*, vol. 54, no. 1, pp. 48–52, 1970.

[46] J. J. Wille and A. Kydonieus, "Palmitoleic acid isomer (C16:1Δ6) in human skin sebum is effective against gram-positive bacteria," *Skin Pharmacology and Applied Skin Physiology*, vol. 16, no. 3, pp. 176–187, 2003.

[47] A. Hinton Jr. and K. D. Ingram, "Microbicidal activity of tripotassium phosphate and fatty acids toward spoilage and pathogenic bacteria associated with poultry," *Journal of Food Protection*, vol. 68, no. 7, pp. 1462–1466, 2005.

[48] M. E. Stewart and D. T. Downing, "Measurement of sebum secretion rates in young children," *Journal of Investigative Dermatology*, vol. 84, no. 1, pp. 59–61, 1985.

[49] Y. Saino, J. Eda, and T. Nagoya, "Anaerobic coryneforms isolated from human bone marrow and skin. Chemical, biochemical and serological studies and some of their biological activities," *Japanese Journal of Microbiology*, vol. 20, no. 1, pp. 17–25, 1976.

[50] N. Hayashi, K. Togawa, M. Yanagisawa, J. Hosogi, D. Mimura, and Y. Yamamoto, "Effect of sunlight exposure and aging on skin surface lipids and urate," *Experimental Dermatology*, vol. 12, supplement 2, pp. 13–17, 2003.

[51] T. Q. Do, S. Moshkani, P. Castillo et al., "Lipids including cholesteryl linoleate and cholesteryl arachidonate contribute to the inherent antibacterial activity of human nasal fluid," *Journal of Immunology*, vol. 181, no. 6, pp. 4177–4187, 2008.

[52] C. B. Huang, B. George, and J. L. Ebersole, "Antimicrobial activity of n-6, n-7 and n-9 fatty acids and their esters for oral microorganisms," *Archives of Oral Biology*, vol. 55, no. 8, pp. 555–560, 2010.

[53] Y. Katsuta, T. Iida, S. Inomata, and M. Denda, "Unsaturated fatty acids induce calcium influx into keratinocytes and cause abnormal differentiation of epidermis," *Journal of Investigative Dermatology*, vol. 124, no. 5, pp. 1008–1013, 2005.

[54] K. Moriyama, S. Yokoo, H. Terashi, and T. Komori, "Cellular fatty acid composition of stratified squamous epithelia after transplantation of ex vivo produced oral mucosa equivalent," *Kobe Journal of Medical Sciences*, vol. 56, no. 6, pp. E253–E262, 2010.

[55] J. W. Fluhr, J. Kao, M. Jain, S. K. Ahn, K. R. Feingold, and P. M. Elias, "Generation of free fatty acids from phospholipids regulates stratum corneum acidification and integrity," *Journal of Investigative Dermatology*, vol. 117, no. 1, pp. 44–51, 2001.

[56] M. Y. Sheu, A. J. Fowler, J. Kao et al., "Topical peroxisome proliferator activated receptor-α activators reduce inflammation in irritant and allergic contact dermatitis models," *Journal of Investigative Dermatology*, vol. 118, no. 1, pp. 94–101, 2002.

[57] G. Siegenthaler, R. Hotz, D. Chatellard-Gruaz, L. Didierjean, U. Hellman, and J. H. Saurat, "Purification and characterization of the human epidermal fatty acid-binding protein: localization during epidermal cell differentiation in vivo and in vitro," *Biochemical Journal*, vol. 302, no. 2, pp. 363–371, 1994.

[58] G. Slegenthaler, R. Hotz, D. Chatellard-Gruaz, S. Jaconi, and J. H. Saurat, "Characterization and expression of a novel human fatty acid-binding protein: the epidermal type (E-FABP)," *Biochemical and Biophysical Research Communications*, vol. 190, no. 2, pp. 482–487, 1993.

[59] H. C. Chen, R. Mendelsohn, M. E. Rerek, and D. J. Moore, "Effect of cholesterol on miscibility and phase behavior in binary mixtures with synthetic ceramide 2 and octadecanoic acid. Infrared studies," *Biochimica et Biophysica Acta*, vol. 1512, no. 2, pp. 345–356, 2001.

[60] C. H. Chen, Y. Wang, T. Nakatsuji et al., "An innate bactericidal oleic acid effective against skin infection of methicillin-resistant *Staphylococcus aureus*: a therapy concordant with evolutionary medicine," *Journal of Microbiology and Biotechnology*, vol. 21, no. 4, pp. 391–399, 2011.

[61] E. M. Gribbon, W. J. Cunliffe, and K. T. Holland, "Interaction of Propionibacterium acnes with skin lipids in vitro," *Journal of General Microbiology*, vol. 139, no. 8, pp. 1745–1751, 1993.

[62] D. Yang, D. Pornpattananangkul, T. Nakatsuji et al., "The antimicrobial activity of liposomal lauric acids against Propionibacterium acnes," *Biomaterials*, vol. 30, no. 30, pp. 6035–6040, 2009.

[63] A. Pupe, R. Moison, P. de Haes et al., "Eicosapentaenoic acid, a n-3 polyunsaturated fatty acid differentially modulates TNF-α, IL-1α, IL-6 and PGE2 expression in UVB-irradiated human keratinocytes," *Journal of Investigative Dermatology*, vol. 118, no. 4, pp. 692–698, 2002.

[64] A. Storey, F. McArdle, P. S. Friedmann, M. J. Jackson, and L. E. Rhodes, "Eicosapentaenoic acid and docosahexaenoic acid reduce UVB- and TNF-α-induced IL-8 secretion in keratinocytes and UVB-induced IL-8 in fibroblasts," *Journal of Investigative Dermatology*, vol. 124, no. 1, pp. 248–255, 2005.

[65] B. Yu, C. Y. Dong, P. T. C. So, D. Blankschtein, and R. Langer, "In vitro visualization and quantification of oleic acid induced changes in transdermal transport using two-photon fluorescence microscopy," *Journal of Investigative Dermatology*, vol. 117, no. 1, pp. 16–25, 2001.

[66] S. J. Jiang and X. J. Zhou, "Examination of the mechanism of oleic acid-induced percutaneous penetration enhancement: an ultrastructural study," *Biological and Pharmaceutical Bulletin*, vol. 26, no. 1, pp. 66–68, 2003.

[67] S. Ben-Shabat, N. Baruch, and A. C. Sintov, "Conjugates of unsaturated fatty acids with propylene glycol as potentially less-irritant skin penetration enhancers," *Drug Development and Industrial Pharmacy*, vol. 33, no. 11, pp. 1169–1175, 2007.

[68] M. J. Kim, H. J. Doh, M. K. Choi et al., "Skin permeation enhancement of diclofenac by fatty acids," *Drug Delivery*, vol. 15, no. 6, pp. 373–379, 2008.

[69] Y. Sun, W. Lo, S. J. Lin, S. H. Jee, and C. Y. Dong, "Multiphoton polarization and generalized polarization microscopy reveal oleic-acid-induced structural changes in intercellular lipid layers of the skin," *Optics Letters*, vol. 29, no. 17, pp. 2013–2015, 2004.

[70] M. I. Hoopes, M. G. Noro, M. L. Longo, and R. Faller, "Bilayer structure and lipid dynamics in a model stratum corneum with oleic acid," *Journal of Physical Chemistry B*, vol. 115, no. 12, pp. 3164–3171, 2011.

[71] A. Conti, J. Rogers, P. Verdejo, C. R. Harding, and A. V. Rawlings, "Seasonal influences on stratum corneum ceramide 1 fatty acids and the influence of topical essential fatty acids," *International Journal of Cosmetic Science*, vol. 18, no. 1, pp. 1–12, 1996.

[72] K. Motoyoshi, "Enhanced comedo formation in rabbit ear skin by squalene and oleic acid peroxides," *British Journal of Dermatology*, vol. 109, no. 2, pp. 191–198, 1983.

[73] E. H. Choi, S. K. Ahn, and S. H. Lee, "The changes of stratum corneum interstices and calcium distribution of follicular

epithelium of experimentally induced comedones (EIC) by oleic acid," *Experimental Dermatology*, vol. 6, no. 1, pp. 29–35, 1997.

[74] Y. Katsuta, T. Iida, K. Hasegawa, S. Inomata, and M. Denda, "Function of oleic acid on epidermal barrier and calcium influx into keratinocytes is associated with N-methyl d-aspartate-type glutamate receptors," *British Journal of Dermatology*, vol. 160, no. 1, pp. 69–74, 2009.

[75] A. Berton, V. Rigot, E. Huet et al., "Involvement of fibronectin type II repeats in the efficient inhibition of gelatinases A and B by long-chain unsaturated fatty acids," *Journal of Biological Chemistry*, vol. 276, no. 23, pp. 20458–20465, 2001.

[76] E. Huet, J. H. Cauchard, A. Berton et al., "Inhibition of plasmin-mediated prostromelysin-1 activation by interaction of long chain unsaturated fatty acids with kringle 5," *Biochemical Pharmacology*, vol. 67, no. 4, pp. 643–654, 2004.

[77] J. H. Cauchard, A. Berton, G. Godeau, W. Hornebeck, and G. Bellon, "Activation of latent transforming growth factor beta 1 and inhibition of matrix metalloprotease activity by a thrombospondin-like tripeptide linked to elaidic acid," *Biochemical Pharmacology*, vol. 67, no. 11, pp. 2013–2022, 2004.

[78] J. L. Burton, "Dietary fatty acids and inflammatory skin disease," *Lancet*, vol. 1, no. 8628, pp. 27–31, 1989.

[79] S. Wright, "Essential fatty acids and the skin," *Prostaglandins Leukotrienes and Essential Fatty Acids*, vol. 38, no. 4, pp. 229–236, 1989.

[80] S. Monpoint, B. Guillot, F. Truchetet, E. Grosshans, and J. J. Guilhou, "Essential fatty acids in dermatology," *Annales de Dermatologie et de Venereologie*, vol. 119, no. 3, pp. 233–239, 1992.

[81] K. Perisho, P. W. Wertz, K. C. Madison, M. E. Stewart, and D. T. Downing, "Fatty acids of acylceramides from comedones and from the skin surface of acne patients and control subjects," *Journal of Investigative Dermatology*, vol. 90, no. 3, pp. 350–353, 1988.

[82] V. M. Sardesai, "The essential fatty acids," *Nutrition in Clinical Practice*, vol. 7, no. 4, pp. 179–186, 1992.

[83] P. M. Elias, B. E. Brown, and V. A. Ziboh, "The permeability barrier in essential fatty acid deficiency: evidence for a direct role for linoleic acid in barrier function," *Journal of Investigative Dermatology*, vol. 74, no. 4, pp. 230–233, 1980.

[84] W. Chen, C. C. Zouboulis, and C. E. Orfanos, "The 5α-Reductase system and its inhibitors. Recent development and its perspective in treating androgen-dependent skin disorders," *Dermatology*, vol. 193, no. 3, pp. 177–184, 1996.

[85] R. L. Rosenfield, A. Kentsis, D. Deplewski, and N. Ciletti, "Rat preputial sebocyte differentiation involves peroxisome proliferator-activated receptors," *Journal of Investigative Dermatology*, vol. 112, no. 2, pp. 226–232, 1999.

[86] C. C. Zouboulis and M. Böhm, "Neuroendocrine regulation of sebocytes—a pathogenetic link between stress and acne," *Experimental Dermatology*, vol. 13, no. 4, pp. 31–35, 2004.

[87] H. L. Yu and N. Salem Jr., "Whole body distribution of deuterated linoleic and α-linolenic acids and their metabolites in the rat," *Journal of Lipid Research*, vol. 48, no. 12, pp. 2709–2724, 2007.

[88] C. Grattan, J. L. Burton, M. Manku, C. Stewart, and D. F. Horrobin, "Essential-fatty-acid metabolites in plasma phospholipids in patients with ichthyosis vulgaris, acne vulgaris and psoriasis," *Clinical and Experimental Dermatology*, vol. 15, no. 3, pp. 174–176, 1990.

[89] S. Chung, S. Kong, K. Seong, and Y. Cho, "γ-linolenic acid in borage oil reverses epidermal hyperproliferation in guinea pigs," *Journal of Nutrition*, vol. 132, no. 10, pp. 3090–3097, 2002.

[90] M. M. McCusker and J. M. Grant-Kels, "Healing fats of the skin: the structural and immunologic roles of the Ω-6 and Ω-3 fatty acids," *Clinics in Dermatology*, vol. 28, no. 4, pp. 440–451, 2010.

[91] J. W. Hopewell, M. E. C. Robbins, G. J. M. J. Van den Aardweg et al., "The modulation of radiation-induced damage to pig skin by essential fatty acids," *British Journal of Cancer*, vol. 68, no. 1, pp. 1–7, 1993.

[92] D. Wu, M. Meydani, L. S. Leka, Z. Nightingale, G. J. Handelman, and J. B. Blumberg, "Effect of dietary supplementation with black currant seed oil or the immune response of healthy elderly subjects," *American Journal of Clinical Nutrition*, vol. 70, no. 4, pp. 536–543, 1999.

[93] V. A. Ziboh, C. C. Miller, and Y. Cho, "Metabolism of polyunsaturated fatty acids by skin epidermal enzymes: generation of antiinflammatory and antiproliferative metabolites," *American Journal of Clinical Nutrition*, vol. 71, supplement 1, pp. 361S–366S, 2000.

[94] Y. C. Chen, W. T. Chiu, and M. S. Wu, "Therapeutic effect of topical gamma-linolenic acid on refractory uremic pruritus," *American Journal of Kidney Diseases*, vol. 48, no. 1, pp. 69–76, 2006.

[95] Z. Fu and A. J. Sinclair, "Increased α-linolenic acid intake increases tissue α-linolenic acid content and apparent oxidation with little effect on tissue docosahexaenoic acid in the guinea pig," *Lipids*, vol. 35, no. 4, pp. 395–400, 2000.

[96] K. S. Bjerve, S. Fischer, F. Wammer, and T. Egeland, "α-Linolenic acid and long-chain ω-3 fatty acid supplementation in three patients with ω-3 fatty acid deficiency: effect on lymphocyte function, plasma and red cell lipids, and prostanoid formation," *American Journal of Clinical Nutrition*, vol. 49, no. 2, pp. 290–300, 1989.

[97] C. C. Miller, W. Tang, V. A. Ziboh, and M. P. Fletcher, "Dietary supplementation with ethyl ester concentrates of fish oil (n-3) and borage oil (n-6) polyunsaturated fatty acids induces epidermal generation of local putative anti-inflammatory metabolites," *Journal of Investigative Dermatology*, vol. 96, no. 1, pp. 98–103, 1991.

[98] R. W. Lacey and V. L. Lord, "Sensitivity of staphylococci to fatty acids: novel inactivation of linolenic acid by serum," *Journal of Medical Microbiology*, vol. 14, no. 1, pp. 41–49, 1981.

[99] K. S. Bjerve, L. Thoresen, I. L. Mostad, and K. Alme, "Alpha-linolenic acid deficiency in man: effect of essential fatty acids on fatty acid composition," *Advances in Prostaglandin, Thromboxane, and Leukotriene Research*, vol. 17, pp. 862–865, 1987.

[100] C. H. Yen, Y. S. Dai, Y. H. Yang, L. C. Wang, J. H. Lee, and B. L. Chiang, "Linoleic acid metabolite levels and transepidermal water loss in children with atopic dermatitis," *Annals of Allergy, Asthma and Immunology*, vol. 100, no. 1, pp. 66–73, 2008.

[101] E. Fehling, D. J. Murphy, and K. D. Mukherjee, "Biosynthesis of triacylglycerols containing very long chain monounsaturated acyl moieties in developing seeds," *Plant Physiology*, vol. 94, no. 2, pp. 492–498, 1990.

[102] J. Alezones, M. Ávila, A. Chassaigne, and V. Barrientos, "Fatty acids profile characterization of white maize hybrids grown in venezuela," *Archivos Latinoamericanos de Nutricion*, vol. 60, no. 4, pp. 397–404, 2010.

[103] N. B. Cater and M. A. Denke, "Behenic acid is a cholesterol-raising saturated fatty acid in humans," *American Journal of Clinical Nutrition*, vol. 73, no. 1, pp. 41–44, 2001.

[104] R. Westerberg, J. E. Månsson, V. Golozoubova et al., "ELOVL3 is an important component for early onset of lipid recruitment in brown adipose tissue," *Journal of Biological Chemistry*, vol. 281, no. 8, pp. 4958–4968, 2006.

[105] A. Schroeter, M. A. Kiselev, T. Hauß, S. Dante, and R. H. H. Neubert, "Evidence of free fatty acid interdigitation in stratum corneum model membranes based on ceramide [AP] by deuterium labelling," *Biochimica et Biophysica Acta*, vol. 1788, no. 10, pp. 2194–2203, 2009.

[106] A. M. Hall, B. M. Wiczer, T. Herrmann, W. Stremmel, and D. A. Bernlohr, "Enzymatic properties of purified murine fatty acid transport protein 4 and analysis of Acyl-CoA synthetase activities in tissues from FATP4 null mice," *Journal of Biological Chemistry*, vol. 280, no. 12, pp. 11948–11954, 2005.

[107] B. Janůšová, J. Zbytovská, P. Lorenc et al., "Effect of ceramide acyl chain length on skin permeability and thermotropic phase behavior of model stratum corneum lipid membranes," *Biochimica et Biophysica Acta*, vol. 1811, no. 3, pp. 129–137, 2011.

[108] L. Norlén, I. Nicander, A. Lundsjö, T. Cronholm, and B. Forslind, "A new HPLC-based method for the quantitative analysis of inner stratum corneum lipids with special reference to the free fatty acid fraction," *Archives of Dermatological Research*, vol. 290, no. 9, pp. 508–516, 1998.

[109] J. Rogers, C. Harding, A. Mayo, J. Banks, and A. Rawlings, "Stratum corneum lipids: the effect of ageing and the seasons," *Archives of Dermatological Research*, vol. 288, no. 12, pp. 765–770, 1996.

Cryoglobulinaemia in Egyptian Patients with Extrahepatic Cutaneous Manifestations of Chronic Hepatitis C Virus Infection

Doaa Salah Hegab[1] and Mohammed Abd El Rahman Sweilam[2]

[1]Faculty of Medicine, Dermatology and Venereology Department, Tanta University Hospitals, El Geish Street, Tanta, Gharbia Governorate 31111, Egypt
[2]Faculty of Medicine, Clinical Pathology Department, Tanta University Hospitals, El Geish Street, Tanta, Gharbia Governorate 31111, Egypt

Correspondence should be addressed to Doaa Salah Hegab; doaasalahhegab@yahoo.com

Academic Editor: Elizabeth Helen Kemp

Background. Hepatitis C is a global major health problem with extremely variable extrahepatic manifestations. Mixed cryoglobulinaemia (MC) shows a striking association with hepatitis C virus (HCV) infection, and it is sometimes asymptomatic. The skin is a frequently involved target organ in MC. *Objective.* To investigate the prevalence of cryoglobulinaemia in a sample of Egyptian patients with cutaneous manifestations of chronic HCV infection and to correlate its presence with clinical criteria and liver function tests. *Methods.* One hundred and eighteen patients with skin manifestations of chronic compensated hepatitis C were included. Venous blood was tested for liver function tests and serum cryoglobulins. *Results.* Twelve patients (10.169%) were positive for serum cryoglobulins (2 with pruritus, 4 with vasculitic lesions, 3 with livedo reticularis, one with oral lichen, one with chronic urticaria, and another with Schamberg's disease). Vasculitic lesions and livedo reticularis of the legs showed higher prevalence in cryoglobulin-positive than in cryoglobulin-negative patients. Presence of serum cryoglobulins did not relate to patients' demographic or laboratory findings. *Conclusions.* Fortunately, MC is not markedly prevalent among Egyptians with cutaneous lesions of chronic hepatitis C, and cryopositivity was commonly, but not exclusively, detected with cutaneous vasculitis and livedo reticularis. Laboratory testing for cryoglobulins in every HCV patient is advisable for earlier MC detection and management.

1. Introduction

Chronic hepatitis C virus (HCV) infection is a major public health problem that affects approximately 300 million people worldwide. Egypt has the highest and devastating prevalence of HCV in the world, amounting to 14–20% [1, 2].

Patients with chronic HCV infection frequently present with extrahepatic manifestations involving different organ systems leading to the concept of systemic HCV infection. According to different studies, 40–75% of patients infected with HCV might develop at least one extrahepatic manifestation during the course of the disease, and sometimes these could represent the first and sole signal of HCV infection [3].

These manifestations include autoimmune phenomena, low-grade chronic systemic inflammation, and frank autoimmune and/or rheumatic diseases [4, 5].

There are many cutaneous manifestations of chronic HCV infection including necrolytic acral erythema, livedo reticularis, cutaneous leukocytoclastic vasculitis, porphyria cutanea tarda, pruritus, urticaria, lichen planus, polyarteritis nodosa, erythema nodosum, erythema multiforme, pyoderma gangrenosum, and mixed cryoglobulinaemia (MC) [6].

MC is a systemic vasculitis that is considered the most common extrahepatic manifestation of HCV infection. Clinical manifestations associated with MC include joint involvement, fatigue, myalgia, renal immune-complex disease, cutaneous vasculitis, and peripheral neuropathy [7, 8].

It has been postulated that MC with chronic HCV infection is commonly associated with skin involvement in the form of cutaneous vasculitis ranging from palpable purpura (leukocytoclastic vasculitis) and petechiae in the lower extremities to large necrotic non-healing ulcerations [9]; however, its association with different dermatologic manifestations in Egyptian patients with compensated chronic HCV infection was not clearly studied.

In the present study we sought to investigate the prevalence of cryoglobulinaemia in a sample of Egyptian patients with extrahepatic cutaneous affection in the setting of chronic HCV infection and to correlate its presence with clinical criteria and biochemical measures of liver function.

2. Materials and Methods

2.1. Study Participants. The study involved a group of one hundred and eighteen patients with cutaneous manifestations of chronic compensated HCV infection on follow-up treatment who were referred to the outpatient clinics of Dermatology & Venereology Department or who were collected from inpatient wards and outpatient clinics of Tropical Medicine Department in Tanta University Hospitals. HCV infection was diagnosed by anti-HCV antibodies through third generation enzyme-linked immunosorbent assay (ELISA) and HCV ribonucleic acid by polymerase chain reaction (PCR). Only patients with cutaneous affection who were positive for HCV antibodies within 6 months prior to the study were enrolled. Baseline evaluation included disease history in addition to physical general and dermatological examination. Investigative evaluation included routine biochemical panel, complete hemogram, chest X-ray, pelvic-abdominal U/S, and urine and stool analysis, in addition to liver function tests. Patients with acute hepatitis C, lymphoma, hepatocellular carcinoma, and decompensated liver cirrhosis (ascites, oesophageal varices, hepatic encephalopathy, or lower limb edema) were excluded. All included patients signed an informed written consent and the study was approved by the institutional ethical committee of Tanta University.

2.2. Blood Sample Collection. Fifteen mL of venous blood was drawn in Vacutainer tubes prewarmed at 37°C and left for 2 hours to clot at the same temperature; then the serum was separated by centrifugation (2500 ×g for 10 min) at 37°C. Samples were dispensed in a graduated tube for cryoglobulins assay.

2.3. Cryoglobulins Detection by the Traditional Method. Serum cryoglobulins were detected through the traditional method [10, 11]. The presence of precipitate in the samples was determined by visual inspection, before centrifugation and after 1, 3, 7, and 15 days of cold incubation at 4°C. Subjective evaluation of cryoprecipitate was done, and absence of cryoprecipitate was scored as negative while cryoprecipitate was scored as positive. On the 15th day of cold incubation, samples were centrifuged at 2500 ×g for 10 min at 4°C and

TABLE 1: Clinical and laboratory criteria of HCV infected patients with cutaneous manifestations ($n = 118$).

Variable	Value in study participants
Age range in years, mean (SD)	24–63, 47.1 (7.5)
Sex, M (%)/F (%)	84 (71.2%)/34 (28.8%)
Liver function test range, mean (SD)	
AST (IU/L)	12–168, 62.6 (32.4)
ALT (IU/L)	10–177, 61 (30.5)
ALP (IU/L)	51–266, 109.6 (34.6)
Serum albumin (g/dL)	3.5–4.8, 4.1 (0.4)
Total serum bilirubin (mg/dL)	0.5–6.4, 1 (0.9)
Prothrombin time	11–18, 13.2 (1)
Skin manifestations of chronic HCV n (%), +ve/−ve cryoglobulins	
Pruritus	74 (62.7%), 2/72
Vasculitic lesions	9 (7.6%), 4/5
Lichen planus (oral ± cutaneous)	8 (6.8%), 1/7
Lichen planus (cutaneous only)	3 (2.5%), 0/3
Melasma	6 (5.1%), 0/6
Urticaria	4 (3.4%), 1/3
Livedo reticularis	3 (2.5%), 3/0
Necrolytic acral erythema	3 (2.5%), 0/3
Erythema nodosum	2 (1.7%), 0/2
Prurigo nodularis	2 (1.7%), 0/2
Vitiligo	2 (1.7%), 0/2
Pigmented purpuric dermatosis (Schamberg's disease)	1 (0.8%), 1/0
Psoriasis	1 (0.8%), 0/1

ALP: alkaline phosphatase; ALT: alanine aminotransferase; AST: aspartate aminotransferase.

the amount of cryoglobulins was estimated. Redissolution of the cryoglobulin precipitate by rewarming to 37°C was done. If the precipitate is not resoluble within a few minutes then the result is negative and no further analysis was adopted, while resolubilization at 37°C confirmed a positive result.

2.4. Statistical Analysis. Statistical presentation and analysis of the present study was conducted using the mean value, standard deviation, Student's t-test, or χ^2-square test (for comparison of qualitative values) by Statistics Package for Social Sciences (SPSS) version 18. Manifestations associated with cryoglobulinaemia were compared by odds ratio (OR) and 95% confidence interval (CI). For all tests a P value < 0.05 was considered statistically significant.

3. Results

Baseline demographic, clinical, and laboratory characteristics of the studied patients are shown in Table 1. Pruritus was the most common skin manifestation among the studied HCV patients. It was noted in 74 patients (62.7%) out of the 118 patients included, and the most commonly affected sites

TABLE 2: Relationship between cryoglobulin-positivity and patients' characteristics.

Characteristic	Cryoglobulin-positive patients ($n = 12$)	Cryoglobulin-negative patients ($n = 106$)	P value (Student's t test or χ^2)	
Age range in years, mean (SD)	29–63, 49.1 (7.1)	24–59, 47.4 (5.1)	0.24	
Gender, n (%)				
Male ($n = 84$)	9 (75%)	75 (70.8%)	0.76	
Female ($n = 34$)	3 (25%)	31 (29.3%)		
Liver function test range, mean (SD)				
AST (IU/L)	28–77, 44.9 (10.6)	12–168, 65.5 (14.6)	0.1	
ALT (IU/L)	31–73, 42.9 (16.5)	10–177, 63.9 (31.3)	0.1	
ALP (IU/L)	92–266, 131 (37.1)	51–200, 96.3 (5.2)	0.1	
Serum albumin (g/dL)	3.6–3.9, 4 (0.5)	3.5–4.8, 4.1 (0.6)	0.7	
Total serum bilirubin (mg/dL)	0.47–1.36, 1.1 (0.7)	0.5–6.4, 1 (0.9)	0.1	
Prothrombin time	11–15.6, 13.2 (0.6)	11–18, 13.3 (1)	0.6	
Cutaneous extrahepatic manifestations associated with MC, n (%)			P value (χ^2)	Odds ratio (95% confidence)
Pruritus ($n = 74$)	2 (16.6%)	72 (67.9%)	0.001*	0.09 (0.02–0.5)
Vasculitic lesions of lower limbs ($n = 9$)	4 (33.3%)	5 (4.7%)	<0.001*	10.1 (2.3–45.2)
Oral lichen planus ($n = 8$)	1 (8.3%)	7 (6.6%)	0.82	1.29 (0.1–11.4)
Chronic urticaria ($n = 4$)	1 (8.3%)	3 (2.8%)	0.32	3.12 (0.3–32.6)
Livedo reticularis ($n = 3$)	3 (25%)	0	<0.001*	—
Pigmented purpuric dermatosis ($n = 1$)	1 (8.3%)	0	0.003*	—

MC: mixed cryoglobulinemia; * significant.

were the legs and the trunk. Vasculitic lesions were noted in 9 patients (7.627%) and appeared as palpable purpura in 5 patients, vesicles and pustules on lower limbs in 1 patient, and erythematous nodules ± ulceration on the legs in 3 patients.

Cryoglobulins were detected in the sera of 12 patients with a total of 10.169%. Among the cryopositive patients, 2 patients had persistent pruritus, 4 had leukocytoclastic vasculitic lesions on the lower limbs (3 with palpable purpura, and 1 with nodules ± ulcerations of lower limbs), 3 had livedo reticularis, one had oral lichen (erosive type), one had chronic urticaria, and another one had pigmented purpuric dermatosis presented as Schamberg's disease (Table 1).

The relationships between the presence of serum cryoglobulins and the clinical and laboratory characteristics of the patients are shown in Table 2. Cryoglobulin-positivity was not significantly related to either patients' age, sex, or any of the performed liver function tests (AST, ALT, ALP, serum albumin, total bilirubin, or prothrombin time) (P value > 0.05 for all).

There was a statistically significant lower association of pruritus with cryoglobulin-positivity than cryoglobulin-negativity (P value = 0.001), while, on the contrary, vasculitic lesions of the lower limbs and livedo reticularis were significantly more prevalent in cryoglobulin-positive than cryoglobulin-negative patients (P value < 0.001 for both) (Table 2).

4. Discussion

MC is a systemic small- and medium-sized vessels vasculitis secondary to vascular deposition of circulating immune-complexes, mainly cryoglobulins and complement [12]. The association between MC and chronic HCV infection has been well established, and unfortunately severe and life threatening complications were reported in up to 10% of MC patients in whom the mortality ranged from 20 to 80% [13]. A previous meta-analysis showed that 44% patients with chronic HCV infection had circulating immune complexes with cryoprecipitating properties [14], and it has been previously reported that the skin is the most frequently involved target organ in MC [15]. However, the association of MC with different extrahepatic manifestations and with cutaneous manifestations in particular has not yet been clearly investigated in Egyptian patients who have an extraordinarily high prevalence of HCV infection.

In our study, pruritus, leukocytoclastic vasculitic lesions (palpable purpura, vesicles, nodules ± ulceration, and crustation) of the lower extremities, and lichen planus were found to be the most frequent skin manifestations of chronic HCV infection among study participants, and that was consistent with the findings of previous studies [16–18].

In the present study, cryoglobulins were isolated in 12 patients (10.169%) out of the included 118 patients with extrahepatic cutaneous affection of HCV infection. It is noticeable that although more than half of the detected cryopositive patients had dermatological manifestations of HCV which were suggestive for cryoglobulinaemia (33.3% of cryopositive patients had vasculitic lesions on lower limbs and 25% had livedo reticularis), several patients were positive for serum cryoglobulins even in the absence of a clear clinical picture suggestive of autoimmune small vascular illness (16.6% of cryopositive patients were associated with intractable pruritus, 8.3% with oral erosive lichen planus, 8.3% with chronic urticaria, and 8.3% with Schamberg's disease). Accordingly, earlier identification of asymptomatic MC is possible through earlier detection of extrahepatic manifestations of HCV infection and particularly the dermatologic manifestations and screening those patients for the presence of serum cryoglobulins.

In a similar context, fatigue was reported to be the most frequent nonspecific clinical symptom of chronic HCV infection [19], and at the same time it is considered a part of the clinical picture of HCV-associated cryoglobulinaemia, since this symptom could be detected more frequently in cryoglobulin-positive than in cryoglobulin-negative patients with hepatitis C as described in a previous study [16]. So, even the nonspecific mild extrahepatic symptoms could act as a signal of a deeper dangerous ongoing vasculitic pathology.

In previous reports, palpable purpura was observed in 10–21% of patients with clinically manifested cryoglobulinemic syndrome [6, 20] and in 7% of all HCV infected patients [21]. In the current study, vasculitic lesions predominantly over the lower extremities were observed in 9 of the 118 included patients (7.627%), with much higher prevalence in cryoglobulin-positive than in cryoglobulin-negative patients (33.33% *versus* 4.71%, OR 10.100, 95% CI 2.255–45.219). Livedo reticularis was observed in 3 out of the 118 included patients (2.542%), and all patients with livedo were positive for serum cryoglobulins with higher prevalence in cryoglobulin-positive than in cryoglobulin-negative patients (25% *versus* 0%, P value < 0.001).

To the best of our knowledge, no previous reports investigating the prevalence of MC in HCV infected patients with skin manifestations were performed, but the frequency of MC in HCV-positive patients varied in the literature. Gad et al. [22] reported that the prevalence of MC in Egyptian patients infected with HCV-genotype 4 was 14%, and that was significantly lower than its prevalence in Japanese patients infected with genotype 1b (40%). It has been reported that 20% of the patients with HCV have MC, but most have cryoglobulins levels of less than 6%, which is not clinically significant and that only 3% of HCV patients have clinically significant MC with cryoglobulins levels of more than 6% [23, 24]. The mean cryocrit levels in HCV patients were determined to be about 2% [25].

Our study detected a lower prevalence of MC among Egyptian patients with cutaneous manifestations of HCV infection (10.169%) than expected. These findings suggest that cryoglobulinaemia in the context of hepatitis C may be less prevalent in Egypt than in other areas and this could be attributed to (1) the apparent protective role of *Schistosoma mansoni* coinfection, which is common in Egypt,

against the development of immune-mediated diseases such as MC in chronic HCV-infected patients [26]. Helminthic infections are characterized by a strong T helper-2 response as well as an overall downregulated immune system which are both beneficial in protecting the host from developing autoimmune diseases and/or relieving symptoms of an established autoimmune disease [27]. (2) There are HCV-related factors, particularly genotype where HCV genotype 4 is the most prevalent in Egypt (90%), while genotype 1 is the most prevalent worldwide followed by genotype 3 (affecting 46.2% and 30.1% of global HCV cases, resp.) [28, 29]. (3) MC shows higher incidence and significantly higher levels of cryoglobulins (>6%) in patients with hepatic cirrhosis and later stages of fibrosis [30], while all the participants in our study were having chronic compensated HCV infection. (4) Different cryoglobulins detection methods from one study to another and difficult detection of cryoglobulins because of their thermolability might cause a heterogeneity in the prevalence results between studies. (5) Finally, there are environmental and/or host genetic factors that might contribute to the pathogenesis of MC [31].

Actually, it is still unknown why only some chronically infected HCV patients develop MC and only some of these exhibit systemic symptoms (MC syndrome). Several studies have investigated the pathogenetic basis of MC and suggested that the virus is able to trigger such a disorder only in the presence of genetic factors that are still unknown [32]. The data that were reported are heterogeneous and sometimes even conflicting. There is a complex relationship between HCV-related MC and the host's genetic background including HLA polymorphisms (as HLA-A9, HLA-B8, HLA-DR3, HLA-DR11, and HLA-DR5-DQ3), cytokine mutations (affecting IL-10 promoter (-1082GG), or BAFF promoter (-871T)), genetic variability of IgG Fc receptors, fibronectin polymorphisms (called *Msp*I and *Hae*IIIb), and low serum levels of vitamin D associated with *CYP27B1* AC or CC genotype [32–37].

The results of the current study detected no significant relation between the presence of serum cryoglobulins in study participants on one side and patients' age, sex, or biochemical parameters of liver functions on the other side.

Some authors had reported that cryoglobulinaemic vasculitis was significantly more common in female population with HCV infection [38], although this association was nonsignificant in another report [39]. Abbas et al. [26] reported that cryoglobulinaemia in their Egyptian patients with HCV was not related to age or progression of cirrhosis; meanwhile it was negatively correlated with serum ALT and serum AST levels, and it was positively correlated with female gender. The discrepancy in the results could be due to variation in sample size and inclusion criteria among different studies.

5. Conclusions

In conclusion, although Egypt still has the highest prevalence of HCV infection worldwide, fortunately, MC is not markedly prevalent among Egyptian patients with cutaneous manifestations of chronic HCV and that might indicate that

Egypt has a lower incidence of MC than other areas. Although a large proportion of cryopositive cases with cutaneous manifestations of HCV present with vasculitic lower limb lesions or livedo reticularis, still some patients with MC could be either asymptomatic or present incidentally with nonspecific lesions. Laboratory testing for cryoglobulins is usually neglected in clinical practice and we think that it should be adopted as a routine test for HCV infected patients even in absence of suggestive manifestations of vasculitis, and that might help in earlier detection and management of MC with HCV before the occurrence of serious internal insult.

Conflict of Interests

The authors declare that there is no conflict of interests regarding the publication of this paper.

Acknowledgments

The authors are grateful to Dr. Nassar S., MD (Professor of Dermatology and Venereology, Faculty of Medicine, Tanta University), and Dr. Elbatae H., MD (Professor of Tropical Medicine, Faculty of Medicine, Tanta University), for their clinical support, cooperation, and generous help in patients' selection and evaluation.

References

[1] H. Wedemeyer, G. J. Dore, and J. W. Ward, "Estimates on HCV disease burden worldwide—filling the gaps," *Journal of Viral Hepatitis*, vol. 22, no. 1, pp. 1–5, 2015.

[2] Y. A. Mohamoud, G. R. Mumtaz, S. Riome, D. Miller, and L. J. Abu-Raddad, "The epidemiology of hepatitis C virus in Egypt: a systematic review and data synthesis," *BMC Infectious Diseases*, vol. 13, no. 1, article 288, 2013.

[3] J. Metts, L. Carmichael, W. Kokor, and R. Scharffenberg, "Hepatitis C: extrahepatic manifestations," *FP Essent*, vol. 427, pp. 32–35, 2014.

[4] E. Rosenthal and P. Cacoub, "Extrahepatic manifestations in chronic hepatitis C virus carriers," *Lupus*, vol. 24, no. 4-5, pp. 469–482, 2015.

[5] A. Antonelli and M. Pistello, "New therapies, markers and therapeutic targets in HCV chronic infection, and HCV extrahepatic manifestations," *Current Drug Targets*, 2015.

[6] A. Akhter and A. Said, "Cutaneous manifestations of viral hepatitis," *Current Infectious Disease Reports*, vol. 17, no. 2, article 452, 2015.

[7] D. Giuggioli, M. Sebastiani, M. Colaci et al., "Treatment of HCV-related mixed cryoglobulinemia," *Current Drug Targets*, In press.

[8] P. Cacoub, C. Comarmond, F. Domont, L. Savey, and D. Saadoun, "Cryoglobulinemia vasculitis," *The American Journal of Medicine*, vol. 128, no. 9, pp. 950–955, 2015.

[9] D. Giuggioli, A. Manfredi, F. Lumetti, M. Sebastiani, and C. Ferri, "Cryoglobulinemic vasculitis and skin ulcers. Our therapeutic strategy and review of the literature," *Seminars in Arthritis & Rheumatism*, vol. 44, no. 5, pp. 518–526, 2015.

[10] P. Vermeersch, K. Gijbels, G. Mariën et al., "A critical appraisal of current practice in the detection, analysis, and reporting of cryoglobulins," *Clinical Chemistry*, vol. 54, no. 1, pp. 39–43, 2008.

[11] R. Sargur, P. White, and W. Egner, "Cryoglobulin evaluation: best practice?" *Annals of Clinical Biochemistry*, vol. 47, no. 1, pp. 8–16, 2010.

[12] K. Krishnamurthy, S. Mohapatra, T. Mishra, and N. Jha, "Early onset mixed cryoglobulinemia in hepatitis C," *Indian Journal of Pathology and Microbiology*, vol. 58, no. 3, pp. 381–383, 2015.

[13] B. Terrier, O. Semoun, D. Saadoun, D. Sène, M. Resche-Rigon, and P. Cacoub, "Prognostic factors in patients with hepatitis C virus infection and systemic vasculitis," *Arthritis & Rheumatism*, vol. 63, no. 6, pp. 1748–1757, 2011.

[14] Z. Kayali, V. E. Buckwold, B. Zimmerman, and W. N. Schmidt, "Hepatitis C, cryoglobulinemia, and cirrhosis: a meta-analysis," *Hepatology*, vol. 36, no. 4 I, pp. 978–985, 2002.

[15] M. Ramos-Casals, J. H. Stone, M. C. Cid, and X. Bosch, "The cryoglobulinaemias," *The Lancet*, vol. 379, no. 9813, pp. 348–360, 2012.

[16] D. V. Stefanova-Petrova, A. H. Tzvetanska, E. J. Naumova et al., "Chronic hepatitis C virus infection: prevalence of extrahepatic manifestations and association with cryoglobulinemia in Bulgarian patients," *World Journal of Gastroenterology*, vol. 13, no. 48, pp. 6518–6528, 2007.

[17] M. Maticic, M. Poljak, T. Lunder, K. Rener-Sitar, and L. Stojanovic, "Lichen planus and other cutaneous manifestations in chronic hepatitis C: pre- and post-interferon-based treatment prevalence vary in a cohort of patients from low hepatitis C virus endemic area," *Journal of the European Academy of Dermatology and Venereology*, vol. 22, no. 7, pp. 779–788, 2008.

[18] L. Shengyuan, Y. Songpo, W. Wen, T. Wenjing, Z. Haitao, and W. Binyou, "Hepatitis C virus and lichen planus: a reciprocal association determined by a meta-analysis," *Archives of Dermatology*, vol. 145, no. 9, pp. 1040–1047, 2009.

[19] S. Monaco, S. Mariotto, S. Ferrari et al., "Hepatitis C virus-associated neurocognitive and neuropsychiatric disorders: advances in 2015," *World Journal of Gastroenterology*, vol. 21, no. 42, pp. 11974–11983, 2015.

[20] J. J. Germer, P. N. Rys, J. N. Thorvilson, and D. H. Persing, "Determination of hepatitis C virus genotype by direct sequence analysis of products generated with the amplicor HCV test," *Journal of Clinical Microbiology*, vol. 37, no. 8, pp. 2625–2630, 1999.

[21] P. Cacoub, C. Renou, E. Rosenthal et al., "Extrahepatic manifestations associated with hepatitis C virus infection. A prospective multicenter study of 321 patients. The GERMIVIC. Groupe d'Etude et de Recherche en Medecine Interne et Maladies Infectieuses sur le Virus de l'Hepatite C," *Medicine*, vol. 79, pp. 47–56, 2000.

[22] A. Gad, E. Tanaka, A. Matsumoto et al., "Factors predisposing to the occurrence of cryoglobulinemia in two cohorts of Egyptian and Japanese patients with chronic hepatitis C infection: ethnic and genotypic influence," *Journal of Medical Virology*, vol. 70, no. 4, pp. 594–599, 2003.

[23] P. Cacoub, L. Gragnani, C. Comarmond, and A. L. Zignego, "Extrahepatic manifestations of chronic hepatitis C virus infection," *Digestive and Liver Disease*, vol. 46, supplement, pp. S165–S173, 2014.

[24] P. Cacoub, T. Poynard, P. Ghillani et al., "Extrahepatic manifestations of chronic hepatitis C. MULTIVIRC Group. Multidepartment Virus C," *Arthritis & Rheumatology*, vol. 42, no. 10, pp. 2204–2212, 1999.

[25] B. Dedania and G. Y. Wu, "Dermatologic extrahepatic mani-
festations of hepatitis C," *Journal of Clinical and Translational Hepatology*, vol. 3, no. 2, pp. 127–133, 2015.

[26] O. M. Abbas, N. A. Omar, H. E. Zaghla, and M. F. Faramawi, "Schistosoma mansoni coinfection could have a protective effect against mixed cryoglobulinaemia in hepatitis C patients," *Liver International*, vol. 29, no. 7, pp. 1065–1070, 2009.

[27] E. van Riet, F. C. Hartgers, and M. Yazdanbakhsh, "Chronic helminth infections induce immunomodulation: consequences and mechanisms," *Immunobiology*, vol. 212, no. 6, pp. 475–490, 2007.

[28] S. C. Ray, R. R. Arthur, A. Carella, J. Bukh, and D. L. Thomas, "Genetic epidemiology of hepatitis C virus throughout Egypt," *The Journal of Infectious Diseases*, vol. 182, no. 3, pp. 698–707, 2000.

[29] J. P. Messina, I. Humphreys, A. Flaxman et al., "Global distribu-tion and prevalence of hepatitis C virus genotypes," *Hepatology*, vol. 61, no. 1, pp. 77–87, 2015.

[30] M. Ramos-Casals, J. H. Stone, M. C. Cid, and X. Bosch, "The cryoglobulinaemias," *The Lancet*, vol. 379, no. 9813, pp. 348–360, 2012.

[31] G. Lauletta, S. Russi, V. Conteduca, and L. Sansonno, "Hepatitis C virus infection and mixed cryoglobulinemia," *Clinical and Developmental Immunology*, vol. 2012, Article ID 502156, 11 pages, 2012.

[32] L. Gragnani, E. Fognani, A. Piluso, and A. L. Zignego, "Hepatitis C virus-related mixed cryoglobulinemia: is genetics to blame?" *World Journal of Gastroenterology*, vol. 19, no. 47, pp. 8910–8915, 2013.

[33] M. W. Ayad, A. A. Elbanna, D. A. Elneily, and A. S. Sakr, "Association of BAFF −871C/T promoter polymorphism with hepatitis C-related cryoglobulinemia a cohort of Egyptian patients," *Molecular Diagnosis & Therapy*, vol. 19, no. 2, pp. 99–106, 2015.

[34] S.-J. Hwang, C.-W. Chu, D.-F. Huang, K.-H. Lan, F.-Y. Chang, and S.-D. Lee, "Genetic predispositions for the presence of cryo-globulinemia and serum autoantibodies in Chinese patients with chronic hepatitis C," *Tissue Antigens*, vol. 59, no. 1, pp. 31–37, 2002.

[35] P. Fallahi, C. Ferri, S. M. Ferrari, A. Corrado, D. Sansonno, and A. Antonelli, "Cytokines and HCV-related disorders," *Clinical and Developmental Immunology*, vol. 2012, Article ID 468107, 10 pages, 2012.

[36] D. Vassilopoulos, Z. M. Younossi, E. Hadziyannis et al., "Study of host and virological factors of patients with chronic HCV infection and associated laboratory or clinical autoimmune manifestations," *Clinical and Experimental Rheumatology*, vol. 21, no. 6, pp. S101–S111, 2003.

[37] B. Terrier, F. Jehan, M. Munteanu et al., "Low 25-hydroxyvit-amin D serum levels correlate with the presence of serum cryo-globulins in patients with chronic hepatitis C," *Rheumatology*, vol. 51, no. 11, pp. 2083–2090, 2012.

[38] R. H. A. Mohammed, H. I. Elmakhzangy, A. Gamal et al., "Prevalence of rheumatologic manifestations of chronic hepati-tis C virus infection among Egyptians," *Clinical Rheumatology*, vol. 29, no. 12, pp. 1373–1380, 2010.

[39] B. Terrier, F. Jehan, M. Munteanu et al., "Low 25-hydroxyvit-amin D serum levels correlate with the presence of extra-hepatic manifestations in chronic hepatitis C virus infection," *Rheumatology*, vol. 51, no. 11, pp. 2083–2090, 2012.

3

Management of Pruritus in Chronic Liver Disease

Angeline Bhalerao[1] and Gurdeep S. Mannu[2]

[1]General Practice, Ipswich, Suffolk IP4 5PD, UK
[2]Oxford University Hospitals, Oxford OX3 9DU, UK

Correspondence should be addressed to Gurdeep S. Mannu; gurdeepmannu@gmail.com

Academic Editor: Luigi Naldi

Background. There continues to be uncertainty on the ideal treatment of pruritus in chronic liver disease. The aim of this study was to gather the latest information on the evidence-based management of pruritus in chronic liver disease. *Methodology.* A literature search for pruritus in chronic liver disease was conducted using Pubmed and Embase database systems using the MeSH terms "pruritus," "chronic liver disease," "cholestatic liver disease," and "treatment." *Results.* The current understanding of the pathophysiology of pruritus is described in addition to detailing research into contemporary treatment options of the condition. These medical treatments range from bile salts, rifampicin, and opioid receptor antagonists to antihistamines. *Conclusion.* The burden of pruritus in liver disease patients persists and, although it is a common symptom, it can be difficult to manage. In recent years there has been greater study into the etiology and treatment of the condition. Nonetheless, pruritus remains poorly understood and many patients continue to suffer, reiterating the need for further research to improve our understanding of the etiology and treatment for the condition.

1. Introduction

Pruritus or itch is a common symptom seen in a number of illnesses. It is an unpleasant sensation of irritation of the skin. Pruritus can further be classified as localised or generalised depending on the affected area and acute or chronic depending on the duration of the symptom. Chronic pruritus is defined as presence of pruritus for more than 6 weeks. Pruritus associated with liver disease has been well described as early as the 2nd century BC when the Greek physician Aretaeus the Cappadocian observed an association between pruritus and jaundice [1]. Pruritus is a common clinical feature seen in most liver diseases but particularly frequently in cholestatic liver disease. Cholestatic liver disease can be further classified into intra- and extrahepatic disease. Chronic pruritus is more frequently seen in intrahepatic cholestatic diseases such as primary biliary cirrhosis (PBC), intrahepatic cholestasis of pregnancy, chronic hepatitis B and C, familial intrahepatic cholestasis, and Alagille syndrome. However, pruritus is also seen in extrahepatic cholestatic liver diseases such as primary sclerosing cholangitis (PSC) and cancer of the head of pancreas [2].

Pruritus contributes a large symptomatic burden to those suffering from liver diseases. A recent survey reported that pruritus occurs in 69% of PBC sufferers and, for 75% of these patients, pruritus was present before the diagnosis of PBC, possibly suggesting pruritus as a diagnostic criterion. Pruritus in PBC can be very debilitating as approximately 65% of PBC sufferers report itching to occur especially at night time, thus affecting sleep. In some PBC patients, pruritus is worse after meals and premenstrually [3]. Cholestasis, pruritus, and jaundice are the main clinical features of progressive familial intrahepatic cholestasis [4]. Furthermore, 15–31% of hepatitis C sufferers complain of chronic pruritus. In all of these cases, pruritus in chronic liver disease tends to be generalised, chronic, intermittent, and of varying severity. It adversely affects patient's quality of life by frequently disrupting sleep [5], their daily activities, and personal relationships. It can also lead to depression and even suicidal intent in extreme cases [6]. Due to the subjective nature of pruritus there is an added difficulty in determining its severity and in treating it. Due to incompletely understood etiology and various different treatments available for pruritus, there remains ambiguity regarding the ideal approach to the treatment of this condition. In light of this, this review aimed to collate all published literature on the pathophysiology and management of pruritus in chronic liver disease in order to address this issue.

2. Methodology

A literature search for pruritus in chronic liver disease was conducted using Pubmed and Embase database systems using the MeSH terms "pruritus," "chronic liver disease," "cholestatic liver disease," and "treatment." This is summarised in supplementary figure 1 in Supplementary Material available online at http://dx.doi.org/10.1155/2015/295891.

2.1. Eligibility Criteria. All prospective and retrospective studies that recruited patients of any age and identified pruritus through clinical assessment were selected. Relevant studies needed to have a longitudinal follow-up of at least 24 hours duration and to report on pathophysiology, treatment, or outcomes. Papers were restricted to patients with chronic liver disease alone.

2.2. Information Sources and Search Strategy. In January 2014 a systematic search utilising PubMed/Medline and OVID search engines was conducted. The initial search was undertaken using MESH search for "pruritus" and "liver disease" and key phrases as listed in supplementary Figure 1. To capture the most recent literature in the field and to ensure that our analysis was based on contemporary datasets, the time period of literature search was limited to the past 20 years (January 1994–January 2014). The results of papers focusing on management were limited to papers focusing on human subjects and in the English language.

2.3. Study Selection. The abstracts were screened and relevant articles meeting the above criteria were selected. Searches were conducted by the authors who independently checked titles and abstracts against the eligibility criteria and subsequently obtained full-text versions of all potentially relevant papers, which were then further considered for final inclusion.

3. Results

3.1. Pathophysiology. The exact pathogenesis of pruritus in chronic liver disease is unknown; however, several hypotheses have been suggested. Pruritus induced by certain substances known as pruritogens is one of the implicated theories. Several pruritogens have been identified over the years. The "bile salts theory" proposes bile salts as the pruritogen. Cholestatic liver disease increases levels of bile salt which accumulate under the skin causing itch. This theory is further supported by studies showing that ingestion of bile salts in cholestatic patients worsens pruritus [6, 7] and intradermal injection of bile salts causes pruritus in healthy persons [8, 9]. Additionally, when bile is removed through nasobiliary drainage or partial external biliary diversion in a cholestatic patient, pruritus is significantly reduced [10, 11]. However, there still exists no established correlation between the bile salt concentration and severity of pruritus [12, 13]. Furthermore, not all cholestatic patients with elevated levels of bile

salts experience pruritus [14] and, additionally, pruritus also occurs in patients with normal levels of bile salts [12].

Histamine is also one of the strong contenders as a pruritogen in cholestatic pruritus. Raised histamine levels are found in cholestatic pruritus sufferers [15]; however, again there is no correlation between histamine concentrations and severity of pruritus [16] and antihistamines are often ineffective in treating pruritus in this setting [17]. Opioids, serotonin, and female sex hormones have all been implicated in the etiology of pruritus. Increased levels of endogenous opioids are reported in chronic liver disease [18, 19] and treatment with an opioid antagonist is shown to reduce pruritus [20–22]. Serotonin is believed to induce pruritus by altering itch perception [17] and so serotonin reuptake inhibitors such as sertraline have reported to be effective in managing pruritus [23].

Female hormonal influence on cholestatic pruritus is seen in different liver diseases. The intrahepatic cholestatic pruritus of pregnancy is self-limiting and often resolves after pregnancy. In addition, symptoms in preexisting primary biliary cirrhosis and primary sclerosing cholangitis female sufferers can sometimes worsen during pregnancy when there are raised female sex hormones [7]. Generally, increased itch sensation is apparent during pregnancy and in women taking hormone replacement therapy [8].

Recent research on cholestatic pruritus have identified another pruritogen called lysophosphatidic acid (LPA). Lysophosphatidic acid is a phospholipid which affects a range of cellular functions. Autotaxin (ATX) is an enzyme which cleaves lysophospholipase to form LPA. Both LPA and autotaxin levels are raised in patients with cholestatic pruritus. Additionally, studies on mice reveal that intradermal injections of LPA produce a dose-dependent induction of pruritus [16, 24]. Pregnane X receptor (PXR) which is a nuclear steroid receptor is believed to have a vital role in ATX synthesis; however, the mechanism still remains unclear. In vitro studies have shown that the PXR agonist rifampicin reduces ATX synthesis and hence reduces pruritus [9].

In terms of the transduction of pruritus sensation, there are two main theories. The first is the intensity theory which proposes that the same neuronal pathways carry both the itch and pain stimuli. As a result, a weaker stimulus gives an itch perception and an increased stimulus gives the perception of pain. The second is the specificity theory, which suggests that a different group of nerves carries the itch and pain perception separately and factors such as genetics, diet, and environment may be responsible for varying susceptibility for pruritus between individuals.

3.2. Management of Pruritus. There has been a plethora of work investigating possible treatment options for pruritus in the setting of chronic liver disease. These medical treatments range from bile salts, rifampicin, andopioid receptor antagonists to antihistamines. Additionally nonpharmacological management such as skin moisturisers, avoidance of skin irritants, and avoiding hot environments can also prove to be very beneficial in reducing pruritus.

Bile salt resins such as cholestyramine are usually the first line treatment for pruritus in cholestatic disease. Several studies have shown the efficacy of bile salt resins in symptom control of pruritus [10, 11]. Cholestyramine is an effective medication with minimal side effects, which include gastrointestinal upset, unpleasant taste, and rarely fat malabsorption. Ursodeoxycholic acid (UDCA) is one of the bile acids which has been shown to improve jaundice, improve ascites, and improve liver function in primary biliary cirrhosis [12], however, has little benefit on pruritus [13]. It is, however, highly effective in intrahepatic cholestasis of pregnancy (ICP) [14] and hence UDCA is currently only indicated in the treatment of ICP in light of a recent randomised control trial which showed that UDCA improves pruritus and is safe to use during pregnancy [18]. More recent research has explored farnesoid X nuclear receptors in maintaining homeostasis in bile acid synthesis and farsenoid X receptor agonists may prove to be an upcoming treatment option for PBC [19].

Rifampicin is another effective treatment option for cholestatic pruritus, especially in pruritus refractory to therapy and in malignant cholestasis [20, 21]. A recent meta-analysis of randomized controlled trials highlighted the safety of rifampicin in the treatment of cholestatic pruritus [22]. However, regular blood test monitoring is still needed for patients on rifampicin treatment owing to the risk of hepatotoxicity [16]. μ-Opioid receptor antagonists such as naloxone or naltrexone are also shown to be effective in the management of cholestatic pruritus [15, 24, 25]. However, opiate withdrawal reaction is one of the common side effects and hence this treatment option should be avoided in patients with drug addiction issues [25]. It should also be avoided in patients with acute hepatitis and liver failure. Finally, in a placebo-controlled trial, selective serotonin reuptake inhibitor sertraline was shown to be more effective than placebo group in controlling pruritus [23].

Contrary to established doctrine, a recent review has shown that topical antihistamines are not very effective in the treatment of pruritus [26]. There are still new emerging therapeutic options for pruritus treatment for patients who remain refractory to the abovementioned treatments. Although further evidence is needed to further test their efficacy. Albumin dialysis using molecular adsorbent recirculating system is one of them. A multicentric analysis concluded that the dialysis was significantly effective in pruritus management [27]. Similarly plasmapheresis is suggested as a treatment option for primary biliary cirrhosis in pregnant woman [28].

There are several other potentially useful agents in the management of chronic liver disease-associated pruritus but to date have only been confined to isolated case reports and small-scale series and so cannot be recommended. However, these are discussed here for completeness and include thalidomide, ondansetron, phenobarbital, and stanozolol. Thalidomide is an example of a primary antipruritic agent which has shown promise in primary biliary sclerosis. Its side effects can include significant drowsiness, suggesting a central depressant mechanism underlying it action [1, 2]. Ondansetron is a serotonin 5-HT3 receptor subtype antagonist that is effective in the management of nausea and vomiting. Although it is usually tolerated well with few side effects, there is only anecdotal evidence to support its use in pruritis from chronic liver disease and studies have provided mixed

results [3–5]. Similarly, phenobarbital or phenobarbitone is a long-acting barbiturate and has also been investigated in reducing pruritus in chronic liver disease; however, it also does not appear to have a clear beneficial effect [6, 17]. Stanozolol is a synthetic anabolic steroid derived from dihydrotestosterone. Although it relieves pruritus, it also worsens cholestasis and so cannot be recommended [23].

4. Discussion

The impact of pruritus on the quality of life of patients suffering from chronic liver failure is often underestimated by physicians. Although the severity of pruritus is variable between patients, it can have significant implications on a patient's mental health and psychological well-being. The paucity of clinical literature addressing pruritus in liver patients demonstrates the lack of focused research on the topic and in turn highlights the difficulty faced by the physician when confronted with treatment-resistant patients with pruritus.

The underlying pathophysiology is unclear and is likely to be a result of a number of interrelated complex pathways with multifactorial etiologies [29]. The European Association for the Study of the Liver (EASL) has established guidelines for the initial clinical assessment, investigation, and management of pruritus in cholestatic liver diseases [30]. The approach to management should be in a step-wise fashion starting with the simple agents listed above and then escalating to more experimental treatments in resistant cases. An appropriate approach would be to start with UDCA and then cholestyramine followed by rifampicin and naltrexone and if symptoms persist this may be followed by therapies such as sertraline [31]. Experimental therapies such as UVA/B light therapy or other experimental drug therapies can be reserved for cases resistant to conventional therapy [32].

Hence it is clear that, due to poorly understood pathophysiology, there is no one single ideal treatment for all chronic liver disease patients suffering from pruritus. Although there are several treatment options available, achieving optimum symptom control may require a trial and error process to find the best regime for each patient. Nonetheless, despite available treatments a small number of sufferers may not respond to any therapy and this group may require liver transplant, even in the absence of liver failure, to treat their symptoms [30, 33, 34].

This review was restricted to published literature in the English language and confined to the eligibility criteria described in the methods section. Due to the heterogeneity of the outcomes measured in the literature and the wide remit of this review a quantitative analysis was not feasible. Nonetheless the general conclusions from the current evidence base have been presented. The future of experimental research in this field will focus on novel agents in the treatment of pruritus; however, basic research into understanding the underlying etiology and signaling of pruritus is paramount for pharmacological progress in this field. Nonetheless there is also a clear need for focused work in phase III and IV studies comparing the clinical effectiveness of established agents and combinations thereof in different etiologies of liver disease and different patient subgroups in order to strengthen the evidence base upon which clinical guidelines can be set.

5. Conclusion

The burden of pruritus in liver disease patients persists and although it is a common symptom, it can be difficult to manage. Despite there being a large body of research into the etiology and treatment of the condition, pruritus remains poorly understood and many patients continue to suffer. What is known has been presented in this review but the field requires continued basic science research to help broaden our knowledge of the etiology of pruritus and more clinical research on treatment options to help improve the quality of life of chronic liver disease patients.

Ethical Approval

Ethical approval was not required for this work.

Conflict of Interests

The authors have no conflict of interests.

Authors' Contribution

Angeline Bhalerao and Gurdeep S. Mannu contributed equally.

References

[1] F. Adams, *The Extant Works of Aretaeus, the Cappadocian,* Sydenham Society, London, UK, 1865.

[2] H. Wang and G. Yosipovitch, "New insights into the pathophysiology and treatment of chronic itch in patients with end-stage renal disease, chronic liver disease, and lymphoma," *International Journal of Dermatology,* vol. 49, no. 1, pp. 1–11, 2010.

[3] E. Rishe, A. Azarm, and N. V. Bergasa, "Itch in primary biliary cirrhosis: a patients' perspective," *Acta Dermato-Venereologica,* vol. 88, no. 1, pp. 34–37, 2008.

[4] E. Jacquemin, "Progressive familial intrahepatic cholestasis," *Clinics and Research in Hepatology and Gastroenterology,* vol. 36, supplement 1, pp. S26–S35, 2012.

[5] S. Montagnese, L. M. Nsemi, N. Cazzagon et al., "Sleep-Wake profiles in patients with primary biliary cirrhosis," *Liver International,* vol. 33, no. 2, pp. 203–209, 2013.

[6] M. Huesmann, T. Huesmann, N. Osada, N. Q. Phan, A. E. Kremer, and S. Ständer, "Cholestatic pruritus: a retrospective analysis on clinical characteristics and treatment response," *Journal of the German Society of Dermatology,* vol. 11, no. 2, pp. 158–169, 2013.

[7] R. Chapman, J. Fevery, A. Kalloo et al., "Diagnosis and management of primary sclerosing cholangitis," *Hepatology,* vol. 51, no. 2, pp. 660–678, 2010.

[8] S. Kunzmann, G. A. Kullak-Ublick, A. Greiner, R. Jeschke, and H. Hebestreit, "Effective opiate-receptor antagonist therapy of cholestatic pruritus induced by an oral contraceptive," *Journal of Pediatric Gastroenterology and Nutrition,* vol. 40, no. 5, pp. 596–599, 2005.

[9] A. E. Kremer, R. van Dijk, P. Leckie et al., "Serum autotaxin is increased in pruritus of cholestasis, but not of other origin, and responds to therapeutic interventions," *Hepatology,* vol. 56, no. 4, pp. 1391–1400, 2012.

[10] C. di Padova, R. Tritapepe, P. Rovagnati, and S. Rossetti, "Double-blind placebo-controlled clinical trial of microporous cholestyramine in the treatment of intra- and extra-hepatic cholestasis: relationship between itching and serum bile acids," *Methods and Findings in Experimental and Clinical Pharmacology,* vol. 6, no. 12, pp. 773–776, 1984.

[11] J. S. Duncan, H. J. Kennedy, and D. R. Triger, "Treatment of pruritus due to chronic obstructive liver disease," *British Medical Journal,* vol. 288, no. 6436, p. 22, 1984.

[12] Y. Gong, Z. B. Huang, E. Christensen, and C. Gluud, "Ursodeoxycholic acid for primary biliary cirrhosis," *The Cochrane Database of Systematic Reviews,* vol. 3, Article ID CD000551, 2008.

[13] C. O. Zein and K. D. Lindor, "Latest and emerging therapies for primary biliary cirrhosis and primary sclerosing cholangitis," *Current Gastroenterology Reports,* vol. 12, no. 1, pp. 13–22, 2010.

[14] A. Glantz, S.-J. Reilly, L. Benthin, F. Lammert, L.-Å. Mattsson, and H.-U. Marschall, "Intrahepatic cholestasis of pregnancy: amelioration of pruritus by UDCA is associated with decreased progesterone disulphates in urine," *Hepatology,* vol. 47, no. 2, pp. 544–551, 2008.

[15] F. H. J. Wolfhagen, E. Sternieri, W. C. J. Hop, G. Vitale, M. Bertolotti, and H. R. Van Buuren, "Oral naltrexone treatment for cholestatic pruritus: a double-blind, placebo-controlled study," *Gastroenterology,* vol. 113, no. 4, pp. 1264–1269, 1997.

[16] M. I. Prince, A. D. Burt, and D. E. J. Jones, "Hepatitis and liver dysfunction with rifampicin therapy for pruritus in primary biliary cirrhosis," *Gut,* vol. 50, no. 3, pp. 436–439, 2002.

[17] O. Hagermark, "Peripheral and central mediators of itch," *Skin Pharmacology,* vol. 5, no. 1, pp. 1–8, 1992.

[18] T. Joutsiniemi, S. Timonen, R. Leino, P. Palo, and U. Ekblad, "Ursodeoxycholic acid in the treatment of intrahepatic cholestasis of pregnancy: a randomized controlled trial," *Archives of Gynecology and Obstetrics,* vol. 289, no. 3, pp. 541–547, 2014.

[19] K. D. Lindor, "Farnesoid X receptor agonists for primary biliary cirrhosis," *Current Opinion in Gastroenterology,* vol. 27, no. 3, pp. 285–288, 2011.

[20] C. Levy and K. D. Lindor, "Current management of primary biliary cirrhosis and primary sclerosing cholangitis," *Journal of Hepatology,* vol. 38, supplement 1, pp. S24–S37, 2003.

[21] T. J. Price, W. K. Patterson, and I. N. Olver, "Rifampicin as treatment for pruritus in malignant cholestasis," *Supportive Care in Cancer,* vol. 6, no. 6, pp. 533–535, 1998.

[22] S. Khurana and P. Singh, "Rifampin is safe for treatment of pruritus due to chronic cholestasis: a Meta-analysis of prospective randomized-controlled trials," *Liver International,* vol. 26, no. 8, pp. 943–948, 2006.

[23] M. J. Mayo, I. Handem, S. Saldana, H. Jacobe, Y. Getachew, and A. J. Rush, "Sertraline as a first-line treatment for cholestatic pruritus," *Hepatology,* vol. 45, no. 3, pp. 666–674, 2007.

[24] N. V. Bergasa, D. W. Ailing, T. L. Talbot et al., "Effects of naloxone infusions in patients with the pruritus of cholestasis: a double-blind, randomized, controlled trial," *Annals of Internal Medicine,* vol. 123, no. 3, pp. 161–167, 1995.

[25] N. Q. Phan, J. D. Bernhard, T. A. Luger, and S. Ständer, "Antipruritic treatment with systemic μ-opioid receptor antagonists: a

review," *Journal of the American Academy of Dermatology*, vol. 63, no. 4, pp. 680–688, 2010.

[26] D. C. Eschler and P. A. Klein, "An evidence-based review of the efficacy of topical antihistamines in the relief of pruritus," *Journal of Drugs in Dermatology*, vol. 9, no. 8, pp. 992–997, 2010.

[27] A. Parés, M. Herrera, J. Avilés, M. Sanz, and A. Mas, "Treatment of resistant pruritus from cholestasis with albumin dialysis: combined analysis of patients from three centers," *Journal of Hepatology*, vol. 53, no. 2, pp. 307–312, 2010.

[28] A. Alallam, D. Barth, and E. J. Heathcote, "Role of plasmapheresis in the treatment of severe pruritus in pregnant patients with primary biliary cirrhosis: case reports," *Canadian Journal of Gastroenterology*, vol. 22, no. 5, pp. 505–507, 2008.

[29] R. Poupon, "Pruritus in liver disease: introductory remarks," *Clinics and Research in Hepatology and Gastroenterology*, vol. 35, no. 2, pp. 79–80, 2011.

[30] European Association for the Study of the Liver, "EASL Clinical Practice Guidelines: management of cholestatic liver diseases," *Journal of Hepatology*, vol. 51, no. 2, pp. 237–267, 2009.

[31] A. E. Kremer, R. P. J. Oude Elferink, and U. Beuers, "Pathophysiology and current management of pruritus in liver disease," *Clinics and Research in Hepatology and Gastroenterology*, vol. 35, no. 2, pp. 89–97, 2011.

[32] N. V. Bergasa, M. J. Link, M. Keogh, G. Yaroslavsky, R. N. Rosenthal, and M. McGee, "Pilot study of bright-light therapy reflected toward the eyes for the pruritus of chronic liver disease," *The American Journal of Gastroenterology*, vol. 96, no. 5, pp. 1563–1570, 2001.

[33] E. J. Heathcote, "Management of primary biliary cirrhosis. The American Association for the Study of Liver Diseases practice guidelines," *Hepatology*, vol. 31, no. 4, pp. 1005–1013, 2000.

[34] S. C. Abraham, P. S. Kamath, B. Eghtesad, A. J. Demetris, and A. M. Krasinskas, "Liver transplantation in precirrhotic biliary tract disease: portal hypertension is frequently associated with nodular regenerative hyperplasia and obliterative portal venopathy," *American Journal of Surgical Pathology*, vol. 30, no. 11, pp. 1454–1461, 2006.

4

Effect of Narrow-Band Ultraviolet B Phototherapy and Methotrexate on MicroRNA (146a) Levels in Blood of Psoriatic Patients

Asmaa M. Ele-Refaei and Fatma M. El-Esawy

Dermatology & Andrology Department, Faculty of Medicine, Benha University, Benha, Egypt

Correspondence should be addressed to Fatma M. El-Esawy; fatmaelesawy99@yahoo.com

Academic Editor: Markus Stucker

Background. Recently, some miRNAs have been proven to show aberrant expression in psoriasis and play a role in the pathogenesis of the disease. *Objective.* To find out whether NB-UVB or methotrexate treatment affects whole blood levels of human miRNA (146a) in patients with psoriasis and demonstrate its correlation with disease severity. *Methods.* Blood samples were obtained from healthy control and from psoriatic patients before and 12 weeks after treatment with NB-UVB, methotrexate. Quantification of human miRNA (146a) by Real Time PCR (RT-PCR). *Results.* Blood human miRNA (146a) levels were higher in patients with psoriasis than those in healthy controls ($P = 0.001$); it had no significant positive relation with PASI scores in patients ($r = 0.2$, $P = 0.107$). Real Time PCR showed that, after 12 weeks of treatment with NB-UVB phototherapy or treatment with methotrexate, there was significantly decreased level of miR146a ($P = 0.001$; $P = 0.002$, resp.). *Conclusion.* The expression of miRNA146a is increased in whole blood samples from psoriasis patients, so we can evaluate its possibility to work as a future therapeutic objective in the treatment of psoriasis. With these markers, it is able to screen therapeutics effect or changes to a further aggressive treatment for psoriasis.

1. Introduction

Psoriasis is a common skin disorder affecting about 3% of the world population. It is characterized by relapsing skin lesions displaying epidermal hyperplasia, an inflammatory infiltrate, and angiogenesis. The inflammatory reaction is believed to be largely the result of an interaction between innate immunity (mediated by antigen-presenting cells and natural killer T lymphocytes) and acquired immunity (mediated by T lymphocytes) [1].

MicroRNAs (miRNAs) are short, endogenous, non-protein-coding RNAs with important roles in health and disease. miRNAs negatively regulate gene expression by binding to the $3'$-untranslated regions of mRNAs and initiating either translational repression or cleavage [2, 3].

Several studies have pointed to the involvement of miRNAs in the pathogenesis of psoriasis miR203, miR21, and miR146a that are all increased, whereas miR125b is downregulated compared with healthy skin. This suggests that miRNAs may play a role in psoriasis pathogenesis. Increased miR203 levels are associated with constitutive activation of STAT3 signaling, and this is achieved by direct targeting of SOCS3 for suppression, which is involved in inflammatory response and in keratinocyte functions [4]. So microRNA deregulation is involved in the pathogenesis of psoriasis and contributes to the dysfunction of the cross talk between resident and infiltrating cells [4].

These differentially expressed miRNAs are likely to influence many processes that are involved in psoriasis pathogenesis such as angiogenesis (miR21, miR31, and miR378), epidermal differentiation (miR135b, miR205, and miR203-AS), and inflammation (miR142-3p) [5]. Other miRNAs that are abnormally expressed in psoriasis are miR146a and miR125b. Overexpression of miR146a in psoriasis is controlled by the transcription factor NF-κB, and the NF-κB target genes TRAF6 and IRAK are involved in regulating the TNF-α signaling pathway [6], suggesting that miR146a may control TNF-α signaling in the skin [7]. In human T cells, miR146a is expressed at low levels in naïve T lymphocytes while it is abundantly expressed in memory T cells and it is induced upon TCR stimulation, consistent with its expression being dependent on NF-κB induction [6, 8]. MiR146a has been shown both in vitro and in vivo to directly target two serine/threonine kinases, interleukin-1 receptor-associated kinase 1 (IRAK1) and tumor necrosis factor (TNF) receptor-associated factor 6 (TRAF6), that become associated with the interleukin-1 receptor (IL-1R) upon stimulation and are partially responsible for IL-1-induced upregulation of NF-κB. This binding results in the suppression of the expression of NF-κB's target genes such as the interleukins IL-6, IL-8, and IL-1β, and TNF-alpha (TNF-α) [9].

Narrow-band ultraviolet B (NB-UVB) therapy is associated with suppression of type I and type II IFN signaling, downmodulation of the Th17 pathway, and modulation of genes involved in epidermal differentiation in lesional psoriatic epidermis. In addition, several anti-inflammatory pathways, such as glucocorticoid, vitamin D, peroxisome proliferator activated receptor, and IL-4 signaling, are modulated by NB-UVB therapy [10].

Methotrexate is a successful and popular medicine used for treating severe psoriasis and some other serious or extensive skin conditions. It has anti-inflammatory properties; the precise mechanism of action is not understood, but it may relate to an increase in intracellular adenosine, a purine nucleoside that has anti-inflammatory effect. Methotrexate also has weak immune suppressive effects, also reducing the speed in which skin cells proliferate; it is a folate antagonist, which means it prevents the action of essential B vitamin, folic acid, on cellular function resulting in reduction in pyrimidine, purines, and methylation of DNA [11].

Aim of Work. The aim of this work is to compare the blood levels of miR146a in psoriasis patients and healthy controls and to evaluate the effect of NB-UVB and methotrexate treatment on blood miR146a levels in patients with psoriasis.

2. Patients and Methods

This case control study included forty patients with moderate or severe chronic plaque psoriasis who were selected from the outpatient Dermatology Clinic in Benha University Hospital, starting from January 2013 to October 2013. Patients had not received systemic immunosuppressive treatment or phototherapy, for at least 1 month, and topical therapy for 2 weeks before inclusion in this study. The control group consisted of 20 apparently healthy persons; both patients and control were between 18 and 65 years old. An informed consent was taken from the patients about their acceptance of being in the study, which was approved by Ethics Committee of Benha University.

A common questionnaire was used to complete demographic and characteristic information (e.g., age, sex, onset age, disease course, and family history). The Psoriasis Area and Severity Index (PASI) score of each psoriasis patient was evaluated.

The patients were divided into two groups. Group I had twenty patients with chronic plaque type psoriasis, 11 males

and 9 females, with mean age 39.9 ± 16.9 years; they received methotrexate 12.5 mg Intramuscular once a week for 12 weeks.

Group II had twenty patients diagnosed with plaque-type psoriasis, 11 males and 9 females, with mean age 42.4 ± 14.1; their individual minimum erythema doses were assessed before the NB-UVB treatment. NB-UVB irradiation was administered to the whole body two to three times a week using a cabinet PCL 8000, Puva Combi Light, ARKADE, Heverlee, Belgium, equipped with fluorescent lamps UVB TL100W/01, Philips, Eindhoven, The Netherlands. About 24 sessions were given during a time of 2-3 months, with an initial dose of 0.1–0.3 J/cm^2, increased accordingly depending on skin tolerance and clinical response.

2.1. Molecular Biology Investigations (Quantification of Human miRNA146a) by Real Time PCR (RT-PCR). Blood samples from the patients were collected before and 12 weeks after the initiation of therapy with methotrexate and NB-UVB irradiation. The samples were collected immediately into RNA Protect Animal Blood tubes supplied by Qiagen, Germany. The tubes contain a reagent that lyses blood cells, designed for stabilization of intracellular RNA to preserve the gene expression profile. The samples were then stored at −80°C for further processing.

2.1.1. Total RNA Extraction Including MicroRNA. Total RNA including miRNA was extracted from blood samples stabilized in RNA Protect Animal Blood tubes, using MiRNeasy Protect Animal Blood Kits (Qiagen, GmbH Hilden, Germany) according to manufacturer instructions [12].

2.1.2. Reverse Transcription Step of Quantitative Real Time PCR. Total RNA was reverse transcribed into cDNA using specific reverse transcription (RT) primers (Table 1). The reaction mixture of 20 μL contained 20 ng total RNA, 2 μL of primer, 2 μL of dNTPs, 1 μL of RT enzyme, 2 μL of RT buffer, 0.5 μL (20 units) RNase inhibitor, and nuclease-free water up to 20 μL. The cDNA was diluted to 200 μL.

2.1.3. Real Time PCR for Detection of miRNA146a. For miRNA quantity by real time PCR, the amount of the target miRNA (miRNA146a) was normalized against endogenous reference RNA. In this study we used U6 as normalization control. The relative quantities of the miRNA146a were normalized against the relative quantities of endogenous control (U6). Fold expression changes are calculated using the equation $2^{-\Delta\Delta ct}$ [13]. Real time PCR was performed using super real premix plus (sybr green) kit supplied by (TIANGEN, Biotech, Beijing). The reaction mix contained 10 μL 2x super real premix plus, 1 μL of forward primer, 1 μL of reverse primer, 5 μL of cDNA, 0.4 50x ROX reference dye, and 2.6 RNase-free water. Amplification of miRNA146a and U6 were done in separate PCR tubes.

2.2. Statistical Analysis. The clinical data were recorded on a report form. These data were tabulated and analyzed using the computer program SPSS (Statistical Package for

TABLE 1: Primers used in the reverse transcription and PCR steps.

| RNA | Reverse transcription specific primers | $5'$-$3'$ primer | | |
| | | | PCR primers | |
		Forward primer	Reverse primer
miR146a	*Stem loop primer* GTCGTATCCAGTGCGTGTCGTGGAGT CGGCAATTGCACTGGATACGACaaccca	GGGTGAGAACTGAATTCCA	CAGTGCGTGTCGTGGAGT

TABLE 2: Comparison between patient groups and control group as regards level of miRNA146a.

		Group I $N = 20$	Group II $N = 20$	Control $N = 10$	F-test	P value
miR146a level (RU)	Mean ± SD	(22.6 ± 3.3)	(17.3 ± 1.3)	(9.3 ± 3.8)	75.6	<0.001

Social Science) version 16 (*SPSS Inc., Chicago*) to obtain the following.

Descriptive statistics were calculated for the data in the form of (1) mean and standard deviation (±SD) for quantitative data; (2) frequency and distribution for qualitative data.

In the statistical comparison between the different groups, the significance of difference was tested using one of the following tests: (1) Student's t-test and Mann-Whitney test, used to compare mean of two groups of parametric and nonparametric quantitative data, respectively; (2) ANOVA test (F value), used to compare mean of more than two groups of quantitative data; (3) intergroup comparison of categorical data performed by using Fisher exact test (FET); (4) correlation coefficient, used to find relationships between variables.

3. Results

All the participants were examined and diagnosed by dermatologists. The mean age for group I was 39.9 ± 16.9 years, for group II was 42.4 ± 14.1 years, and was 44.6 ± 17.82 years for the controls ($P = 0.677$); the percentage of men was 55% for group I and for group II and 60.0% for the control ($P = 0.15$). The patients who have a family history of psoriasis are 30% in group I, 15% in group II ($P = 0.02$). The mean disease duration for group I was 2.9 ± 1.2 years, while it was 8 ± 5.6 years for group II ($P = 0.001$). The mean value of PASI score before and after treatment was 26.5 ± 3.8, 9.7 ± 2.9, respectively, in group I ($P = 0.001$), while in group II it was 25.7 ± 2.8, 8.3 ± 1.9, respectively ($P = 0.001$).

The blood levels of miR146a in patients were significantly higher than control (Table 2 and Figure 1). The mean level of miRNA146a before and after therapy was 22.6 ± 3.3 RU, 16.3 ± 1.7 RU correspondingly ($P = 0.001$) in group I, while it was 17.3 ± 1.3, 14.0 ± 1.3 RU correspondingly ($P = 0.002$) in group II (Table 3 and Figure 2).

There was no significant positive correlation between miR146a level before treatment and age and PASI score among all patients ($r = 0.1$, P value = 0.269) ($r = 0.2$, P value = 0.107), respectively. Whereas there was a significant positive correlation between miR146a and disease duration ($r = 0.3$, P value = 0.03) (Table 4 and Figure 3).

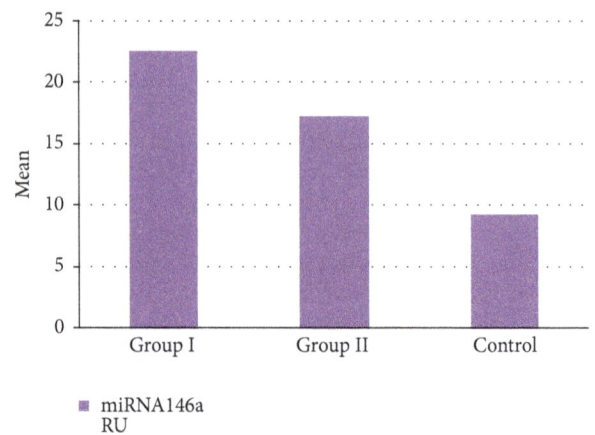

FIGURE 1: Comparison between group I, group II patients and control group as regards level of miRNA146a.

TABLE 3: Comparison between patient groups as regards level of miR146a before and after therapy.

Variable	Group I $n = 20$ Mean ± SD	Group II $n = 20$ Mean ± SD	t-test	P value
miR146a (RU) before	(22.6 ± 3.3)	(17.3 ± 1.3)	6.6	<0.001
miR146a (RU) after	(16.3 ± 1.7)	(14 ± 1.3)	4.8	<0.001
t-test	7.6	8		
P value	<0.001	<0.001		

4. Discussion

Taganov et al. [6] reported that microRNA146a/b (miR146a/b) is induced in response to lipopolysaccharide (LPS) and proinflammatory mediators and that miR146a induction is regulated by NF-κB. They also found that miR146a/b targets were TNF receptor-associated factor 6 (TRAF6) and IL-1 receptor-associated kinase 1 (IRAK1) genes and concluded that miR146 plays a role in fine-tuning innate immune responses by negative feedback, including downregulation of TRAF6 and

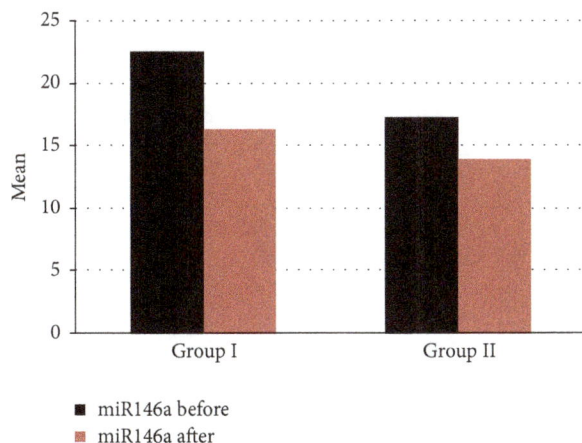

FIGURE 2: Comparison between group I and group II as regards level of miR146a before and after therapy.

■ miR146a before
■ miR146a after

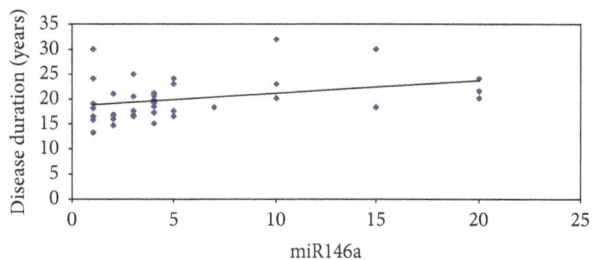

FIGURE 3: Correlation between miR146a level before treatment and disease duration among all patients.

TABLE 4: Correlation between miR146a level before treatment and age, disease duration, and PASI score among all patients.

Variables	miR146a level	
	r	P value
Age	0.1	0.269
Duration of disease	0.3	0.03
PSAI score	0.2	0.107

IRAK1 genes. A recent major observation involving a new role for miRNAs is their ability to determine the efficacy of drugs. These findings gave rise to the field of miRNA pharmacogenomics [14].

Previous studies showed that most of tissue miRNAs could be detected in body fluid. Circulating miRNA in serum has been postulated as reliable biomarkers for disease prediction, diagnosis, and severity assessment. Under normal conditions, miRNAs are released mostly from circulating blood cells in serum, while under diseased conditions, miRNAs expression profiles are different and depend on the types and natures of the diseases [15].

The results of the present study showed that there were increased blood levels of miR146a in psoriatic patients higher than the control group. This was in agreement with the results of other studies [16–18]. miR146a is possibly involved in pathogenesis of psoriasis by modulating functions of macrophage [19], dendritic cells [20], Th1 cells [6], T reg cells [21], and Th17 cells [22]. Xia et al. [16] reported that increased miR146a with impaired function failed to repress the expression of *IRAK1*, thus inducing IL-17 persistence in psoriatic skin lesions.

In the current study, there was significant decrease of miR146a levels after therapy with methotrexate; this was in concurrence with the results of Pivarcsi et al. [17]; they found that anti-TNF-alpha therapy, etanercept, and methotrexate altered serum miRNA level in psoriatic patients. This may be due to the effect of methotrexate on DNA synthesis in epidermal cells and also due to its immunosuppressive effects on activated T cells that control psoriasis [23].

Also there was decrease in miR146a level in patients treated with NB-UVB in this study; this was in accordance with the results of Gu et al. [24]. This was due to the effect of NB-UVB leading to cell cycle arrest, T cell apoptosis, and apoptosis upon DNA damage as stated by Menter et al. [25] and Gu et al. [24].

There was no significant positive correlation between PASI score and the levels of correlation between miRNAs and PASI score, while there was a significant positive correlation between the disease duration and the levels of miR146a. This was in agreement of the results of Xia et al. [16]; this can be due to associated comorbidities including hypertension, atherosclerosis, and diabetes mellitus.

5. Conclusion

In conclusion, we have shown significant changes in blood levels of miR146a subsequent treatment with methotrexate and NB-UVB phototherapy, indicating considerable roles for these molecules in treatment of the disease. Early prediction of response to therapy using mRNA is an opportunity for effective individual medication and therefore allows preventing side effects by reducing the costs.

Conflict of Interests

The authors declare that there is no conflict of interests regarding the publication of this paper.

References

[1] J. Wohlrab, G. Fiedler, S. Gerdes et al., "Recommendations for detection of individual risk for comorbidities in patients with psoriasis," *Archives of Dermatological Research*, vol. 305, no. 2, pp. 91–98, 2013.

[2] I. Alvarez-Garcia and E. A. Miska, "MicroRNA functions in animal development and human disease," *Development*, vol. 132, no. 21, pp. 4653–4662, 2005.

[3] R. Visone and C. M. Croce, "MiRNAs and cancer," *The American Journal of Pathology*, vol. 174, no. 4, pp. 1131–1138, 2009.

[4] E. Sonkoly, T. Wei, P. C. J. Janson et al., "MicroRNAs: novel regulators involved in the pathogenesis of psoriasis?" *PLoS ONE*, vol. 2, no. 7, article e610, 2007.

[5] C.-Z. Chen, L. Li, H. F. Lodish, and D. P. Bartel, "MicroRNAs modulate hematopoietic lineage differentiation," *Science*, vol. 303, no. 5654, pp. 83–86, 2004.

[6] K. D. Taganov, M. P. Boldin, K.-J. Chang, and D. Baltimore, "NF-κB-dependent induction of microRNA miR-146, an inhibitor targeted to signaling proteins of innate immune responses," *Proceedings of the National Academy of Sciences of the United States of America*, vol. 103, no. 33, pp. 12481–12486, 2006.

[7] E. Tili, J.-J. Michaille, A. Cimino et al., "Modulation of miR-155 and miR-125b levels following lipopolysaccharide/TNF-α stimulation and their possible roles in regulating the response to endotoxin shock," *The Journal of Immunology*, vol. 179, no. 8, pp. 5082–5089, 2007.

[8] G. Curtale, F. Citarella, C. Carissimi et al., "An emerging player in the adaptive immune response: microRNA-146a is a modulator of IL-2 expression and activation-induced cell death in T lymphocytes," *Blood*, vol. 115, no. 2, pp. 265–273, 2010.

[9] M. A. Nahid, K. M. Pauley, M. Satoh, and E. K. L. Chan, "MiR-146a is critical for endotoxin-induced tolerance: implication in innate immunity," *The Journal of Biological Chemistry*, vol. 284, no. 50, pp. 34590–34599, 2009.

[10] E. Rácz, E. P. Prens, D. Kurek et al., "Effective treatment of psoriasis with narrow-band UVB phototherapy is linked to suppression of the IFN and Th17 pathways," *Journal of Investigative Dermatology*, vol. 131, no. 7, pp. 1547–1558, 2011.

[11] S. Shen, T. O'Brien, L. M. Yao, H. M. Prince, and C. J. McCormack, "The use of methotrexate in dermatology: a review," *Australasian Journal of Dermatology*, vol. 53, no. 1, pp. 1–18, 2012.

[12] W. W. Wilfinger, K. Mackey, and P. Chomczynski, "Effect of pH and ionic strength on the spectrophotometric assessment of nucleic acid purity," *BioTechniques*, vol. 22, no. 3, pp. 474–481, 1997.

[13] K. J. Livak and T. D. Schmittgen, "Analysis of relative gene expression data using real-time quantitative PCR and the $2^{-\Delta\Delta C_T}$ method," *Methods*, vol. 25, no. 4, pp. 402–408, 2001.

[14] N. Shomron, "MicroRNAs and pharmacogenomics," *Pharmacogenomics*, vol. 11, no. 5, pp. 629–632, 2010.

[15] X. Chen, Y. Ba, L. Ma et al., "Characterization of microRNAs in serum: a novel class of biomarkers for diagnosis of cancer and other diseases," *Cell Research*, vol. 18, no. 10, pp. 997–1006, 2008.

[16] P. Xia, X. Fang, Z.-H. Zhang et al., "Dysregulation of miRNA146a versus IRAK1 induces IL-17 persistence in the psoriatic skin lesions," *Immunology Letters*, vol. 148, no. 2, pp. 151–162, 2012.

[17] A. Pivarcsi, F. Meisgen, N. Xu, M. Stahle, and E. Sonkoly, "Changes in the level of serum microRNAs in patients with psoriasis after antitumor necrosis factor-α therapy," *British Journal of Dermatology*, vol. 169, pp. 563–570, 2013.

[18] W. Zhang, X. Yi, S. Guo et al., "A single-nucleotide polymorphism of miR-146a and psoriasis: an association and functional study," *Journal of Cellular and Molecular Medicine*, vol. 18, no. 11, pp. 2225–2234, 2015.

[19] O. Ichii, S. Otsuka, N. Sasaki, Y. Namiki, Y. Hashimoto, and Y. Kon, "Altered expression of microRNA miR-146a correlates with the development of chronic renal inflammation," *Kidney International*, vol. 81, no. 3, pp. 280–292, 2012.

[20] M. L. Turner, F. M. Schnorfeil, and T. Brocker, "MicroRNAs regulate dendritic cell differentiation and function," *The Journal of Immunology*, vol. 187, no. 8, pp. 3911–3917, 2011.

[21] L.-F. Lu, M. P. Boldin, A. Chaudhry et al., "Function of miR-146a in controlling treg cell-mediated regulation of Th1 responses," *Cell*, vol. 142, no. 6, pp. 914–929, 2010.

[22] T. Niimoto, T. Nakasa, M. Ishikawa et al., "MicroRNA-146a expresses in interleukin-17 producing T cells in rheumatoid arthritis patients," *BMC Musculoskeletal Disorders*, vol. 11, article 209, 2010.

[23] R. A. Gottlieb, H. A. Giesing, J. Y. Zhu, R. L. Engler, and B. M. Babior, "Cell acidification in apoptosis: granulocyte colony-stimulating factor delays programed cell death in neutrophils by up-regulating the vacuolar H$^+$-ATPase," *Proceedings of the National Academy of Sciences of the United States of America*, vol. 92, no. 13, pp. 5965–5968, 1995.

[24] X. Gu, E. Nylander, P. J. Coates, and K. Nylander, "Effect of narrow-band ultraviolet B phototherapy on p63 and MicroRNA (miR-21 and miR-125b) expression in psoriatic epidermis," *Acta Dermato-Venereologica*, vol. 91, no. 4, pp. 392–397, 2011.

[25] A. Menter, N. J. Korman, C. A. Elmets et al., "Guidelines of care for the management of psoriasis and psoriatic arthritis: section 5. Guidelines of care for the treatment of psoriasis with phototherapy and photochemotherapy," *Journal of the American Academy of Dermatology*, vol. 62, no. 1, pp. 114–135, 2010.

5

Study of the Etiological Causes of Toe Web Space Lesions in Cairo, Egypt

Hussein Mohamed Hassab-El-Naby,[1,2] Yasser Fathy Mohamed,[1,2] Hamed Mohamed Abdo,[1,2] Mohamed Ismail Kamel,[1,2] Wael Refaat Hablas,[1,3] and Osama Khalil Mohamed[1,2]

[1]*Al-Hussein University Hospital, Gawhar Al Qaed Street, El Darrasa, Cairo 11633, Egypt*
[2]*Dermatology, Venereology and Andrology, Faculty of Medicine, Al-Azhar University, Cairo 11823, Egypt*
[3]*Clinical and Chemical Pathology, Faculty of Medicine, Al-Azhar University, Cairo 11823, Egypt*

Correspondence should be addressed to Hamed Mohamed Abdo; hamed392@yahoo.com

Academic Editor: Iris Zalaudek

Background. The etiology of foot intertrigo is varied. Several pathogens and skin conditions might play a role in toe web space lesions. *Objective.* To identify the possible etiological causes of toe web space lesions. *Methods.* 100 Egyptian patients were enrolled in this study (72 females and 28 males). Their ages ranged from 18 to 79 years. For every patient, detailed history taking, general and skin examinations, and investigations including Wood's light examination, skin scraping for potassium hydroxide test, skin swabs for bacterial isolation, and skin biopsy all were done. *Results.* Among the 100 patients, positive Wood's light fluorescence was observed in 24 and positive bacterial growth was observed in 85. With skin biopsy, 52 patients showed features characteristic for eczema, 25 showed features characteristic for fungus, 19 showed features characteristic for callosity, and 3 showed features characteristic for wart while in only 1 patient the features were characteristic for lichen planus. *Conclusion.* Toe web space lesions are caused by different etiological factors. The most common was interdigital eczema (52%) followed by fungal infection (25%). We suggest that patients who do not respond to antifungals should be reexamined for another primary or secondary dermatologic condition that may resemble interdigital fungal infection.

1. Introduction

Toe web intertrigo may present as a relatively asymptomatic, mild scaling but it also can be seen as a painful, exudative, macerated, erosive, inflammatory process which is sometimes malodorous [1].

Foot intertrigo is mostly caused by dermatophytes and yeasts and less frequently by Gram-negative and Gram-positive bacteria. Gram-negative infection is relatively common and may represent a secondary infection of tinea pedis. With time, a "complex" may develop in the setting of moisture and maceration that contains multiple fungal and bacterial organisms [2, 3]. Frequently, these interdigital lesions are often diagnosed as tinea pedis or eczematous dermatitis. However, in some patients, the macerated eruption is unresponsive to treatment with antifungal agents or anti-inflammatory agents such as topical steroids [4].

Other less common conditions may also affect the web space such as erythrasma [5]. Because the texture of soft corn is macerated, it may be misdiagnosed clinically as a mycotic infection of the interdigital space [6]. Interdigital psoriasis ("white psoriasis" or "psoriasis alba") is a distinct but atypical form of psoriasis that is often missed as it is commonly mistaken for interdigital fungal infection [7]. A report of Bowen's disease [8] and a case of *Verrucous* carcinoma in the third and fourth toe web space which is presented by intractable intertrigo has been reported [9]. Also, malignant melanoma in the interdigital space has been diagnosed [10].

It is apparent that several pathogens and factors might play a role in toe web space lesions. Therefore, clinical and microbiologic studies are suggested to assist in the selection of appropriate treatment and the prevention of important complications [3]. In this study, we aimed to determine the different etiological causes of pedal web space lesions.

2. Patients and Methods

This study included 100 Egyptian patients living in Cairo who presented at Dermatology Departments of Al-Azhar University Hospitals with toe web space lesions. The study was approved by the Al-Azhar University Medical Ethics Committee, and written prior informed consent was obtained from every participant. Patients who have received systemic and/or topical antifungal and/or antibiotic treatments in the past 6 weeks were excluded.

Every patient was subjected to the following: (1) full history taking; (2) general and local examinations; (3) Wood's light examination for possible fluorescence; (4) skin scraping for direct potassium hydroxide (KOH) test: scraping of lesions was done with a blunt scalpel then a drop of 20% KOH/40% dimethyl sulfoxide (DMSO) mixture was added to the specimen (DMSO increases sensitivity of the preparation and softens keratin more quickly than KOH alone in the absence of heat [11]); the slide was then examined for fungus using low power field ×10 then high power field ×40; (5) skin swabs for bacterial isolation: cotton swabs were taken from the lesions and incubated for 24 hours at 37°C in blood and MacConkey (BIOTEC Lab. Ltd., UK) and nutrient (Oxoid Ltd., England) agars; the bacterial cultures were considered negative if there was no growth after 48 hours of incubation; the suspected colony was picked up for morphological and biochemical reactions for their identifications; (6) a 3 mm punch biopsy was taken from the lesion. Specimens were fixed in 10% formalin then sectioned and stained with haematoxylin and eosin stain (as a routine) and PAS stain (to highlight fungal elements).

All involved toe web spaces were examined with Wood's light while KOH test, skin swabs for bacterial isolation, and skin biopsy were done from the most affected web space showing intensive erythema and desquamation (almost the 4th web space). Wood's light examination aimed to show the characteristic coral red fluorescence with erythrasma [12].

The goal of mycological workup in this study was to demonstrate just the presence of fungi (regardless of its nature) as an etiologic cause of web space lesions; so we thought that KOH test (supported by PAS-stained tissue sections) will suffice this aim. The recognition of fungal organisms as dermatophyte, mould, or yeast by KOH is presumptive although it is highly probable [13]. We relied upon the WHO guidelines on standard operating procedures for microbiology [14]. These guidelines document that dermatophyte has regular, small hyphae (2-3 μm) with some branching, sometimes with rectangular arthrospores. *Candida* has hyphae/pseudohyphae (with distinct points of constriction) with budding yeast forms. *Aspergillus* species had hyphae that are usually small (3–6 μm) and regular in size, dichotomously branching at 45-degree angles with distinct cross septa.

The histopathological examination aimed to correlate with and confirm the clinical diagnosis. A diagnosis of lichen planus is established when the biopsy showed the following criteria: dense, band-like infiltrate of lymphocytes that is strictly confined to the subepidermal area. The lymphocytes attack and destroy the basic part of the epidermis, giving rise to characteristic sawtooth like rete ridges. The cell infiltrate in the dermis consists of lymphocytes with a mixture of some mast cells and macrophages; there is also a variable amount of melanin pigment which has leaked from the injured epidermis. There are no plasma cells or eosinophils [15].

In biopsies stained with PAS, fungal elements are highlighted, with hyphae and spores stained red. Dermatophytes produce septate hyphae and arthrospores [15].

Biopsy from patients with eczema demonstrates that epidermis shows moderate to marked acanthosis and hyper/parakeratosis. There may be areas of inter- and intracellular edema and rarely scattered small vesicles. The inflammatory cell infiltrates mainly consist of lymphocytes. Edema in the dermis is not prominent. Sometimes the pattern is psoriasis-like and shows long, slender rete ridges and papillae, which are covered by thin epidermis and contain thin-walled dilated venules filled with erythrocytes [15].

Acanthosis, papillomatosis, and hyperkeratosis are observed in biopsies from patients with warts, with confluence of the epidermal ridges in the centre of the lesion and koilocytes [16].

A thickened compact stratum corneum with slight cup-shaped depression of the underlying epidermis is seen in patients with callosity. The granular layer, in contrast to corn, may be thickened. There may be some parakeratosis overlying the dermal papillae, but much less than in a corn [17].

3. Results

3.1. Demographic and Clinical Findings. Of 100 patients with toe web space lesions, 72 were females and 28 were males. Their ages ranged from 18 to 79 years (mean 43.94 years; SD ±14.94). Regarding the presenting symptoms, 64 patients complained of pruritus while only 2 complained of pain and 34 were asymptomatic. The 4th web space was the commonest space affected in both right and left feet, followed by 3rd space, 2nd space, and 1st space (79%, 62%, 33%, and 7% versus 76%, 63%, 30%, and 8%, resp.) (Table 1). Of the 100 patients, 8 patients had lesion in 1 web space, 21 had lesion in 2 web spaces, 26 had lesion in 3 web spaces, 17 had lesion in 4 web spaces, 6 had lesion in 5 web spaces, 18 had lesion in 6 web spaces, 1 had lesion in 7 toe web spaces, and 3 had lesion in 8 web spaces.

3.2. Wood's Light Examination. Among the 100 patients, positive Wood's light fluorescence was observed in 24; of them, 20 were females and 4 were males. All revealed coral red fluorescence characteristic for erythrasma.

3.3. Microbiological Findings. Positive KOH results were noticed in 66 patients; 50 were females and 16 were males. 57 KOH mounts were highly typical of yeast species (yeast

TABLE 1: Distribution of toe web space lesions in the 100 patients.

Toe web space	Right foot		Left foot	
	Frequency	%	Frequency	%
1st space	7	7.0	8	8.0
2nd space	33	33.0	30	30.0
3rd space	62	62.0	63	63.0
4th space	79	79.0	76	76.0

TABLE 2: Microbiological findings in the 100 patients.

	Positive KOH mount	Positive bacterial cultures	
		G+ve cocci	G−ve bacilli
Female	50	36	28
Male	16	11	10
Total	66	47	38
%	66.0	47.0	38.0

TABLE 3: Frequency of histological diagnosis among the 100 patients.

Histopathological diagnosis	Frequency		Total	%
	Female	Male		
Eczema	40	12	52	52.0
Fungus	20	5	25	25.0
Callosity	10	9	19	19.0
Wart	1	2	3	3.0
Lichen planus	1	0	1	1.0
Total	72	28	100	100.0

cells alone or with pseudohyphae with distinct points of constrictions) while 9 were typical of mold/dermatophytes (arthrospores and hyphae of uniform diameter). Positive bacterial growth was observed in 85 patients (64 females and 21 males). These were 47 Gram-positive cocci (36 females and 11 males) and 38 Gram-negative bacilli (28 females and 10 males) (Table 2). No combined presence of Gram-positive cocci and Gram-negative bacilli was detected in any case but both were associated with other microbial and nonmicrobial states.

3.4. Histopathological Findings. Of the 100 skin biopsy sections, 52 (40 females and 12 males) showed features characteristic for eczema (Figure 1), 25 (20 females and 5 males) showed features characteristic for fungus (Figure 2), KOH was also positive in 22 of these patients (18 yeasts and 4 dermatophytes), 19 (10 females and 9 males) showed features characteristic for callosity (Figure 3), 3 (2 males and 1 female) showed features characteristic for wart (Figure 4), and only 1 section (female) showed features characteristic for lichen planus (Figure 5) (Table 3).

Most of the patients showed more than one etiological factor for the intertrigo. 50 cases presented with 2 diseases, 38 cases presented with 3 diseases, 9 cases presented with 4 diseases, and only 3 patients showed a single disease. Positive Wood's light fluorescence (erythrasma) was associated with 14 KOH-positive cases, 15 cases with Gram-positive cocci, 6 cases with Gram-negative bacilli, 12 cases with biopsy proven eczema, 8 cases with biopsy proven fungus, and 3 cases with biopsy proven callosity. Gram-positive cocci were associated with 36 KOH-positive cases, 15 positive Wood's light fluorescence (erythrasma) cases, 10 biopsy proven fungi, 26 eczema cases, 6 callosities, and 1 wart. Gram-negative bacilli were associated with 22 KOH-positive cases, 6 positive Wood's light fluorescence (erythrasma) cases, 11 biopsy proven fungi, 20 eczema cases, 7 callosities, and 1 lichen planus.

4. Discussion

Foot intertrigo may present as a chronic erythematous desquamative eruption. This is often diagnosed as tinea pedis or eczematous dermatitis. However, in some patients, the macerated eruption is unresponsive to treatment with antifungals or anti-inflammatory agents [4]. Therefore, clinical and microbiological studies are suggested to assist in the selection of appropriate treatment and the prevention of important complications [3]. This study was planned to verify the etiological causes of toe web space lesions in randomly selected 100 Egyptian patients. All of the patients were adults between 18–79 years of age (mean 43. 94 yrs). This is in agreement with other similar reports [18, 19].

In our study, 72 (72%) were females; the majority of them were housewives. Household work including kitchen work, duties for cleaning, washing, caring for children and other domestic activities, and shopping may explain the increased incidence of microbial intertrigo especially tinea pedis in this sector of population. On the contrary, Ahmad et al. [19] in Pakistan reported higher rate in males (56.7%). They attributed this to wearing closed shoes most of the time in hot and humid climate. In our patients, the 4th (lateral) toe web space was the most commonly affected in both right (79%) and left (76%) foot. This is in agreement with several reports [18–20]. This could be related to anatomical considerations (potentially occluded space).

Many authors refer to web space infection as tinea pedis or "foot ringworm" and some consider it to be purely dermatophytes induced [21–23]. However, other studies have demonstrated that recovery of dermatophytes from macerated webs is low. Generally, it ranges from 7.5% to 61% [1, 24–26]. The lower incidence of dermatophyte infection in these studies may be explained by the fact that, in mixed intertrigo, bacterial production of methanethiol and other sulfur compounds can lead to inhibition of dermatophytes [1].

Depending on KOH mount, this study showed that tinea pedis was observed in 66 (66%) patients; 50 of them were females (75.76%) and 16 were males (24.24%). This agrees with Morales-Trujillo et al. [5] who declared that fungi were positive in 62.5% of 70 cases. Using KOH, Ahmad et al. [19] out of 118 cases reported higher rate of positivity where 90% had positive direct microscopy while only 50.8% had positive cultures. On the other hand, Pau et al. [27] in a study on 1568 patients reported lower rate of tinea pedis infection (14.79%). This disagreement may be due to difference in life styles (e.g.,

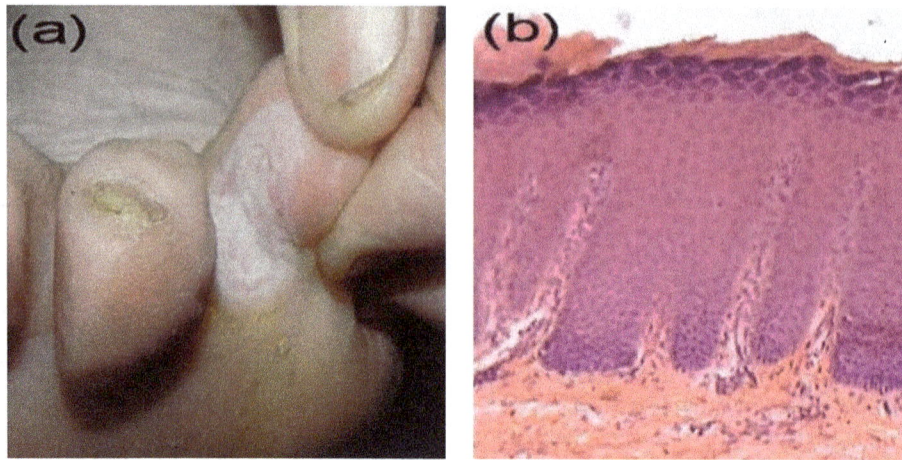

FIGURE 1: Interdigital eczema. (a) Interdigital whitish plaque with an ill-defined border. (b) Histopathological features of subacute spongiotic dermatitis (H&E, ×100).

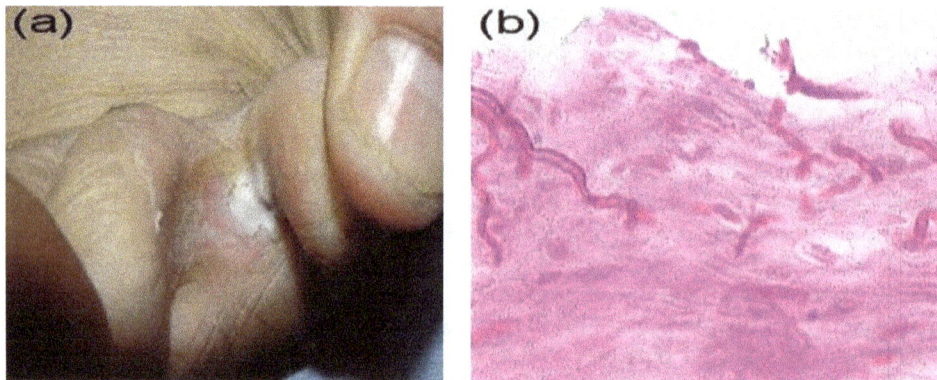

FIGURE 2: Interdigital fungal intertrigo. (a) Interdigital whitish plaques with macerated, sodden skin. (b) Biopsy from the lesion showing fungal pseudohyphae in the stratum corneum (PAS, ×400).

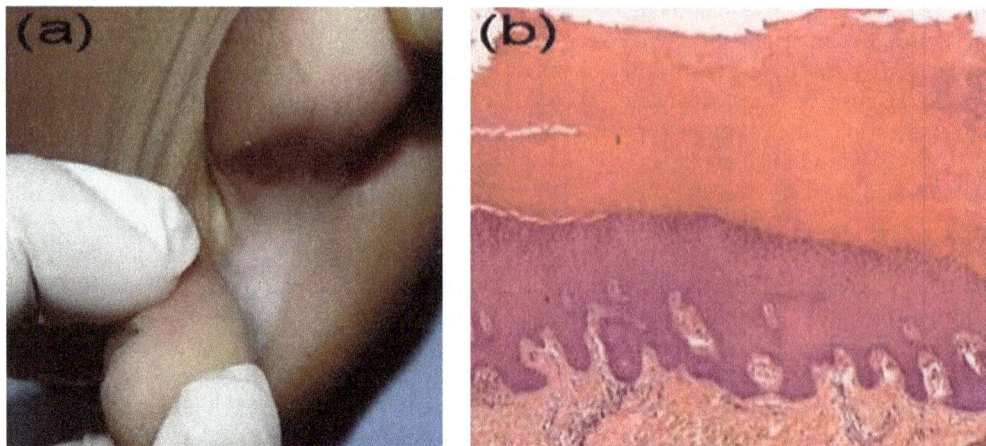

FIGURE 3: Interdigital callosity. (a) Interdigital whitish plaque with well-defined border. (b) Histopathological picture showing compact hyperkeratosis and moderate acanthosis (H&E, ×100).

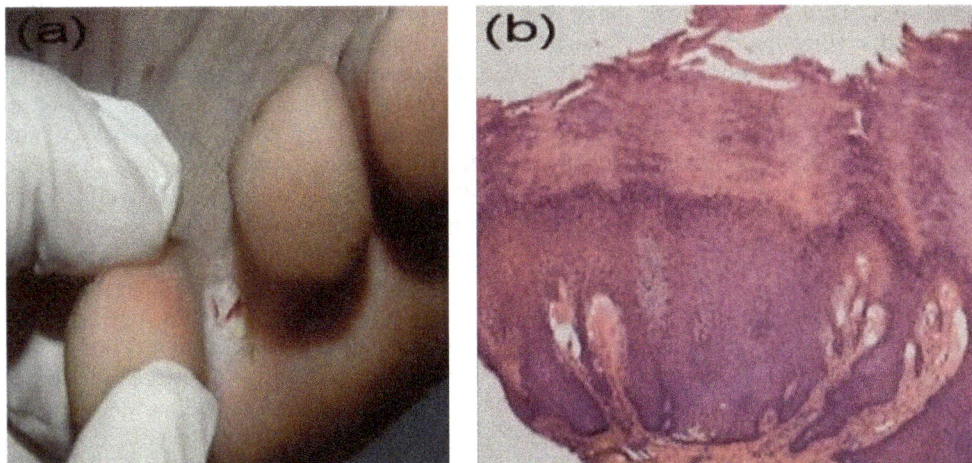

FIGURE 4: Interdigital wart. (a) Interdigital whitish plaque with well-defined border. (b) The punch biopsy shows changes characteristic for a common wart (H&E, ×100).

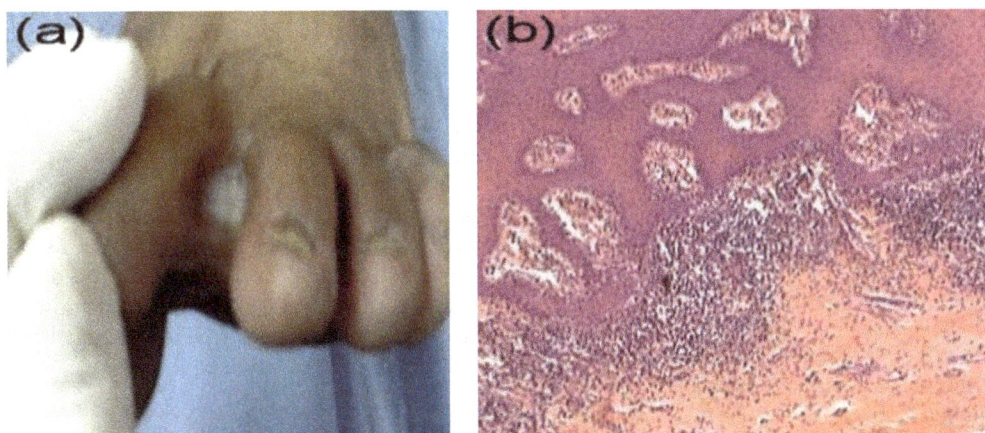

FIGURE 5: Interdigital lichen planus. (a) Interdigital whitish plaque with well-defined border. (b) The biopsy shows acanthosis, band-like lymphocytic infiltrate in the papillary dermis and vacuolar alteration of basal cell layer (H&E, ×100).

type of shoes worn), weather conditions such as humidity, and the varying number of cases in each study.

Cases with erythrasma can be diagnosed by positive Wood's lamp examination and/or Gram staining/culture [28]. In the present study, positive coral red fluorescence with Wood's light, which is characteristic for erythrasma, was found in 24% of the patients. The prevalence of erythrasma varies greatly from one study to another. Sariguzel et al. [29] reported a prevalence of 19.6% in 121 patients with interdigital foot lesions. Allen et al. [30] reported that, in 300 patients, 18.7% were determined to have erythrasma. Morales-Trujillo et al. [5] examined 73 patients, of whom 24 (32.8%) were diagnosed with erythrasma. Inci et al. [28] concluded that the rate of erythrasma was found to be 46.7% among 122 patients with interdigital foot lesions. Svejgaard et al. [31] reported a prevalence of 51.3%, (prior to military service) and 77.1% (reexamined at the end of military service) in a group of Danish military recruits.

This discrepancy may be attributed to the type of population studied, environmental conditions such as heat and humidity that increased the risk for developing erythrasma, and the methods used in diagnosis, for example, Wood's light examination, culture, and/or direct microscopy with Gram staining. In Polat and İlhan [32] study, using only Wood's lamp examination or Gram's staining resulted in 31 (42.5%) or 14 (19.2%) positive patients, respectively. Using Wood's lamp examination and Gram's staining concurrently resulted in 28 positive patients (38.4%). Interestingly, Inci et al. [28] reported no growth for *C. minutissimum* in bacteriological cultures from all patients with interdigital lesions. However, they found that using only Wood's lamp examination or Gram staining resulted in 11 (9%) and 19 positive patients (15.6%), respectively, whereas using both Wood's lamp examination and Gram staining concurrently resulted in 27 positive patients (22.1%). This suggests that bacteriological cultures have no or limited role in diagnosing erythrasma.

In this study, interdigital erythrasma was demonstrated more in females (83.3%) than males (16.7%). This finding agrees with Morales-Trujillo et al. [5] who stated that interdigital erythrasma was more common in women than men

(83.3% versus 16.7%). Also, Polat and İlhan [32] stated that most of their patients with erythrasma were women (56.2%). The exact cause of this female predominance is unknown but may be attributed to occupational factors including household duties and exposure to more heat and humidity.

The interdigital space is typically colonized by polymicrobial flora. Dermatophytes may damage the stratum corneum and produce substances with antibiotic properties. Gram-negative bacteria may resist antibiotic-like substances and proliferate. This process may progress to Gram-negative foot intertrigo [4]. In this study, no combined presence of Gram-positive cocci and Gram-negative bacilli was detected in any case. Although the lack of this association is unreasonable, it could not be exactly explained. Gram-positive cocci were associated with 36 KOH and 10 biopsy proven fungi. Gram-negative bacilli were associated with 22 KOH and 11 biopsy proven fungi. Gram-negative bacterial infection may represent a secondary invasion of web space lesions. With time, in the presence of local humidity and maceration, other Gram-positive bacterial (and fungal) organisms may proliferate. So, the web space infection may represent a single or polymicrobial etiology.

Based on bacterial cultures, 47 patients (47%) were harboring Gram-positive cocci, while 38 (38%) were harboring Gram-negative bacilli. This agrees with Karaca et al. [3] who concluded that the most common pathogen was Gram-positive cocci (17.9%), followed by *P. aeruginosa* (16.7%). Also the bacteria isolated by Ahmad et al. [19] were *S. aureus* (Gram-positive cocci) in 83.4%, *P. aeruginosa* in 10%, *Proteus* spp. in 3.3%, and β-hemolytic streptococci in 3.3% (Gram-negative bacteria). This disagrees with Aste et al. [2] who concluded that *P. aeruginosa* was found to be the prevailing pathogen, both alone and associated with other Gram-negative bacteria (such as *E. coli*, *Proteus mirabilis*, and *Morganella morganii*) and Gram-positive bacteria.

Twenty-eight females were suffering from Gram-negative bacterial web space lesion versus only 10 males with female to male ratio 2.8 : 1. This disagrees with Aste et al. [2] who reported that Gram-negative interweb foot infection represents a male-to-female ratio of 4 : 1. Also Lin et al. [4] reported that foot bacterial intertrigo was more common in men (82%). The more prevalence in male gender can be related to the more frequent use of closed shoes for occupational and nonoccupational activities such as during the practice of sports.

Generally speaking, the routine diagnosis of interdigital lesions depends mainly upon history and clinical appearance with or without the need for direct microscopy of a KOH preparation, bacterial cultures, and/or Wood's light examination while web space biopsy is not routinely used. Yet this study declared the additional value of web space histopathology with clinical correlation in definitive diagnosis of interdigital lesions.

Despite the great clinical similarities, after clinicopathological correlations, we have diagnosed a lot of cases of interdigital eczema (52% of cases). These were clinically manifested as pruritic macerated glazed skin usually limited to the interdigital space. PAS-positive cases (interdigital fungal intertrigo) which constituted 25% of cases were clinically

presented as pruritic, wet, and macerated interdigital space which usually extended to the plantar and/or dorsal surface of the foot. Some cases were associated with fungal infection of other parts of the body. Cases of callosity of toe web space (19%) were characterized by a well-defined white plaque limited to the web space. Three cases of interdigital warts were diagnosed (3%): two cases were asymptomatic while the third case was complaining of painful lesion. All of the 3 cases were associated with planter warts.

In this study, we found a healthy 49-year-old female clinically presented with pruritic interdigital lesions of 3 weeks' duration. Examination revealed bilateral and symmetrical whitish ill-defined plaques in the second and the third web spaces of both feet. Biopsy was characteristic for lichen planus. This is a very rare site for lichen planus. We think that it is important to recall such underestimated variant of lichen planus and other uncommon dermatoses in this site.

5. Conclusion

Many cases of web space lesions can be overdiagnosed, underdiagnosed, or misdiagnosed. These may be caused by different conditions including eczema, fungal intertrigo, erythrasma, callosity, wart, or even lichen planus. Although fungal foot infection is common, we suggest that patients who do not respond to topical and/or systemic antifungal therapy should be reexamined for another primary or secondary dermatologic condition that may resemble pedal fungal intertrigo. The diagnostic procedures in this work can be complementary to each other and can be used as an investigative workup tailored to individual patients who have resistant to treat or have atypical interdigital lesions.

Conflict of Interests

The authors declare that there is no conflict of interests regarding the publication of this paper.

References

[1] J. L. Leyden, "Tinea pedis pathophysiology and treatment," *Journal of the American Academy of Dermatology*, vol. 31, no. 3, part 2, pp. S31–S33, 1994.

[2] N. Aste, L. Atzori, M. Zucca, M. Pau, and P. Biggio, "Gram-negative bacterial toe web infection: a survey of 123 cases from the district of Cagliari, Italy," *Journal of the American Academy of Dermatology*, vol. 45, no. 4, pp. 537–541, 2001.

[3] S. Karaca, M. Kulac, Z. Cetinkaya, and R. Demirel, "Etiology of foot intertrigo in the district of Afyonkarahisar, Turkey: a bacteriologic and mycologic study," *Journal of the American Podiatric Medical Association*, vol. 98, no. 1, pp. 42–44, 2008.

[4] J.-Y. Lin, Y.-L. Shih, and H.-C. Ho, "Foot bacterial intertrigo mimicking interdigital tinea pedis," *Chang Gung Medical Journal*, vol. 34, no. 1, pp. 44–49, 2011.

[5] M. L. Morales-Trujillo, R. Arenas, and S. Arroyo, "Interdigital erythrasma: clinical, epidemiologic, and microbiologic findings," *Actas Dermo-Sifiliográficas*, vol. 99, no. 6, pp. 469–473, 2008.

[6] R. K. Snider, "Corns and calluses," in *Essentials of Musculoskeletal Care*, W. B. Greene, Ed., pp. 437–441, American Academy of Orthopaedic Surgeons, Rosemont, Ill, USA, 2nd edition, 2001.

[7] J. M. R. Mommers, M. M. B. Seyger, C. J. M. van der Vleuten, and P. C. M. van de Kerkhof, "Interdigital psoriasis (psoriasis alba): renewed attention for a neglected disorder," *Journal of the American Academy of Dermatology*, vol. 51, no. 2, pp. 317–318, 2004.

[8] G. T. Liu, M. O. Lovell, and J. S. Steinberg, "Digital syndactylization for the treatment of interdigital squamous cell carcinoma in situ (Bowen disease)," *Journal of Foot and Ankle Surgery*, vol. 43, no. 6, pp. 419–422, 2004.

[9] C. McKay, P. McBride, and J. Muir, "Plantar verrucous carcinoma masquerading as toe web intertrigo," *Australasian Journal of Dermatology*, vol. 53, no. 2, pp. e20–e22, 2012.

[10] O. M. Rashid, J. C. Schaum, L. G. Wolfe, N. K. Brinster, and J. P. Neifeld, "Prognostic variables and surgical management of foot melanoma: review of a 25-year institutional experience," *ISRN Dermatology*, vol. 2011, Article ID 384729, 8 pages, 2011.

[11] N. Zaias, B. Glick, and G. Rebell, "Diagnosing and treating onychomycosis," *The Journal of Family Practice*, vol. 42, no. 5, pp. 513–518, 1996.

[12] P. Asawanonda and C. R. Taylor, "Wood's light in dermatology," *International Journal of Dermatology*, vol. 38, no. 11, pp. 801–807, 1999.

[13] H. W. Walling, "Subclinical onychomycosis is associated with tinea pedis," *British Journal of Dermatology*, vol. 161, no. 4, pp. 746–749, 2009.

[14] World Health Organization, "Mycological techniques," in *Guidelines on Standard Operating Procedures for Microbiology*, chapter 21, World Health Organization, Regional Office for South-East Asia, New Delhi, India, 2000, http://apps.searo.who .int/PDS_DOCS/B0217.pdf?ua=1.

[15] E. Brehmer-Andersson, Ed., *Dermatopathology*, Springer, Berlin, Germany, 1st edition, 2006.

[16] L. Requena and C. Requena, "Histopathology of the more common viral skin infections," *Actas Dermo-Sifiliograficas*, vol. 101, no. 3, pp. 201–216, 2010.

[17] J. W. Patterson, Ed., *Weedon's Skin Pathology: Expert Consult*, Elsevier Health Sciences, 4th edition, 2014.

[18] G. D. Masri-Fridling, "Dermatophytosis of the feet," *Dermatologic Clinics*, vol. 14, no. 1, pp. 33–40, 1996.

[19] S. Ahmad, S. Aman, I. Hussain, and T. S. Haroon, "A clinico-etiological study of toe web fungal infection," *Journal of Pakistan Association of Dermatologists*, vol. 13, no. 4, pp. 62–66, 2003.

[20] A. G. Martin and G. S. Kobayashi, "Superficial fungal infection," in *Dermatology in General Medicine*, I. M. Freedberg, A. Z. Eisen, K. Wolff et al., Eds., pp. 2337–2357, McGraw-Hill, New York, NY, USA, 5th edition, 1999.

[21] J. J. Leyden and A. M. Kligman, "Interdigital athlete's foot: new concepts in pathogenesis," *Postgraduate Medicine*, vol. 61, no. 6, pp. 113–116, 1977.

[22] A. K. Gupta, A. R. Skinner, and E. A. Cooper, "Interdigital tinea pedis (dermatophytosis simplex and complex) and treatment with ciclopirox 0.77% gel," *International Journal of Dermatology*, vol. 42, supplement 1, pp. 23–27, 2003.

[23] M. Al Hasan, S. M. Fitzgerald, M. Saoudian, and G. Krishnaswamy, "Dermatology for the practicing allergist: tinea pedis and its complications," *Clinical and Molecular Allergy*, vol. 2, article 5, 2004.

[24] J. J. Leyden and A. M. Kligman, "Interdigital Athlete's foot: interaction of dermatophytes and resident bacteria," *Archives of Dermatology*, vol. 114, no. 10, pp. 1466–1472, 1978.

[25] S. G. Kates, K. M. Nordstrom, K. J. McGinley, and J. J. Leyden, "Microbial ecology of interdigital infections of toe web spaces," *Journal of the American Academy of Dermatology*, vol. 22, no. 4, pp. 578–582, 1990.

[26] N. El Fekih, I. Belghith, S. Trabelsi, H. Skhiri-Aounallah, S. Khaled, and B. Fazaa, "Epidemiological and etiological study of foot mycosis in Tunisia," *Actas Dermo-Sifiliograficas*, vol. 103, no. 6, pp. 520–524, 2012.

[27] M. Pau, L. Atzori, N. Aste, R. Tamponi, and N. Aste, "Epidemiology of Tinea pedis in Cagliari, Italy," *Giornale Italiano di Dermatologia e Venereologia*, vol. 145, no. 1, pp. 1–5, 2010.

[28] M. Inci, G. Serarslan, B. Ozer et al., "The prevalence of interdigital erythrasma in southern region of Turkey," *Journal of the European Academy of Dermatology and Venereology*, vol. 26, no. 11, pp. 1372–1376, 2012.

[29] F. M. Sariguzel, A. Nedret Koc, G. Yagmur, and E. Berk, "Interdigital foot infections: *Corynebacterium minutissimum* and agents of superficial mycoses," *Brazilian Journal of Microbiology*, vol. 45, no. 3, pp. 781–784, 2014.

[30] S. Allen, T. I. Christmas, W. McKinney, D. Parr, and G. F. Oliver, "The Auckland skin clinic tinea pedis and erythrasma study," *The New Zealand Medical Journal*, vol. 103, no. 896, pp. 391–393, 1990.

[31] E. Svejgaard, J. Christophersen, and H. M. Jelsdorf, "Tinea pedis and erythrasma in Danish recruits. Clinical signs, prevalence, incidence, and correlation to atopy," *Journal of the American Academy of Dermatology*, vol. 14, no. 6, pp. 993–999, 1986.

[32] M. Polat and M. N. İlhan, "The prevalence of interdigital erythrasma—a prospective study from an outpatient clinic in Turkey," *Journal of the American Podiatric Medical Association*, vol. 105, no. 2, pp. 121–124, 2015.

6

Relationship between Vitamin D Status and Striae Distensae: A Case-Referent Study

Rafaela Koehler Zanella,[1] **Denis Souto Valente,**[2] **Leo Francisco Doncatto,**[3]
Daniele Dos Santos Rossi,[4] **Aline Grimaldi Lerias,**[4] **and Alexandre Vontobel Padoin**[2]

[1]*Mãe de Deus Health System, Rua Soledade 569, 90470-340 Porto Alegre, RS, Brazil*
[2]*Graduate Program in Medicine and Health Sciences, School of Medicine, PUCRS (FAMED), Avenida Ipiranga 6681, 90619-900 Porto Alegre, RS, Brazil*
[3]*ULBRA School of Medicine, Lutheran University of Brazil (ULBRA), Avenida Farroupilha 8001, 92425-900 Canoas, RS, Brazil*
[4]*School of Medicine, PUCRS (FAMED), Avenida Ipiranga 6681, 90619-900 Porto Alegre, RS, Brazil*

Correspondence should be addressed to Denis Souto Valente; denisvalentedr@gmail.com

Academic Editor: Lajos Kemény

Vitamin D (VD) plays a role in the skin regulation. Striae Distensae (SD) are manifestations of epidermal atrophy that occurs after tissue tearing due to overstretching or rapid growth. The objective of this study was to investigate the relation between serum VD and occurrence of SD in women who had undergone mammaplasty with silicone implants. A case-referent study was conducted. The blood values of 25-hydroxyvitamin D (25OHD) were measured before the surgery. For each patient postoperatively diagnosed with SD, four other participants submitted to the same surgery, without the development of SD, were enrolled as the healthy controls. 67 women with SD after the surgery entered the study. 268 formed the control group. In the serum of healthy controls 25OHD mean was 27 ng/mL, and SD cases presented 20 ng/mL ($P = 0.01$). Scarce values of VD have been observed in 56.71% of the cases presenting SD and in 39.91% without SD ($P = 0.002$). Chance of having VD values lower than 20 ng/mL amongst cases with SD is 2.38 ($P = 0.0001$). Lower serum levels of VD are linked to a higher occurrence of SD.

1. Introduction

It is nowadays proven that the physiological significance of vitamin D (VD) status spreads far beyond the bone metabolism regulation [1]. Lately, a huge rise in the number of clinical studies explaining the VD decisive role in a plenty of physiological functions and associating lower levels of VD with lots of diseases has been observed. Deficit of VD is currently recognized as a worldwide pandemic [2, 3]. VD deficit major cause is the absence of appraisement that the major source of VD in all ages is sun exposure. Throughout life, VD plays a decisive role in the maintenance and development of a healthy body. A controversy still remains in relation to the serum level of 25-hydroxyvitamin D (25OHD) that must be attained for both bone health and reducing risk for VD deficit associated illness and how much VD must be supplemented [4, 5]. Having normal VD in the skin helps reduce acne, boost cutaneous elasticity, stimulate the dermal collagen production, and probably reduce skin cancer incidence [6–8].

Striae Distensae (SD), also known as stretch marks, are manifestations of an epidermal atrophy occurring after tissue tearing due to overstretching or rapid growth and are characterized by distinct microstructural features. Atrophic, linear, and parallel lesions usually characterize SD. The lesions are usually running perpendicular to Langer's lines, which represent the direction of minimum extensibility [9, 10]. The literature review performed using PUBMED and SciELO finds a 7.06% to 4.60% frequency of occurrence of SD following augmentation mammoplasty [11, 12].

The main objective of the present study has been to investigate the relation between serum VD and occurrence of SD in women who had undergone breast augmentation surgery with silicone implants.

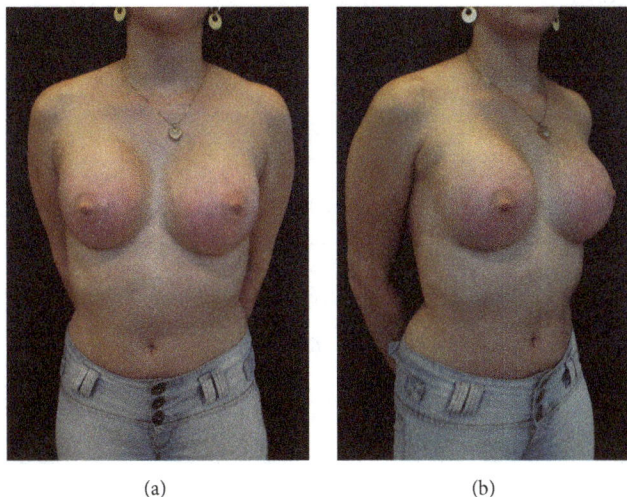

FIGURE 1: SD 9 weeks after 350 mL breast implants placement in a 29-year-old woman. (a) Frontal view, (b) oblique view.

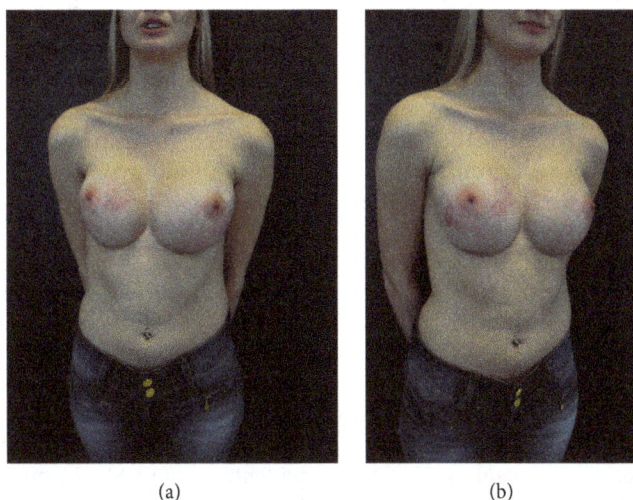

FIGURE 2: SD 6 weeks after 425 mL breast implants placement in a 24-year-old woman. (a) Frontal view, (b) oblique view.

2. Patients and Methods

A case-referent study has been conducted and the data of individuals who underwent breast augmentation surgery with silicone implants in a private clinic was analyzed. Data has been collected from patients' electronic records stored in RMD Clinic Software (RDTI Systems, Brazil) starting from January 2005 to March 2015. The protocol of the study has been approved by the Human Research Ethics Committee of the Lutheran University of Brazil (ULBRA) and is registered in the National Ministry of Health. This experiment did not affect the medical assistance provided to the patients because it was an analytical review of their medical records. All participants were made aware of the study and provided written consent before the surgery, so that their data, as well as blood level of 25OHD, could be used in research.

The inclusion criteria have been patients aged between 18 and 60 years who had undergone breast augmentation surgery with placement of silicone implants and who underwent a follow-up appointment that was performed at least 2 months after the breast augmentation surgery.

The exclusion criteria have been consumption of supplements with VD or drugs modulating serum 25OHD values, concomitant mastopexy, incomplete medical records, absence of postoperative photos, use of corticosteroids, and previous breast surgery.

The criteria to define SD included the presence of cutaneous atrophy with acquired, reddish lesions of linear appearance and with a minimum width of 2 mm. Figures 1 and 2 show these findings. White or silver SD was considered old and was not accounted for by this study.

For each patient diagnosed with SD, four other participants submitted to the same surgery performed by the same surgeon, without the development of SD after breast augmentation surgery, were enrolled as the healthy controls.

TABLE 1: Comparison of cases in Striae Distensae and non-Striae Distensae groups.

Parameter	Striae Distensae group ($n = 67$)	Healthy controls ($n = 268$)	P value
25OHD (ng/mL)	20 (2.9)	27 (2.2)	0.01
Age (years)	25 (4.2)	26 (4.1)	0.51
BMI (kg/m^2)	22.24 (1.59)	21.96 (1.52)	0.39
Current smoker (%)	8.95	7.46	0.27
Implant volume (cc)	327.28 (64.1)	324.91 (61.9)	0.61

TABLE 2: Confrontation of serum 25OHD status in Striae Distensae and non-Striae Distensae groups.

Vitamin D status	Striae Distensae group ($n = 67$)	Healthy controls ($n = 268$)	P value
Scarce (<20 ng/mL)	38 (56.71%)	107 (39.91%)	
Inadequate (20–30 ng/mL)	16 (23.88%)	56 (20.88%)	0.002
Normal (>30 ng/mL)	13 (19.41%)	105 (39.21%)	

Prior to the surgery, blood samples from the patients have been collected by venous puncture. 25OHD values ≥30 ng/mL have been designated as normal, among 20 to 30 ng/mL as inadequate and lower than 20 ng/mL as scarce [13, 14]. 25OHD serum concentration was assayed with an electrochemiluminescence (ECL) method. Data regarding blood level of 25OHD prior to the surgery and SD onset were collected from the electronic records in which information had been entered by the surgeon who performed the procedures.

The obtained data have been evaluated applying Kruskal-Wallis test, one way ANOVA, Student's t-test, and Chi-square (linear by linear correlation), as applicable (considering a preset probability of $P < 0.05$). The quantitative data were stated as mean ± standard deviation. The statistical analysis was performed with SPSS (IBM, USA) and Epi Info (CDC, USA) software. The Independent t-test has been employed to equate different quantitative variables (including 25OHD serum level, age, body mass index, and implant volume) among SD cases and patients without SD. Farther, the simultaneous effects of the confounding variables like age, implant volume, and body mass index (BMI) have been calculated using simple, multiple, and logistic regression analysis. Kolmogorov-Smirnov test was used to check normality assumptions of distributions. VD values have not reached a normal distribution in the two groups; thus, only logarithmic transformation of VD levels has been compared in both groups.

From an ethical point of view, this study did not affect the medical assistance provided to the patients because it was a simple analytical review of their medical records. Medical confidentiality was assured because the only person responsible for data collection, having access to the identities of the patients, was allowed only to copy information regarding the variables included in this study.

3. Results

67 Caucasian women with recognized SD after the surgery entered the study constituting Group I. To form the control group, 268 Caucasian women without recognized SD after the same surgery were enrolled for the study composing Group II.

Comparative analyses between the groups are shown in Table 1. There was no difference in age, BMI, smoking, or implant volume between SD patients and the healthy controls. A statistically significant difference has been detected among the groups regarding the values of 25OHD. In the serum of healthy controls, mean was 27 ng/mL, and SD cases presented a 20 ng/mL serum mean ($P = 0.01$, 95% CI, 1.46–3.86).

Confrontation of serum 25OHD status in Striae Distensae and non-Striae Distensae groups is shown in Table 2. Scarce values of VD have been observed in 38 (56.71%) cases presenting SD and 107 (39.91%) without SD ($P = 0.002$). 16 (23.88%) of SD patients and 56 (20.88%) of the group without SD had inadequate values of VD. Normal values of VD have been detected in 13 (19.41%) SD patients and in 105 (39.21%) patients without SD. Comparing with patients without SD, the chance of having VD values lower than 20 ng/mL amongst cases with SD is 2.38 (95% CI, 1.46–3.86, $P = 0.0001$).

4. Discussion

Vitamin D supply is changeable, being sourced from skin synthesis following solar exposure, which is curtailed seasonally in high latitude countries, and from oral intake of natural foodstuffs, fortified foodstuffs, and supplements. Although sunlight exposure is the predominant natural source of vitamin D, the primacy of oral intake over sunlight exposure in both the prevention and correction of vitamin D deficiency has been known for some time. This is apposite given the concerns about sunlight exposure and skin cancer. For these reasons, the Institute of Medicine (IOM) 2011 Report specified dietary reference vitamin D intakes for those with minimal or no sunlight exposure [15]. Individuals with intentional or inadvertent sunlight exposure have lesser dependence on oral sources. The recommended daily allowances specified by IOM in 2011 are between 30% and threefold higher compared to 1997 [16]. Noting the trend for unsubstantiated claims regarding vitamin D, IOM cautioned against exceeding recommended intakes [17].

The IOM gave guidance about the interpretation of the 25OHD result. According to the IOM, 25OHD is a measure of risk: a concentration below 30 nmol/L (12 ng/mL) indicates increased risk of vitamin D deficiency; a concentration of 40 nmol/L (16 ng/mL) corresponds to the estimated average requirement (EAR) satisfying the needs of half the population; a concentration above 50 nmol/L (20 ng/mL) meets the requirements of 97.5% of the population; a concentration above 125 nmol/L (50 ng/mL) indicates risk of harm [13–17]. In our study, we did not found any hypervitaminosis D.

The samples were obtained along all seasons of the year, avoiding a sun exposure bias. Notably, in this study, the sample was obtained from a private clinic, corresponding to a specific social group that does not represent the general population. Therefore, the obtained results and their interpretation must take into account this specificity. The fact that 100% of the sample studied was Caucasian precludes extrapolation of the obtained results to the general population; however, it makes the external validity of this study higher for populations similar to the one used in the study [11].

The physiopathology of SD remains unclear. Excessive skin distention, prolonged exposure to cortisol, and genetics may all have a role. The aetiological mechanisms proposed relate to hormones, and structural alterations to the integument. However, it may involve stretching of the skin, causing lesions in microfibrils, which in younger women are likely to be more fragile and are therefore more susceptible to rupture [11]. Some diseases from the connective tissue, such as congenital contractural arachnodactyly or Marfan syndrome, are also known to be related to SD. Rapid mechanical stretch produced by implant introduction seems to be the main factor leading to SD in the population of our study [12].

Histopathologically, SD shows loss of the supporting material, that is, the collagen and the elastin fibers compared to normal skin, which reduces the thickness and stability of the dermis. Though striae do not present any significant medical issues, they are a cause of cosmetic concern. Many therapeutic modalities have been tried including topical tretinoin, microdermabrasion, radiofrequency, photothermolysis, intense pulsed light, fractional lasers, and ablative and nonablative lasers; but no consistently effective modality is available yet [9, 11].

Hormonal receptor expression is increased under certain conditions suggesting that regions undergoing greater mechanical stretching of the skin may express greater hormonal receptor activity. This fact may influence the metabolism of the extracellular matrix, causing SD formation. Alterations in hormone receptors occur within a well-defined period during the formation of SD. However, the functionality of hormone receptors varies during the different stages of SD development. Estrogen receptors doubled in skin with SD compared with healthy skin. The androgen and glucocorticoid receptors in the SD skin are also increased [11, 18]. Recent evidence supports a positive role for VD in reproductive hormone biosynthesis and ovarian reserve and also a negative role in estrogen receptors; thus, hypovitaminosis D leads to an increase in the estrogen receptors [19, 20]. Probably, this increase in the estrogen receptors observed in hypovitaminosis D can be the explanation to the higher incidence of SD amongst women with lower levels of VD.

We choose to conduct a case-referent study because it is good for studying rare conditions, needs less time to conduct the study because the condition has already occurred, and is useful as an initial study to establish an association. Knowing its disadvantages, we avoid recall bias doing patients' electronic records review to find a suitable control group four times bigger than the SD group. We have used our own previously published work [11], as a basis for this paper; the novel contribution beyond those of the previous paper is the levels of VD study. In our prior study, we did not mention vitamin D along the manuscript. Further studies with VD measurement must be performed in other groups with increased risk to develop SD (during pregnancy, hormonal growth spurts, obesity, or rapid weight gain).

5. Conclusion

Lower serum levels of VD are linked to a higher occurrence of SD. Further studies are needed to elucidate a potentially different impact of hypovitaminosis D on SD.

Conflict of Interests

The authors declare that they do not have any commercial associations or financial disclosures that might pose or create a conflict of interests with information presented in this submitted paper. There is no conflict of interests in this research.

References

[1] I. R. Reid, M. J. Bolland, and A. Grey, "Effects of vitamin D supplements on bone mineral density: a systematic review and meta-analysis," *The Lancet*, vol. 383, no. 9912, pp. 146–155, 2014.

[2] A. Sahbaz, O. Aynioglu, H. Isik, K. Gulle, M. Akpolat Ferah, and H. Cicekler Sahbaz, "Cholecalciferol (vitamin D3) prevents postoperative adhesion formation by inactivating the nuclear factor kappa B pathway: a randomized experimental study," *Journal of Surgical Research*, vol. 198, no. 1, pp. 252–259, 2015.

[3] S. Upala, A. Sanguankeo, and N. Permpalung, "Significant association between vitamin D deficiency and sepsis: a systematic review and meta-analysis," *BMC Anesthesiology*, vol. 15, no. 1, article 84, 2015.

[4] Z. Samochocki, J. Bogaczewicz, R. Jeziorkowska et al., "Vitamin D effects in atopic dermatitis," *Journal of the American Academy of Dermatology*, vol. 69, no. 2, pp. 238–244, 2013.

[5] M. Wacker and M. F. Holiack, "Vitamin D—effects on skeletal and extraskeletal health and the need for supplementation," *Nutrients*, vol. 5, no. 1, pp. 111–148, 2013.

[6] K. K. Reddy and B. A. Gilchrest, "The role of vitamin D in melanoma prevention: evidence and hyperbole," *Journal of the American Academy of Dermatology*, vol. 71, no. 5, pp. 1004–1005, 2014.

[7] C. Curiel-Lewandrowski, J. Y. Tang, J. G. Einspahr et al., "Pilot study on the bioactivity of vitamin D in the skin after oral supplementation," *Cancer Prevention Research (Phila)*, vol. 8, no. 6, pp. 563–569, 2015.

[8] T. Soleymani, T. Hung, and J. Soung, "The role of vitamin D in psoriasis: a review," *International Journal of Dermatology*, vol. 54, no. 4, pp. 383–392, 2015.

[9] G. N. Stamatas, A. Lopes-DaCunha, A. Nkengne, and C. Bertin, "Biophysical properties of striae distensae evaluated in vivo using non-invasive assays," *Skin Research and Technology*, vol. 21, no. 2, pp. 254–258, 2015.

[10] G. Lemperle, M. Tenenhaus, D. Knapp, and S. M. I. Lemperle, "The direction of optimal skin incisions derived from striae distensae," *Plastic and reconstructive surgery*, vol. 134, no. 6, pp. 1424–1434, 2014.

[11] D. S. Valente, R. K. Zanella, L. F. Doncatto, and A. V. Padoin, "Incidence and risk factors of striae distensae following breast augmentation surgery: a cohort study," *PLoS ONE*, vol. 9, no. 5, Article ID e97493, 2014.

[12] P. A. M. Guimarães, A. Haddad, M. Sabino Neto, F. C. Lage, and L. M. Ferreira, "Striae distensae after breast augmentation: treatment using the nonablative fractionated 1550-nm erbium glass laser," *Plastic and Reconstructive Surgery*, vol. 131, no. 3, pp. 636–642, 2013.

[13] J. C. Gallagher, V. Yalamanchili, and L. M. Smith, "The effect of vitamin D supplementation on serum 25OHD in thin and obese women," *The Journal of Steroid Biochemistry and Molecular Biology*, vol. 136, pp. 195–200, 2013.

[14] R. Bouillon, N. M. Van Schoor, E. Gielen et al., "Optimal vitamin D status: a critical analysis on the basis of evidence-based medicine," *The Journal of Clinical Endocrinology & Metabolism*, vol. 98, no. 8, pp. E1283–E1304, 2013.

[15] Committee to Review Dietary Reference Intakes for Vitamin D and Calcium. Institute of Medicine, *Dietary Reference Intakes for Calcium and Vitamin D*, The National Academies Press, Washington, DC, USA, 2011.

[16] Institute of Medicine, *Dietary Reference Intakes for Calcium, Phosphorus, Magnesium, Vitamin D and Fluoride*, National Academies Press, Washington, DC, USA, 1997.

[17] A. C. Ross, J. E. Manson, S. A. Abrams et al., "The 2011 report on dietary reference intakes for calcium and vitamin D from the institute of medicine: what clinicians need to know," *Journal of Clinical Endocrinology and Metabolism*, vol. 96, no. 1, pp. 53–58, 2011.

[18] R. C. T. Cordeiro, K. G. Zecchin, and A. M. de Moraes, "Expression of estrogen, androgen, and glucocorticoid receptors in recent striae distensae," *International Journal of Dermatology*, vol. 49, no. 1, pp. 30–32, 2010.

[19] E. M. Chang, Y. S. Kim, H. J. Won, T. K. Yoon, and W. S. Lee, "Association between sex steroids, ovarian reserve, and vitamin D levels in healthy nonobese women," *The Journal of Clinical Endocrinology & Metabolism*, vol. 99, no. 7, pp. 2526–2532, 2014.

[20] C. J. Narvaez, D. Matthews, E. LaPorta, K. M. Simmons, S. Beaudin, and J. Welsh, "The impact of vitamin D in breast cancer: genomics, pathways, metabolism," *Frontiers in Physiology*, vol. 5, article 213, 2014.

7

Tamarind Seed Xyloglucans Promote Proliferation and Migration of Human Skin Cells through Internalization via Stimulation of Proproliferative Signal Transduction Pathways

W. Nie and A. M. Deters

Westfalian Wilhelms University of Muenster, Institute for Pharmaceutical Biology and Phytochemistry, Hittorfstraße 56, 48149 Muenster, Germany

Correspondence should be addressed to A. M. Deters; adeters@uni-muenster.de

Academic Editor: Lajos Kemeny

Xyloglucans (XGs) of *Tamarindus indica* L. Fabaceae are used as drug vehicles or as ingredients of cosmetics. Two xyloglucans were extracted from *T. indica* seed with cold water (TSw) and copper complex precipitation (TSc). Both were analyzed in regard to composition and influence on cell viability, proliferation, cell cycle progression, migration, MAPK phosphorylation, and gene expression of human skin keratinocytes (NHEK and HaCaT) and fibroblasts (NHDF) *in vitro*. TSw and TSc differed in molecular weight, rhamnose content, and ratios of xylose, arabinose, galactose, and glucose. Both XGs improved keratinocytes and fibroblast proliferation, promoted the cell cycle, and stimulated migration and intracellular enzyme activity of NHDF after endosomal uptake. Only TSw significantly enhanced HaCaT migration and extracellular enzyme activity of NHDF and HaCaT. TSw and TSc predominantly enhanced the phosphorylation of molecules that referred to Erk signaling in NHEK. In NHDF parts of the integrin signaling and SAPK/JNK pathway were affected. Independent of cell type TSw marginally regulated the expression of genes, which referred to membrane proteins, cytoskeleton, cytokine signaling, and ECM as well as to processes of metabolism and transcription. Results show that *T. indica* xyloglucans promote skin regeneration by a direct influence on cell proliferation and migration.

1. Introduction

The tamarind is a bushy tree in family Fabaceae and native to tropical Africa. The main components of tamarind seed are xyloglucans. Xyloglucans are one of the two major hemicelluloses in plant primary walls. In general, xyloglucans have a cellulose-like backbone consisting of β-1,4-glucosyl residues distributed by short side chains containing fucosyl, arabinosyl, galactosyl, and xylosyl residues [1]. Niemann et al. 1997 [2] characterized the oligosaccharide mixtures after enzymatic digestion of the tamarind seed xyloglucan by endo-$(1 \rightarrow 4)$-β-D-glucanase (*Aspergillus niger*) and described that in addition to β-D-glucosyl, α-D-xylosyl and β-D-galactosyl residues some oligosaccharides also contained α-L-arabinosyl, and β-D-galactosyl-$(1 \rightarrow 5)$-α-L-arabinosyl residues.

In ayurvedic pharmacopeia of India (Part I, Vol IV) the fruits (Ciña) have been noted as laxative. In traditional African medicine the bark and leaves have been often used for treatment of wounds and diarrhea. Tamarind seeds have been powdered and orally administered to treat digestive disorder [2]. Nowadays Tamarind extracts were used for cosmetic preparations [3] and drug vehicles. Tamarind xyloglucans are used in mucoadhesive buccal film [4], microspheres [5], hydrogels [6], and eyedrops [7]. Using tamarind xyloglucans improves percutaneous transport [8], regulates release [9], enhances bioavailability [8], and prolongs systemic absorption [5] of various drugs. Furthermore various investigations were done to lighten the activity of these special xyloglucans on different *in vivo* and *in vitro* models far of the traditional use against digestive disorders. Tamarind seed xyloglucans were shown to reduce UV-induced repression of the delayed-type hypersensitivity response as well as the production of IL-10 in mice [10]. Additionally *in vitro* and *in vivo* studies are available dealing with the antitumor and immune stimulating activity [11, 12], NO production [13], healing properties of dry eye syndrome [14, 15], and cutaneous wounds [16]. Moreover tamarind xyloglucans protected human skin from immune suppression by inhibition of UV-radiation-induced dendritic cell loss from the epidermis [17].

The *in vivo* studies underline the effect and benefit of tamarind xyloglucan use in drug delivery systems and in cosmetics the background of the xyloglucans bioactivity has not been investigated so far. *In vitro* cell cultures are an efficient tool for investigation of cell behavior and its causative cellular response. Proliferation and migration are essential for wound regeneration [18] and can be uncomplicatedly investigated *in vitro*. For the present research human skin keratinocytes and fibroblasts were used. These cells construct the dermis and epidermis of skin and are involved in the regeneration and epithelialization of cutaneous wound healing [19]. During the presented study different *in vitro* tests were carried out analyzing the effect of tamarind seed xyloglucans on proliferation, migration, cell viability, cell cycle, and signal pathways in addition to their interaction with cells. Extraction of studies Tamarind xyloglucans was done in different ways. Since variation in precipitation process of water-soluble polysaccharides or using of different solvents and temperatures results in extracts composed of different polysaccharides [20, 21], tamarind seed xyloglucans were extracted by copper precipitation [22] and with cold water to elucidate a possible difference in structure and bioactivity.

2. Materials and Methods

Chemicals were purchased in analytical quality from Sigma, Taufkirchen, or Merck, Darmstadt, Germany. Water for cell culture and *in vitro* purpose was purified using a Millipore-System from Millipore, Molsheim, France. If not stated otherwise media and supplements were purchased from PAA Laboratories GmbH (Cölbe, Germany). FCS was supplied by PerBio, Bonn, Germany. Cell culture plates and flasks were obtained from Greiner Bio-One, Frickenhausen, Germany or Sarstedt, Nuembrecht, Germany. MCDB153 medium was obtained from Biochrom, Berlin, and KGM_{Gold} was purchased from Lonza, Cologne, both from Germany. The cells were cultivated at $37°C$ in an humidified atmosphere at 5% (KGM_{Gold}, MEM, and MCDB153 complete) and 8% CO_2 (DMEM) according to the suppliers instruction.

2.1. Isolation of TSw and TSc from T. indica Seed. Tamarind Gum (Powder) was kind gift from Professor Dr. Kottapalli Seshagirirao, University of Hyderabad, India. Xyloglucans were isolated according to [22] with a final yield of 27% (w/w) or extracted using cold water as described for Kiwi polysaccharides [23] resulting in 10% water soluble polysaccharide (TSw).

2.2. Characterization of TSw and TSc from T. indica Seed. The amount of neutral sugars was quantified using resorcinol [24]. Amount of accompanying proteins was measured

with Coomassie Brilliant Blue G-250 [25]. The monosaccharide composition was determined by High Performance Anion Exchange Chromatography with Pulsed Amperometric Detection (HPAEC-PAD; Dionex, Idstein, Germany) after hydrolysis with trifluoroacetic acid (TFA, 2 M, at $121°C$ for 1 h), followed by identification of the D/L configuration by capillary electrophoresis (CE). Performance of HPAEC-PAD and CE referred to [26]. Gel-filtration chromatography (GFC) of TSw and TSc was carried out on a Sepharose CL-6B column (Pharmacia Biotech, Sweden) for determining average molecular weight (MW). Elution was conducted with 0.15 M NaCl (0.3 mL/min).

2.3. Labeling of Tamarind Polysaccharides with Fluorescein Isothiocyanate (FITC). 10 mg of TSw and TSc was labeled with FITC as described by [27]. The labeled polysaccharides were purified by ethanol precipitation (80%) followed by dialyzation against Aqua Millipore (MWCO 3500) and GPC on Sepharose CL-6B. Thin-layer chromatography (TLC) of TSw-FITC and TSc-FITC on silica gel G 60_{F254} was performed to verify the absence of unbound FITC.

2.4. Cell Culture Conditions of NHEK, HaCaT, and NHDF. Normal human dermal fibroblasts (NHDF) were isolated from human skin grafts (Pediatric Surgical Clinic, University of Muenster, Germany) of various Caucasian subjects as described by [23, 28]. The studies were approved by the local ethical committee of the University of Muenster (acceptance number 2006-117-f-S). Adherent spontaneously immortalized HaCaT-keratinocytes were kindly provided by Professor Dr. Fusenig from German Cancer Research Center (DKFZ), Heidelberg, Germany.

Stock cultures of NHEK grew in KGM_{Gold}. Subculture of NHDF was performed in MEM high glucose supplemented with 10% FCS, 1% L-glutamine, and 1% Penicillin/Streptomycin. HaCaT keratinocytes were cultured in D-MEM high glucose (10% FCS, L-glutamine, NEAA, and Penicillin/Streptomycin, each 1%). Cells were allowed to grow to a confluence of 80% before splitting. The studies were performed on the 2nd to 6th (NHDF and NHEK) and 45th–56th passage (HaCaT).

Prior to incubation with xyloglucans cells were directly adapted to serum and BPE-starved media; fibroblasts to MEM high glucose supplemented with 10% SerEx (a defined serum alternate of PAA, Colebe, Germany), 1% L-glutamine, and keratinocytes to MCDB 153 complete medium. Incubation with xyloglucans started 24 h after seeding in serum-starved media when the cells had reached a confluence of 50%. Medium was exchanged against fresh serum-starved medium (untreated control), serum-starved medium containing xyloglucans, and medium supplemented with 10% FCS instead of SerEx (positive control). The incubation was quitted by adding BrdU and MTT reagents after 48 h. Medium was not exchanged during this time. Three independent tests were performed in 96-well plates at starting cell densities of 5×10^3 HaCaT and 3×10^3 NHDF in each well. BrdU incorporation, extracellular enzyme activity (WST-1), and LDH release assays were performed according to the manufacturer's instructions (Roche, Penzberg, Germany).

Activity of intracellular reducing enzymes was measured with MTT according to [29]. ATP production of keratinocytes and fibroblasts was quantified using the CellTiter-Glo Luminescent Cell Viability Assay (Promega, USA) and a Fluoroskan Ascent FL (Thermo Scientific, USA).

2.5. Determination of DNA Content Using Flow Cytometer for Cell Cycle Analysis.

Due to the difference of DNA amount in each cell cycle phase, the cell cycle progression was analyzed by determining the DNA content via flow cytometry. First the human skin cells were seeded in 6-well plates with 1.5×10^5 cells/well (NHEK and HaCaT) and 1×10^5 cells/well (NHDF) and treated with 10 μg/mL TSw or TSc after 3, 6, 12, 24, and 48 h. Afterwards cells were trypsinized, centrifuged, and resuspended in 450 μL PBS. For fixation of the cell status 1.05 mL ethanol (96%, −20°C) was added for 2 h at 4°C. The fixed cells were mixed with 500 μL ice-cold PBS and centrifuged for 10 min at 11000 ×g. The resultant pellet was resuspended in 900 μL PBS followed by the addition of 50 μL RNase solution (1 mg/mL). After incubation in darkness at 37°C for 30 min 50 μL of propidium iodide (PI, 1 mg/mL) were added and stored for further 5 min in darkness. Data were acquired with a FACSCalibur flow cytometer (BD, Heidelberg, Germany). The data were analyzed with FlowJo 7.6.5 software (Treestar Inc., USA).

2.6. Scratch Test for Observation of Cell Migration Behavior.

Effect of xyloglucans on human skin cell migration was investigated by forming a "wound" in cell monolayer. HaCaTs (3 × 10^4 cells/well) and NHDF (2 × 10^4 cells/well) were cultured in 24-well plates to 95% confluence. Growth medium was discarded and cells were washed with PBS buffer. A defined area was scratched with a pipette tip through the monolayer. The detached cells were gently washed away with PBS buffer before 10 μg/mL TSw, respectively, TSc were applied to the cell cultures. 5 μg/mL mitomycin C (MMC) was added to inhibit the closure of the monolayer as a result of proliferation [30]. The scratched area was labeled and photographed with a DFC 300FX camera of a DMIL light microscope (Leica, Mannheim, Germany). The size of the area was calculated using ImageJ software (Wayne Rasband, USA). After 24 h of incubation the scratched area was photographed again and the differences of area size before and after the incubation were computed.

2.7. Internalization of TSw-FITC and TSc-FITC into HaCaT and NHDFs.

For fluorescence laser-scanning microscopy removable silicone chambers FlexiPERM (Greiner Bio-one, Frickenhausen, Germany) were attached to polylysine-coated glass slides (Menzel GmbH, Braunschweig, Germany) and to slides with ground colored frosted green (VWR, Darmstadt, Germany). 3 × 10^4 HaCaT were seeded on polylysine-coated slides and 2 × 10^4 NHDF on the others. At 70% confluence the cells were incubated with 50 μg/mL FITC labeled xyloglucans and 100 μg/mL Dextran-TexasRed (Invitrogen, USA) for 3 h, 6 h, 12 h, and 24 h. Cells were counterstained with 1 μg/mL DAPI 30 min before incubation was finished. Then cells were washed thrice with PBS buffer, fixed with Dako fluorescent mounting medium (Dako, USA) and covered with a cover slip. Fluorescence confocal laser-scanning microscopy was performed on a TCS SP2 fluorescence microscope (Leica, Mannheim, Germany). Internalized FITC-labeled xyloglucans were also quantified with a FACSCalibur flow cytometer using CellQuest Pro software (BD, Heidelberg, Germany). For these investigations HaCaT and NHDF were cultivated in 6-well plates. The rate of internalization of 50 μg/mL of FITC-TSw or FITC-TSc was measured over a timeline of 3 h, 6 h, 12 h, 24 h, and 48 h. On purpose to analyze the amount of internalized xyloglucans TSw and TSc were put on the cells in concentrations of 0.01 μg/mL to 100 μg/mL for 48 h. Before data acquisition cells were trypsinized, washed thrice with PBS, and again resuspended in PBS. Discrimination of internalized from attached xyloglucans was conducted with trypan blue (0,25 mg/mL) that quenches the fluorescence of FITC on cell surface [31].

2.8. Gene Expression Analysis.

Three independent cultivations of NHEKs and NHDFs were conducted in 6-well plates. Prior to treatment with xyloglucans the cells were directly adapted to MCDB basal containing neither serum, respectively, BPE nor growth factors. After incubation with the 10 μg/mL TSw in serum and growth factor-starved medium for 6 h, the cells were harvested by trypsinization. Isolation and quantification of total RNA, topic-defined PIQOR Skin Microarray, and bioinformatic calculation of 4-fold replicates and statistical analysis were performed by supplier Miltenyi Biotech GmbH, Cologne, Germany. A laser scanner from Agilent (Agilent Technologies, Böblingen, Germany) was used to detect fluorescence signals of the hybridized PIQOR Microarrays. Signal and background intensities of spots were measured using the ImaGene software (Biodiscovery, Hawthorne, CA, USA). Spots were only taken into consideration for calculation of the Cy5/Cy3 ratio that had at least in one channel a signal intensity that was at least 2-fold higher than the mean background. These spots were analyzed with the PIQOR Analyzer software that allows automated data processing of the raw data text files derived from the ImaGene software. In addition, the provided PIQOR Navigator software together with gene cards databank [32] was used for the search for information about the function of a gene of interest. In regard to [33] only genes were accounted with a minimal fold change of 1.5 respective 1.7.

2.9. Analysis of Protein Phosphorylation Profiles via Proteome Profiler Human Phospho-Kinase Array Kit.

The Proteome Profiler Human Phospho-Kinase Array kit (R&D Systems, Wiesbaden, Germany) determines the relative phosphorylation level of 46 kinases. After culturing in 25 cm^2 flasks for 24 h NHEKs and NHDF were treated with 10 μg/mL TSw and TSc for 6 h, harvested by trypsin treatment, and washed with PBS buffer. Cell number was adjusted to 1 × 10^7 cells that were suspended in 1 mL lysis buffer followed by incubation at 4°C for 30 min with constant shaking. The resultant suspension was centrifuged (11000 ×g, 5 min) and the supernatant was transferred into a clean test tube. The performance and analysis of twice replicated assays from three independent approaches each were done as described by manufacturer.

TABLE 1: Monosaccharide composition of TSw and TSc from *T. indica* seeds determined by HPAEC-PAD and CE after total hydrolysis with TFA (%, w/w). The average MW of TSw and TSc was determined by GFC against dextrans of known molecular weight on Sepharose CL-6B.

	Cold water soluble TSw	Copper precipitated TSc
L rhamnose	2.0	0
L arabinose	6.9	1.9
D galactose	15.0	12.2
D glucose	36.4	57.4
D xylose	39.6	28.5
Average MW [kDa]	437	63

2.10. Statistics. Statistical analysis was performed by use of SigmaPlot 12 (Systat Software GmbH, Erkrath, Germany). Data were calculated with Holm-Sidak test after analysis of variance (ANOVA). Results are presented as the mean ± standard deviation (SD). Data were considered as statistically significant and highly significant, respectively, with P values <0.05 and <0.01.

3. Results

3.1. Characterization of T. indica Seed Xyloglucans. The extraction of TSc, a hot water soluble and copper precipitated xyloglucan, was more complex than the simple extraction of xyloglucan TSw with cold water. It was observed that neither TSw nor Tsc content any protein or uronic acids. As main monosaccharides glucose, xylose, and galactose were determined by HPLC-PAD analysis and capillary electrophoresis. TSw exhibited a seven fold higher molecular weight than TSc and additionally contained slight amounts of rhamnose (Table 1). As well as the arabinose content a closer look revealed that the ratio of glucose and xylose differed.

3.2. Influence of Xyloglucans TSw and TSc on the Cell Viability of Human Skin Cells. The tetrazolium salts MTT and WST-1 were chosen to investigate the activity of reducing enzymes in the cells and as parts of the cell membrane [34]. TSw did not affect the intra- and extracellular metabolic activities of NHEK (Figures 1(a) and 1(d)) whereas the activity of extracellular reducing enzymes of HaCaT keratinocytes was significantly enhanced (Figure 1(b)). Though TSw showed no influence on MTT reduction by HaCaT cells (Figure 1(e)). Contrary to keratinocytes, 0.1 μg/mL–10 μg/mL of TSw significantly increased the extra- and intracellular enzyme activities of NDHF (Figures 1(c) and 1(f)).

0.1 μg/mL, 1 μg/mL, and 10 μg/mL TSc significantly improved the extracellular enzyme activity of NHEK (Figure 1(a)) and intracellular reduction of MTT by NHDF (Figure 1(f)). The extracellular enzyme activity of HaCaT was also enhanced but not significantly compared to untreated cells. Intracellular enzyme activity of keratinocytes was not affected. For elucidation of direct cytotoxic activity the extracellular LDH activity in cell cultures incubated with

tamarind seed xyloglucans was measured. After 48 h of incubation neither TSw nor TSc exhibited no cytotoxic effects in concentrations of 0.01–100 μg/mL. Quite the contrary compared to untreated control cells the amount of extracellular LDH was slightly reduced (Figures 1(g), 1(h), and 1(i)).

Adenosine-5′-triphosphate (ATP) is the molecular unit to save chemical energy. Energy transfer during the metabolism is characterized by conversion of ATP to its precursors and a turnover back to ATP. The level of ATP determines the energy status of a cell. The energy status of normal skin cells was not influenced after incubation with tamarind seed xyloglucans. However 10 μg/mL TSw and TSc slightly increased the ATP amount of immortalized HaCaT keratinocytes in regard to untreated cells (100%) as shown in Table 2.

3.3. Cell Proliferation after Incubation with Tamarind Seed Xyloglucans. The proliferation of NHEK highly significantly increased in a dose-independent manner if TSw was applied with increasing concentration in a range of 0.01–10 μg/mL. 100 μg/mL TSw reduced the NHEK proliferation rates but the differences were not significant (Figure 2(a)). TSw significantly elevated the proliferation of HaCaT keratinocytes but independent of the used dosage (Figure 2(b)). As presented in Figure 2(c) TSw also boosted the proliferation of normal fibroblasts but not dependent of the used concentration. In comparison to NHEK the effect started not with a concentration of 0.01 μg/mL TSw but with 0.1 μg/mL (Figure 2(c)).

Similar to TSw the copper precipitated xyloglucan TSc increased the cell proliferation of fibroblasts and keratinocytes. No dependence on used concentration was observed with NHEK (Figure 2(a)). HaCaT cell proliferation was also enhanced with a visible but not significant step between concentrations below and above 1 μg/mL (Figure 2(b)). TSc mostly effected NHDF proliferation in dosages of 0.1 and 1 μg/mL with a 70% increase of proliferation rates. This effect was significant compared to the results obtained with 0.01, 10, and 100 μg/mL (Figure 2(c)).

In addition the particular cell cycle phases were analyzed when cells were incubated with TSw and TSc. Compared to control cells both xyloglucans triggered keratinocytes and fibroblasts to switch from G_0/G_1 into S- and, respectively, or G_2/M-phases.

The number of NHEK in S-phase increased 30% after 24 h when they had been incubated with both xyloglucans. Also more than 20% of NEHK were in G_2/M-phase at this time. After 6 h, 12 h and 48 h the number of xyloglucan-treated NHEK in G_2/M-phase was twofold enhanced compared to untreated NHEK while the number of NHEK in S-phase remained nearly the same (Figure 3(a)). When TSw and TSc were applied to HaCaT keratinocytes the number of cells in S-phase rose during the first 6 h to a maximum of 53% (TSw), respectively, 52% (TSc) and decreased to a minimum of 28% at 48 h. The amount of cells in G_2/M rose when HaCaT was incubated with TSc and TSw, too, but differences did not exceed 15%. The maximum values of HaCaT in G_2/M-phase were obtained 48 h after incubation. The number of HaCaTs in S- and G_2/M-phase was elevated compared to untreated cells every time (Figure 3(b)). NHDF incubated with TSw

Table 2: Energy status of NHEK, HaCaT keratinocytes, and NHDF after incubation with 10 μg/mL Tamarind xyloglucans TSw and TSc. Shown are mean values ± SD of $n = 8$ replicates of two independent experiments.

| | TSw | | | TSc | |
NHEK	HaCaT	NHDF	NHEK	HaCaT	NHDF
91.78 ± 11.22	124.59 ± 14.56	98.96 ± 14.28	101.86 ± 12.37	108.33 ± 2.72	89.28 ± 8.08

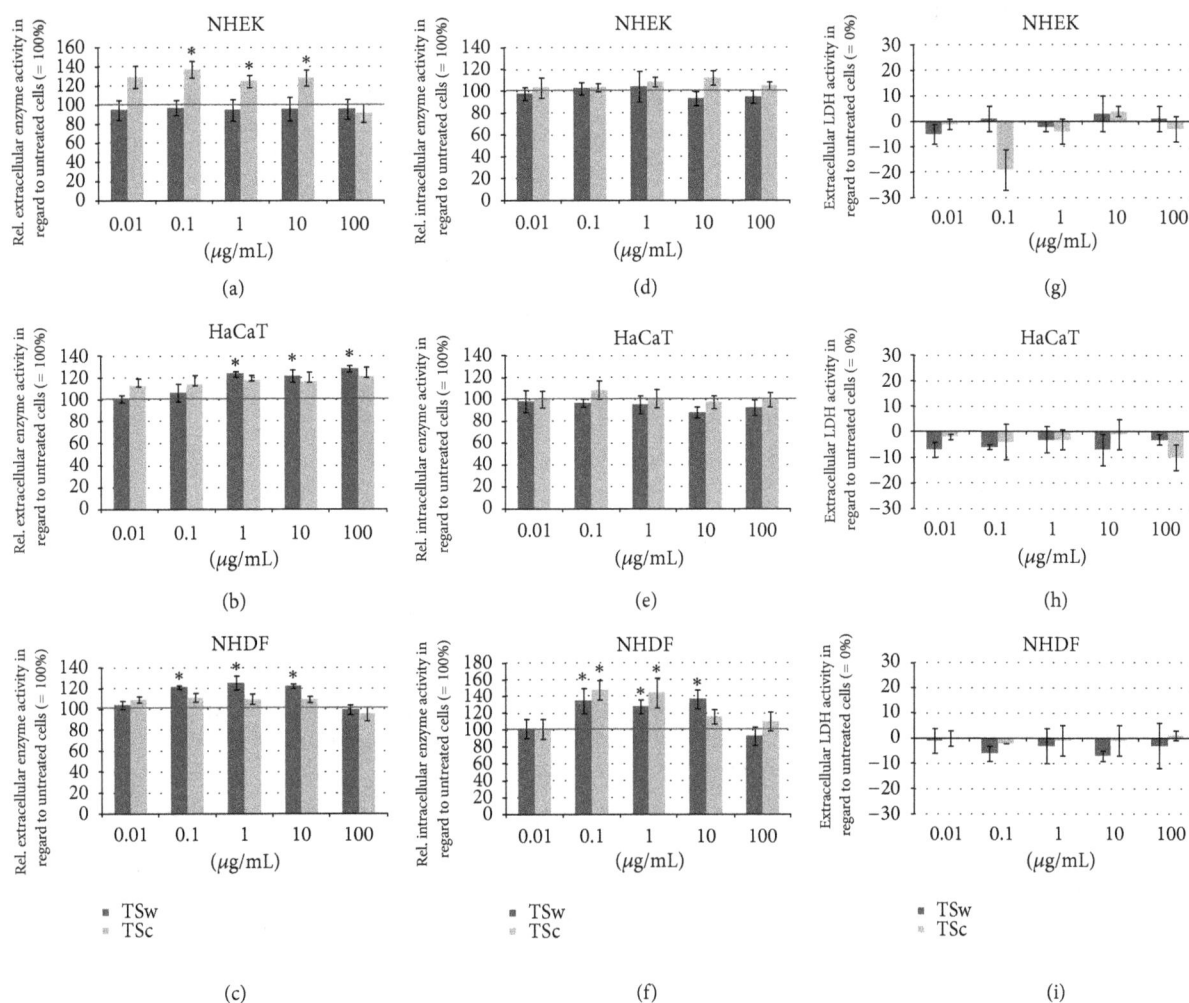

Figure 1: Cell viability of NHEK, HaCaT, and NHDF after incubation with 0.01–100 μg/mL TSw and TSc for 48 h normalized to activity of untreated control cells (black line). Extracellular enzyme activity measured by WST-1 reduction is shown in (a) (NHEK), (b) (HaCaT), and (c) (NHDF). MTT reduction as indicator for intracellular enzyme activity is presented in (d) (NHEK), (e) (HaCaT), and (f) (NHDF). (g), (h), and (i) depict the extracellular LDH activity compared to extracellular LDH activity of untreated cells (=0%). Presented are the mean values ± SD of $n = 8$ replicates of three independent experiments with $^*P < 0.05$ compared to untreated cells.

and TSc for 3 h showed an increase of cells in S-phase and a maximum of cells in G_2/M-phase compared to untreated cells. The most NHDF in S-phase was observed 6 h after incubation of TSw (55%) and TSc (51%). Further incubation resulted in a reduced number of NHDF in S-phase and G_2/M-phase but remained enhanced compared to untreated NHDF (Figure 3(c)).

3.4. Effect of Tamarind Seed Xyloglucans on the Migration of Skin Cells.
Migration analysis of NHEK was not possible when mitomycin C (MMC) was used because NHEK started

to differentiate. Even though the use of different media resulted in a differentiation of NHEK. This effect was not seen with HaCaT cells because they lost the ability to differentiate.

Compared to untreated control and to positive control, the cold water soluble tamarind xyloglucan TSw improved the closure of the scratched area of a HaCaT monolayer. TSc-treated HaCaT-scratched monolayer was not closed and the scratched area was as large as in the culture of untreated cells. The monolayer of scratched NHDF was closed during 24 h when TSc, TSw, or 10% FCS were applied. The tamarind xyloglucans were as active as 10% FCS (Table 3).

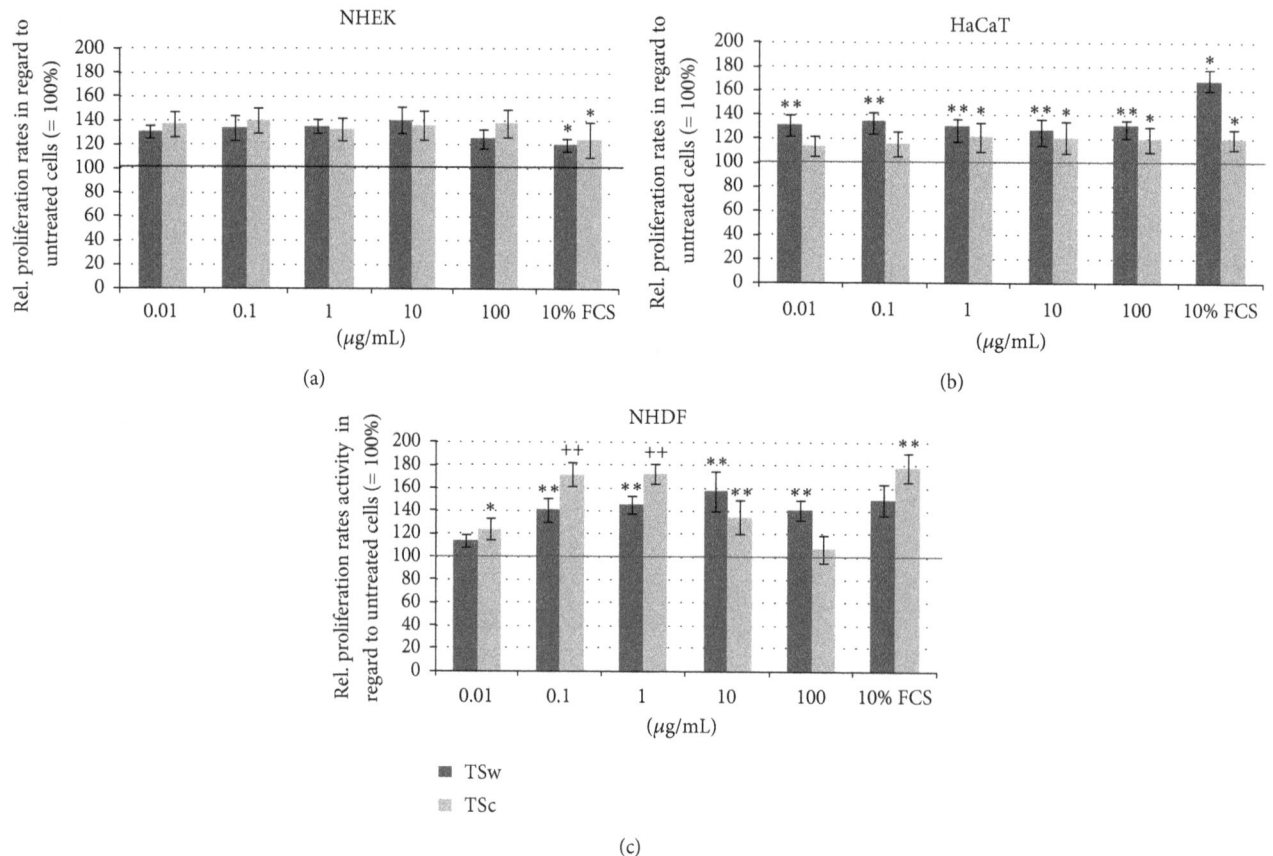

FIGURE 2: BrdU incorporation as marker for cell proliferation. NHEK (a), HaCaT (b), and NHDF (c) were incubated with TSw and TSc in concentrations of 0.01–100 μg/mL for 48 h. Mean values ± SD of n = 8 replicates of three independent experiments are shown with $^*P < 0.05$ and $^{**}P < 0.01$ compared to untreated cells as well as with $^{++}P < 0.01$ compared to cells treated with 0.01 μg/mL and 10 μg/mL TSc; 10% FCS = positive control. Results were normalized to untreated cells (=100%, black line).

TABLE 3: Effect of tamarind xyloglucans on migration of HaCaT and NHDF. Migration was investigated by scratch assay for 24 h.

	TSw (10 μg/mL)	TSc (10 μg/mL)	PC (10% FCS)
HaCaT	310 ± 9%**	104 ± 20%	197 ± 5%**
NHDF	147 ± 12%**	143 ± 7%**	144 ± 17%**

PC: positive control with 10% FCS. Values are mean ± SD related to untreated cells (=100%) of n = 4 replicates of three independent experiments, $^*P < 0.05$, $^{**}P < 0.01$ compared to untreated cells.

3.5. Internalization of TSw and TSc in Human Keratinocytes and Fibroblasts. Previous presented results showed slight differences in composition and in bioactivity of tamarind seed xyloglucans TSw and TSc. Due to the immense difference in molecular weight the question rose according to the way of activity especially of an activity from outside or inside the cells.

The uptake of TSw in HaCaT was already observed after incubation of 3 h. Until 12 h most FITC-labeled TSw was localized in endosomes which were spread over the whole cell. During further incubation green spots got obvious at the periphery of the nucleus (Figure 4). Quantification by flow cytometry revealed that the endosomal uptake of FITC-TSw

reached a maximum at 24 h and decreased during further 24 h as observed by focal laser-scanning microscopy (Figure 6(a)). The overlay of fluorescence images FITC-TSc-treated cells presented an increasing yellow fluorescence 3 h after addition to HaCaT with a maximum at 24 h (Figure 4). Quantification of yellow fluorescence resulted in a stepwise increase until 12 h incubation. When the incubation was prolonged the intensity resisted (Figure 6(b)).

The images of NHDF after treatment with FITC-labeled xyloglucans revealed that FITC-TSw was internalized by endosomes between 3 h and 6 h. After 12 h and 24 h the yellow-colored spots (representing FITC-TSw loaded endosomes) condensed and were spread all over the cell (Figure 5). Additionally an increasing number of red- and green-labeled spots were detected at these times. The decrease of FITC-TSw loaded endosomes and the increase of unloaded endosomes as well as free green fluorescence were measured during flow cytometry after incubation for 24 h and 48 h (Figure 6(c)). Until 12 h a stepwise increase of yellow fluorescence intensity was observed. In case of FITC-TSc an increase of yellow fluorescence was already shown after 3 h. During 24 h the internalization increased and resulted in a condensation of FITC-TSc loaded endosomes at the periphery of the nucleus (Figure 5). But flow cytometric analysis revealed that the

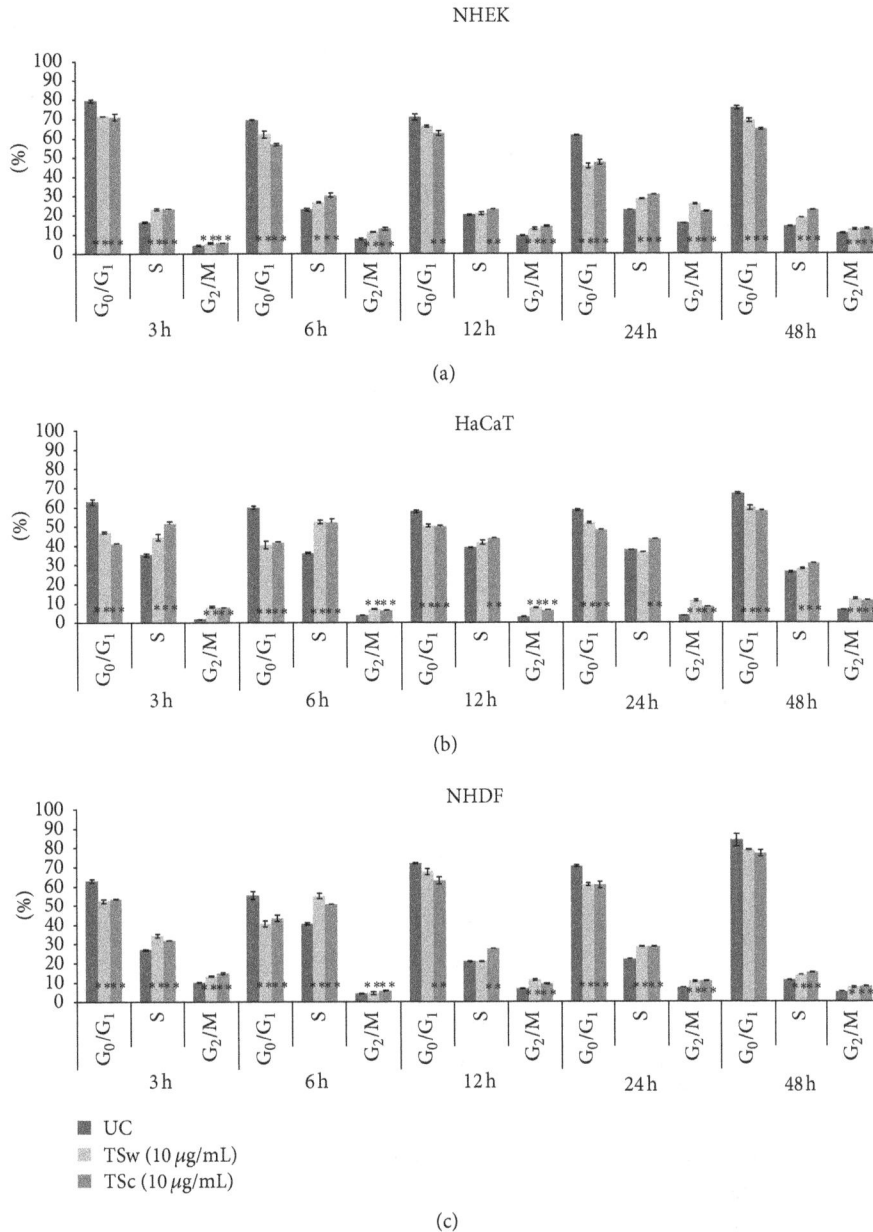

(a)

(b)

(c)

FIGURE 3: Flow cytometric analysis of cell cycle progression. The cells NHEK (a), HaCaT (b), and NHDF (c) were incubated with TSw, respectively, TSc from 3 h to 48 h. The percentage of cells in entire cell cycle was considered as 100%, presented are mean values ± SD with $n = 2$ replicates of two independent experiments; $^*P < 0.05$, $^{**}P < 0.01$ compared to untreated cells. UC: untreated cells.

maximum internalization was reached not before 6 h. The intensity of yellow fluorescence increased only to less extends at an incubation time of 24 h. This intensity level did not change during further 24 h (Figure 6(d)).

The investigations concerning cell viability, proliferation, and migration revealed no significant differences in activity in relation to the used concentration. Furthermore no inhibition or homeostasis of cell physiologic activities was observed when 100 mg/mL xyloglucan was added. For that the capability of cells to internalize different amounts of xyloglucans was studied with FITC-labeled xyloglucans in

a flow cytometric assay. As depicted in Figure 7 an increase of fluorescence intensity was already seen after incubation of 0.01 mg/mL FITC-TSw in HaCaT (A) and NHDF (C). The relationship of fluorescence intensity of internalized FITC-TSw and applied concentration was linear with a coefficient of determination $R^2 > 0.999$ (HaCaT) and $R^2 > 0.997$ (NHDF). In case of FITC-TSc an increase of fluorescence intensity was observed after incubation with 0.1 μg/mL (NHDF), respectively, 1 μg/mL. The linearity of uptake was determined with $R^2 > 0.998$ (HaCaT) and $R^2 > 0.999$ (NHDF). The results exhibit that the capacity of skin cells

TABLE 4: Relative protein phosphorylation levels related to untreated cells after treatment of NHEK and NHDF with 10 mg/mL TSw and TSc for 6 h measured with the Proteome Profiler Human Phospho-Kinase Array kit. An increase or decrease of >20% was considered as significant.

MAPK	NHEK		NHDF	
	TSw	TSc	TSw	TSc
Upstream MAPK				
β-Catenin	**133,06 ± 1,20**	**126,01 ± 2,23**	**141,65 ± 1,13**	**131,62 ± 2,38**
FAK	104,81 ± 0,24	110,06 ± 2,59	100,55 ± 1,28	**127,12 ± 0,93**
Fgr	105,95 ± 0,06	111,22 ± 3,05	98,48 ± 0,56	**127,24 ± 1,56**
Fyn	102,18 ± 0,63	**121,00 ± 0,14**	99,01 ± 0,53	104,46 ± 0,14
Hck	103,86 ± 0,05	105,10 ± 0,99	119,15 ± 1,06	**125,04 ± 0,61**
Lyn	109,22 ± 0,70	**124,27 ± 1,02**	118,27 ± 0,19	110,09 ± 0,25
Yes	110,89 ± 0,11	119,43 ± 1,23	99,64 ± 0,10	**128,49 ± 0,35**
Src	108,57 ± 2,92	**123,20 ± 4,24**	**120,78 ± 0,20**	**129,15 ± 0,74**
PLCγ-1	**128,85 ± 2,99**	**131,00 ± 2,81**	110,24 ± 0,48	102,65 ± 1,22
Downstream MAPK				
MEK1/2	**123,56 ± 2,57**	**125,09 ± 1,56**	101,89 ± 0,97	106,50 ± 4,19
ERK1/2	**135,51 ± 2,21**	**138,77 ± 0,16**	**140,68 ± 1,32**	**174,00 ± 0,20**
p38α	**136,46 ± 0,66**	**123,92 ± 1,74**	**121,99 ± 0,27**	**123,37 ± 0,64**
TOR	**124,83 ± 1,42**	**124,38 ± 1,22**	**121,25 ± 0,11**	113,47 ± 0,27
Akt$_{S473}$	109,47 ± 0,23	114,84 ± 0,76	120,33 ± 0,95	**121,18 ± 0,21**
HSP27	**125,22 ± 0,20**	**123,86 ± 0,98**	**129,28 ± 0,77**	111,02 ± 2,82
MSK1/2	**158,29 ± 1,07**	**147,02 ± 0,32**	**129,84 ± 0,64**	114,41 ± 2,08
RSK1/2	**124,35 ± 0,23**	**129,07 ± 0,81**	**121,93 ± 0,27**	108,05 ± 5,76
RSK1/2/3	**123,08 ± 0,40**	**129,31 ± 0,56**	**127,61 ± 0,59**	**124,46 ± 0,59**
p70 S6$_{T229}$	**122,07 ± 0,77**	**133,79 ± 2,27**	109,13 ± 0,80	107,49 ± 0,31
p70 S6$_{T389}$	**138,98 ± 0,72**	**143,35 ± 6,93**	105,90 ± 1,09	100,43 ± 0,52
p70 S6$_{T421}$	**123,33 ± 0,19**	**130,05 ± 0,16**	**126,00 ± 0,75**	117,22 ± 0,01
JNKpan	118,99 ± 1,41	**154,76 ± 0,24**	102,72 ± 2,12	103,13 ± 1,48
eNOS	**123,01 ± 0,33**	**124,12 ± 3,02**	116,37 ± 0,53	103,72 ± 0,67
Transcription				
c-Jun	**125,84 ± 0,39**	**126,25 ± 0,12**	104,08 ± 0,10	92,42 ± 0,85
CREB	**134,43 ± 0,40**	**131,86 ± 0,62**	98,90 ± 2,15	102,68 ± 2,10
STAT1	**130,79 ± 0,36**	**132,63 ± 0,55**	**126,87 ± 2,15**	111,37 ± 0,92
STAT2	118,20 ± 0,90	**122,22 ± 0,22**	**123,78 ± 0,51**	**126,55 ± 0,61**
STAT3	**121,22 ± 0,86**	115,62 ± 2,41	**121,89 ± 0,18**	**124,50 ± 0,06**
STAT5a	**126,52 ± 0,90**	**125,32 ± 2,02**	**120,40 ± 0,03**	**120,60 ± 0,21**
STAT5a/b	**121,46 ± 0,86**	118,70 ± 0,13	**121,63 ± 0,27**	**120,78 ± 0,24**
STAT5b	109,81 ± 0,78	104,03 ± 0,68	100,65 ± 1,32	**123,94 ± 0,26**
STAT6	105,77 ± 0,22	107,15 ± 3,14	**137,50 ± 0,38**	**132,08 ± 7,89**

to internalize xyloglucans did not depend on the molecular weight of xyloglucans and the capacity is not exhausted with 100 μg/mL.

3.6. Phosphorylation of MAPK after Incubation with TSw and TSc. The effect of Tsw and Tsc on the phosphorylation status of different proteins involved in cell signaling was measured after incubation for 6 h. The proteins are mitogen-activated protein kinases (MAPK) as well as their protein substrates that refer to ERK signaling, SAPK/JNK pathway, Wnt/β-Catenin signaling, and Akt signaling.

Neither NHEK nor NHDF showed a significant inhibition of phosphorylation of the tested proteins 6 h after incubation with TSw and TSc. No influence was observed on the phosphorylation of p53, GSK-3α/β, Chk-2, Lck, Paxillin, p27, STAT4, Akt$_{T308}$, and AMPKα1,2. In response to TSw or TSc MEK1/1, PLC-γ, CREB, JNKpan, c-Jun, p70S6$_{T229}$ and p70S6$_{T289}$, eNOS, Fyn, Lyn, Pyk-2, and STAT4 were phosphorylated in NHEK but not in NHDF. On the other hand Akt$_{S473}$, FAK, Fgr, Hck, Yes, STAT5b, and STAT6 were activated in NHDF and not in NHEK. ERK1/2, RSK1/2, p38α, β-Catenin, and STAT5 were phosphorylated independent of the used xyloglucan and the respective cell type. As shown in Table 4 the incubation of skin cells with TSc resulted in a promotion of the phosphorylation of STAT upstream proteins Fyn, Lyn, Src, and Yes and additionally of the most STATs including STAT1, 2, 3, 5a, and 5a/b in NHEK and NHDF. Furthermore TOR and of p70S6$_{T421}$ (TSw) as well

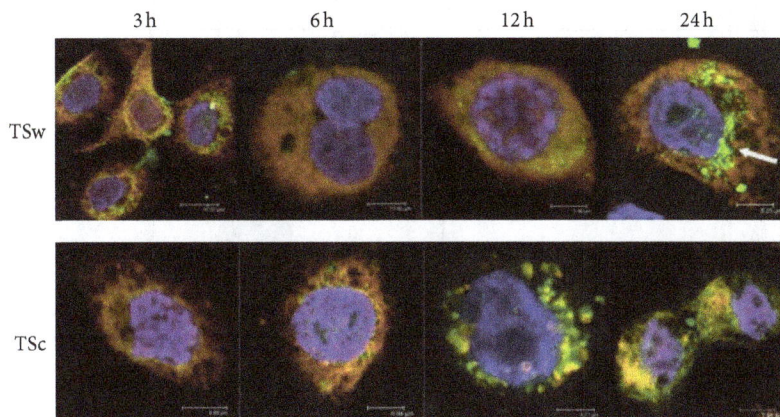

FIGURE 4: Laser-scanning confocal microscopy for internalization of green fluorescent FITC-TSw, respectively, FITC-TSc (50 µg/mL) in HaCaT after incubation of 3 h, 6 h, 12 h, and 24 h. Nuclei were labeled with blue fluorescent DAPI (1 µg/mL). Green spots: FITC-TSw, respectively, FITC-TSc; red spots: Dextran-TexasRed labeled endosomes; yellow spots: Colocalization of FITC-TSw, respectively, FITC-TSc and Dextran-TexasRed labeled endosomes structures. Arrows point to zones of not internalized FITC-labeled xyloglucans.

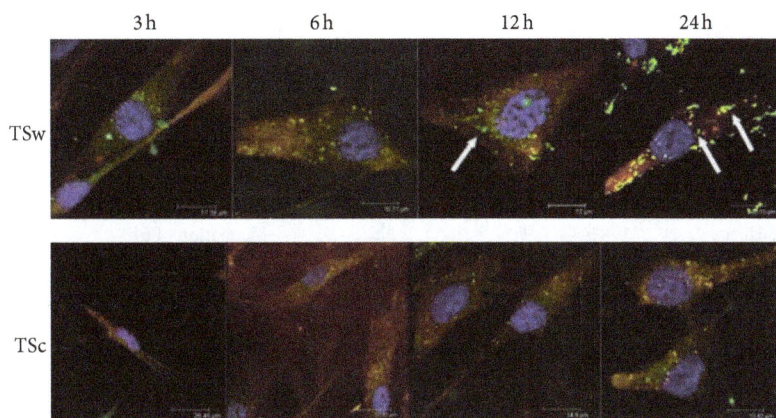

FIGURE 5: Internalization of green fluorescent FITC-TSw, respectively, FITC-TSc (50 µg/mL) by NHDF analyzed via laser-scanning confocal microscopy after incubation of 3 h, 6 h, 12 h, and 24 h. Blue fluorescence: DAPI-stained nuclei; red fluorescence: endosomes labeled with Dextran-TexasRed; yellow fluorescence: colocalization of FITC-TSw, respectively, FITC-TSc and Dextran-TexasRed within the endosomes.

as Akt_{S473} (TSc) were activated in NHDF. With exception of MSK1/2 and JNKpan both tamarind xyloglucans generally induced the phosphorylation of proteins involved in MAPK cascades especially in NHEK. Whereby, incubation with TSw resulted in a predominant phosphorylation of downstream MAPK.

3.7. Gene Expression of Skin Cells after Incubation with Tamarind Xyloglucans. Regulation of gene expression occur in response to extra- or intracellular signals. Close relation had been shown between extra- or intracellular signals and pathways which lead the signals through the cell. In regard to the speed of signal transduction the gene expression mostly starts between 3 h and 6 h, prolongs to 12 h, and decreases after 24 h. Evaluation of NHDF and NHEK gene expression after treatment with 10 µg/mL TSw in serum and growth factor-starved medium for 6 h showed that only 5% (NHEK) and 2% (NHDF) of all 1303 investigated genes were regulated. Furthermore mostly gene expression was inhibited. As presented in Figure 8 the regulated genes

referred to apoptosis-related pathways, extracellular matrix (ECM) proteins, growth factors, MAPK signaling, cytoskeleton, metabolism, cytokine signaling, and membrane proteins in NHEK. Genes related to cytokine signaling, stress or inflammation, immune response, cell cycle, membrane proteins, and metabolism were affected in NHDF. The expression of tumor suppressors, as well as genes of development, protein trafficking, calcium signaling, and translation was not seen as response to the incubation with TSw at this time.

4. Discussion

The intention of the presented study was to investigate the effects of xyloglucans from *T. indica* seeds on cell viability, proliferation, and migration of human skin cells and to study the response in regard to molecular changes in signal transduction and endocytosis.

Investigations were carried out with two xyloglucans differing in molecular weight and composition as cause of extraction method. The diversity of tamarind xyloglucans has

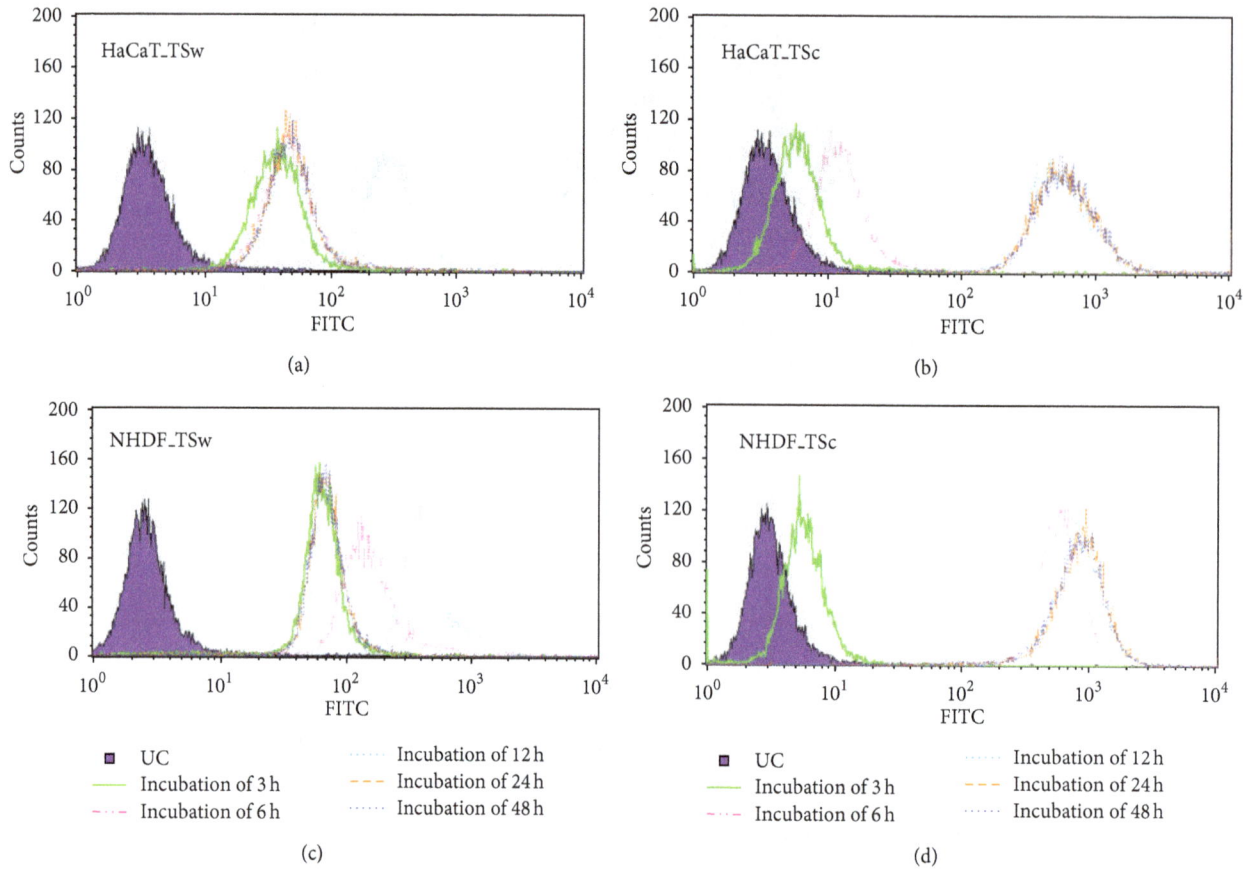

FIGURE 6: Fluorescence intensity of 50 μg/mL FITC-TSw ((a) and (c)) and FITC-TSc ((b) and (d)) in HaCaT and NHDF measured with flow cytometer after incubation for 3 h to 48 h.

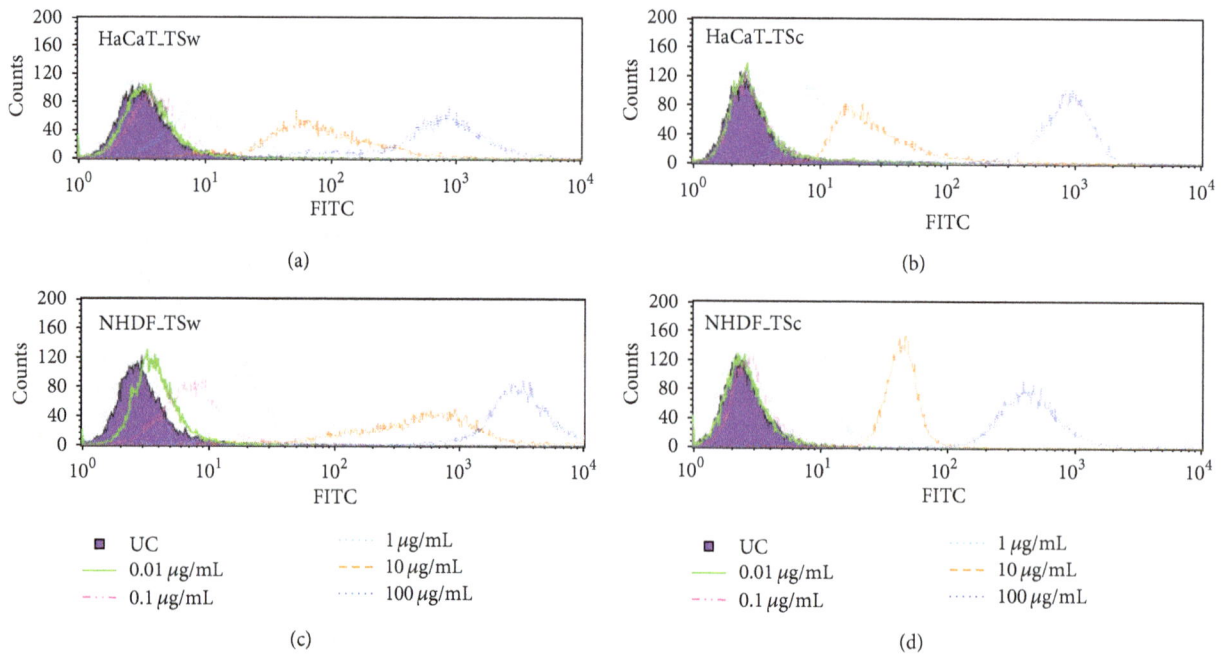

FIGURE 7: Fluorescence intensity of FITC-TSw ((a) and (c)) and FITC-TSc ((b) and (d)) applied to HaCaT ((a) and (b)) and NHDF ((c) and (d)) in concentrations of 0.01 μg/mL–100 μg/mL. Incubation took place for 48 h.

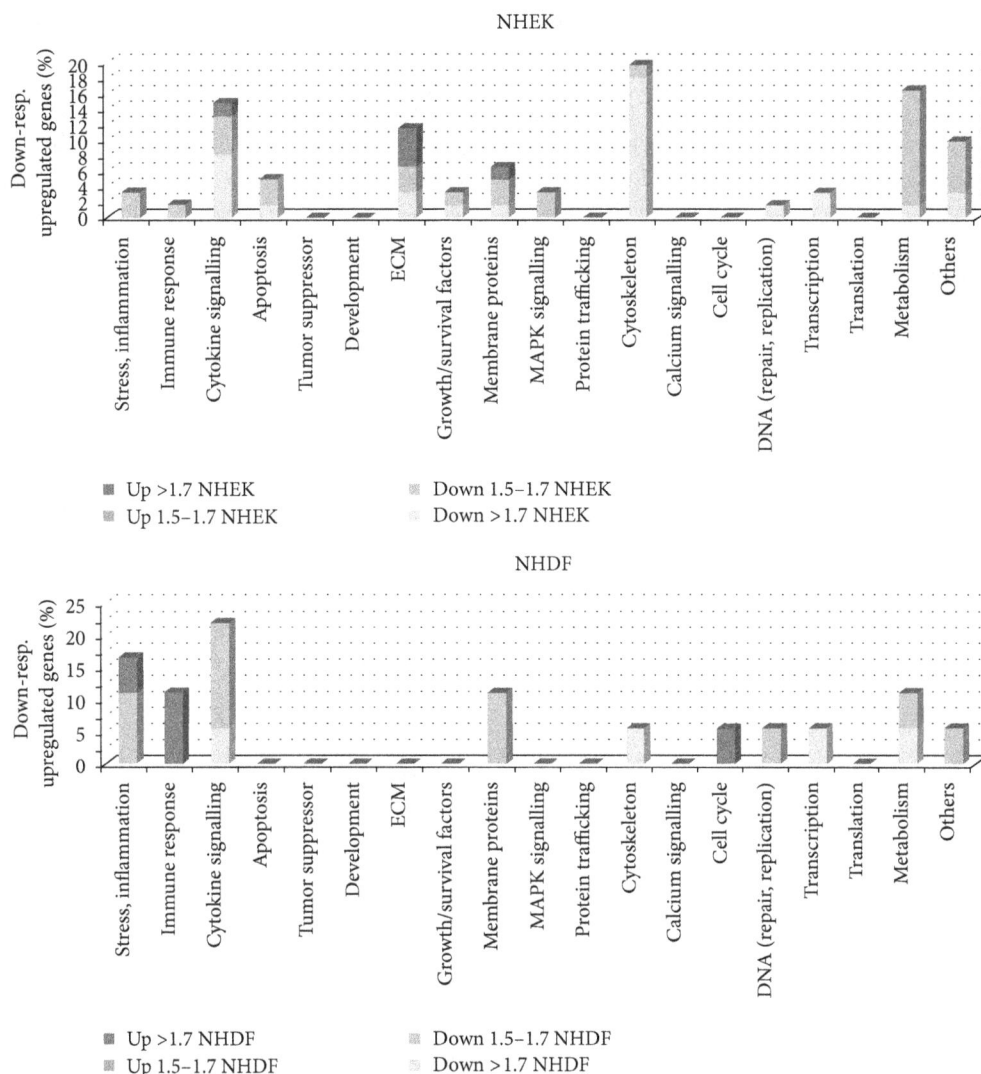

FIGURE 8: Genes regulated in NHEK, respectively, NHDF determined with the topic-defined PIQOR skin microarray after incubation of cells with 10 μg/mL TSw for 6 h. Presented is the ratio of regulated genes in percent in regard to the total number of regulated genes. The amount of not regulated genes is not presented. The minimal fold change is significant if the ratio is >1.7.

been described in a variety of publications [35]. The main sugar composition of TSw with L-arabinose, D-galactose, D-xylose, and D-glucose in ratios of 0.46 : 1 : 2.64 : 2.43 was in line with the report from [36] which also purified the tamarind xyloglucan with water extraction. This xyloglucan was identified as a galactoxyloglucan containing $(1 \rightarrow 4)$-β-D-glucan backbone branched by α-D-xylopyranose and β-D-galactopyranosyl-$(1 \rightarrow 2)$-α-D-xylopyranose through $(1 \rightarrow)$-link; additionally a minority of this xyloglucan possessed not branched $(1 \rightarrow 4)$-beta-D-galactopyranan and branched $(1 \rightarrow 5)$-alpha-L-arabinofuranan residues. The monosaccharide composition of TSc (arabinose : galactose : xylose : glucose 0.16 : 1 : 2.23 : 4.7), which was extracted according to [22], went conform with the xyloglucan that was described by ibid and [2].

The bioactivity of the isolated xyloglucans TSw and TSc resembled at the first sight. Both significantly improved the cell proliferation of keratinocytes and fibroblasts as well as the migration of NHDF. Neither the cold water extracted TSw nor the through copper precipitation isolated TSc offered cytotoxic effects. Both xyloglucans were internalized by endosomes in NHDF and HaCaT and promoted the cell cycle progression. But differences were observed in regard to cell viability, migration of HaCaT, internalization time, signal transduction, and gene expression.

Within 3 h of incubation TSw was rapidly internalized by keratinocytes and fibroblasts. Cell cycle analysis revealed that the TSw-treated cells passed on to S-phase already after 6 h and again after 24 h and 48 h of incubation compared to untreated control cells. The increase of cells in S-phase after 48 explained the results of BrdU test. In both cell types the downstream kinases as well as the transcription factors were phosphorylated. The receptor-related kinases and the other upstream kinases were not activated with exception of PLC-γ

in NHEK, Src in NHDF, and β-catenin in NHDF and NHEK. Kinases like p53 or GSK-3α/β that regulate cellular homeostasis were not affected. The most phosphorylated kinases participate in the Erk pathway. Difference in phosphorylation of MAPK was observed concerning STAT6, STAT2, and Src that were activated in NHDF and PLC-γ, CREB, c-Jun, eNOS, and p70 S6 at T229, respectively, T389 that were solely phosphorylated in NHEK. Phosphorylation of TOR, p70 S6$_{T229}$, and p70S6$_{T389}$ in NHEK as well as p70S6$_{T421}$ and STAT3 in NHDF displayed that contiguous to the Erk signaling different pathways were affected. The protein complex TOR regulates cell survival and growth by activation of p70S6 [37] or STAT3 [38]. Recent publications showed that the STAT6 pathway is involved in nutrient metabolism and regulates insulin sensitivity [39]. STAT2 is commonly involved in IFN-mediated immune response while STAT1 and STAT5 are known to be activated by different growth factors forming dimers STAT2 [32]. Although the startpoint is not clarified, TSw increased phosphorylation of signal molecules of pathways leading to cell survival, proliferation, and migration. The underlying signaling pathway could not be identified owing to the less regulation of genes after 6 h of incubation. Compared to other polysaccharides only a few genes were expressed due to the incubation with TSw [40]. As signal transduction was ongoing, shown by MAPK phosphorylation, regulation of gene expression was marginally started and must be evaluated after longer incubation times. At this early stage gene expression mostly concerned genes that refer to proteins of ECM, cytokine signaling, membrane proteins, and cytoskeleton in NHEK whereas expression of genes involved in stress response or and cytokine signaling were induced in NHDF. Nevertheless MAPK phosphorylation and gene expression results show that the different effect of TSw on cell viability and migration of fibroblasts and keratinocytes depends on a modified signal transduction.

As TSw the copper-precipitated xyloglucan TSc improved skin cell proliferation but only promoted the migration of NHDF. On the other hand TSc was more effective on extracellular reducing enzymes of NHEK and on intracellular reducing enzymes in NHDF. Interestingly, despite the lower molecular weight TSc internalization was prolonged compared to TSw as it required 6 h in keratinocytes and almost 12 h in NHDF. Furthermore the phosphorylation analysis showed that the signal transduction was less advanced in cells that were incubated with TSc. In detail upstream kinases of Src family (FAK, Fgr, Fyn, Hck, and Yes) as well as the STATs, which are commonly activated close to the cell membrane, were phosphorylated in NHEK and NHDF to a higher extent. Differences were observed when cell type was contemplated. Only Fyn was phosphorylated in both cell types whereas TSc mostly activated Fak, Fgr, and Hck in NHDF but not in NHEK. The phosphorylation of downstream MAPK was nearly independent of used xyloglucan in NHEK. But the phosphorylation of c-Jun and JNKpan as well as the inhibition of STAT3 phosphorylation suggests that TSc affected the SAPK/JNK signal cascade additionally to Erk signaling in NHEK [40, 41]. Similar to TSw the growth inhibitory kinases were not phosphorylated in cells incubated with TSc.

An interesting fact was that both xyloglucans with their high molecular weight were internalized by the cells and that the internalization of the huge TSw (437 kDa) was faster than the uptake of TSc (63 kDa). So a high molecular weight did not anticipate the uptake. The yellow color, a result of overlay of Texas Red Dextran labeled endosomes and FITC labeled xyloglucans, reveals that the uptake was done by endosomes. Fluorescence microscopic analysis demonstrated that the colocalization of FITC-TSw and endosomes was abrogated within 12 h (NHDF) and 24 h (HaCaT). So would they be metabolized and used as nutrients and then stimulated the cell proliferation or did they directly affect the signal transduction? The first part of the question must be cleared in further experiments. But results of MAPK phosphorylation might explain the second part. While TSc and TSw were internalized by endosomes, the phosphorylation of MAPK was altered compared to untreated cells. For that it is possible that the signal transduction was influenced through the xyloglucan uptake as it had been described for clathrin-mediated and clathrin-independent endocytosis [42]. The phosphorylation of Lyn, Fyn, Hck, and protein tyrosine kinases (PTK) pointed to a non-clathrin-mediated endocytosis [43] but that has to be investigated in future. That the character of cargo predetermines the endocytotic uptake and the influence on signal transduction [44] might explain the differences in the influence on MAPK phosphorylation. Analysis on MAPK phosphorylation and gene expression could not clearly identify the signal pathways leading to an increase of proliferation and migration of skin cells incubated with xyloglucan. But the presented results limited the number of possible pathways. Reactions to irritation and inflammation are very fast and had been obvious during 6 h on gene expression level. Apoptosis-inducing pathways seemed to be inhibited and cell proliferation inhibiting pathways were affected neither on gene nor on protein or cellular level. Depending on results of MAPK phosphorylation the integrin [45], SAPK/JNK [40, 41, 46], and ERK signaling [40] could be involved in reaction of cells to xyloglucans. The activation of proproliferative pathways and signal molecules known to be involved in cancer might be aware of using Tamarind xyloglucans for wound healing, drug vehicle, digestive disorders, or dry eye syndrome. But concern is appeased with moderate activation of these molecules *in vitro* as well as the results of various *in vivo* studies that proofed the lack of carcinogenicity [11, 47] and the benefit for wound healing [16].

5. Conclusion

TSw and TSc differed immensely in molecular weight but slightly in composition. So it remains open if single monosaccharides of side chains or the molecular weight and overall structure were responsible for differences in internalization and bioactivity. The results showed that the bioactivity of a xyloglucan depends on its extraction and on the cell type that would be affected. Nevertheless, the effectivity of tamarind xyloglucans for wound-healing properties was proved because they improved processes of reepitheliaization and remodeling. In concern of xyloglucan's use in different drug formulations it should be taken in mind that they are not only an inactive excipient but also might affect the cells at the application site even if this effect is beneficial for the cells.

Acknowledgments

This work was supported by German Research foundation (DFG) within the framework of the First Indo-German International Research Training Group on Molecular and Cellular Glyco-Sciences.

References

[1] S. C. Fry, "The structure and functions of xyloglucan," *Journal of Experimental Botany*, vol. 40, no. 1, pp. 1–11, 1989.

[2] C. Niemann, N. C. Carpita, and R. L. Whistler, "Arabinose-containing oligosaccharides from tamarind xyloglucan," *Starch/Staerke*, vol. 49, no. 4, pp. 154–159, 1997.

[3] E. Abraham Tholath and K. S. Ghandroth, "Transparent Xyloglucan/Chitosan Gel and a Process for the Preparation Thereof," US 20120009132 A1, 2012.

[4] A. M. Avachat, K. N. Gujar, and K. V. Wagh, "Development and evaluation of tamarind seed xyloglucan-based mucoadhesive buccal films of rizatriptan benzoate," *Carbohydrate Polymers*, vol. 91, pp. 537–542, 2013.

[5] D. Pal and A. K. Nayak, "Novel tamarind seed polysaccharide-alginate mucoadhesive microspheres for oral gliclazide delivery: *in vitro-in vivo* evaluation," *Drug Delivery*, vol. 19, no. 3, pp. 123–131, 2012.

[6] D. Chen, P. Guo, S. Chen et al., "Properties of xyloglucan hydrogel as the biomedical sustained-release carriers," *Journal of Materials Science*, vol. 23, pp. 955–962, 2012.

[7] G. Uccello-Barretta, S. Nazzi, Y. Zambito, G. Di Colo, F. Balzano, and M. Sansò, "Synergistic interaction between TS-polysaccharide and hyaluronic acid: implications in the formulation of eye drops," *International Journal of Pharmaceutics*, vol. 395, no. 1-2, pp. 122–131, 2010.

[8] A. Takahashi, S. Suzuki, N. Kawasaki et al., "Percutaneous absorption of non-steroidal anti-inflammatory drugs from in situ gelling xyloglucan formulations in rats," *International Journal of Pharmaceutics*, vol. 246, no. 1-2, pp. 179–186, 2002.

[9] H. S. Mahajan, V. Tyagi, G. Lohiya, and P. Nerkar, "Thermally reversible xyloglucan gels as vehicles for nasal drug delivery," *Drug Delivery*, vol. 19, no. 5, pp. 270–276, 2012.

[10] F. M. Strickland, Y. Sun, A. Darvill, S. Eberhard, M. Pauly, and P. Albersheim, "Preservation of the delayed-type hypersensitivity response to alloantigen by xyloglucans or oligogalacturonide does not correlate with the capacity to reject ultraviolet-induced skin tumors in mice," *The Journal of Investigative Dermatology*, vol. 116, no. 1, pp. 62–68, 2001.

[11] S. R. Aravind, M. M. Joseph, S. Varghese, P. Balaram, and T. T. Sreelekha, "Antitumor and immunopotentiating activity of polysaccharide PST001 isolated from the seed kernel of *Tamarindus indica*: an *in vivo* study in mice," *The Scientific World Journal*, vol. 2012, Article ID 361382, 14 pages, 2012.

[12] M. M. T. do Rosário, M. M. Kangussu-Marcolino, A. E. do Amaral, G. R. Noleto, and C. L. D. O. Petkowicz, "Storage xyloglucans: potent macrophages activators," *Chemico-Biological Interactions*, vol. 189, no. 1-2, pp. 127–133, 2011.

[13] T. Komutarin, S. Azadi, L. Butterworth et al., "Extract of the seed coat of *Tamarindus indica* inhibits nitric oxide production by murine macrophages *in vitro* and *in vivo*," *Food and Chemical Toxicology*, vol. 42, no. 4, pp. 649–658, 2004.

[14] S. Burgalassi, L. Raimondi, R. Pirisino, G. Banchelli, E. Boldrini, and M. F. Saettone, "Effect of xyloglucan (tamarind seed polysaccharide) on conjunctival cell adhesion to laminin and on corneal epithelium wound healing," *European Journal of Ophthalmology*, vol. 10, no. 1, pp. 71–76, 2000.

[15] M. Rolando and C. Valente, "Establishing the tolerability and performance of tamarind seed polysaccharide (TSP) in treating dry eye syndrome: results of a clinical study," *BMC Ophthalmology*, vol. 7, article 5, 2007.

[16] M. Y. Bin Mohamad, H. B. Akram, D. N. Bero, and M. T. Rahman, "Tamarind seed extract enhances epidermal wound healing," *International Journal of Biology*, vol. 4, pp. 81–88, 2012.

[17] J. M. Kuchel, R. S. C. Barnetson, L. Zhuang, P. M. Strickland, R. P. Pelley, and G. M. Halliday, "Tamarind inhibits solar-simulated ultraviolet radiation-induced suppression of recall responses in humans," *Letters in Drug Design & Discovery*, vol. 2, no. 2, pp. 165–171, 2005.

[18] T. K. Hunt, "The physiology of wound healing," *Annals of Emergency Medicine*, vol. 17, no. 12, pp. 1265–1273, 1988.

[19] W. Mutschler, "Physiology and pathophysiology of wound healing of wound defects," *Der Unfallchirurg*, vol. 115, pp. 767–773, 2012.

[20] M. Maas, M. Kemper, F. Lamerding, A. Klenke, and A. Deters, "Variations in extraction protocol lead to differences in monosaccharide composition and bioactivity on human keratinocytes as shown by polysaccharides from banana and plum fruits," *Planta Medica*, vol. 72, p. 237, 2006.

[21] C. Junchen, L. Pufu, S. Hengsheng, Z. Hengguang, and F. Rutao, "Effect of extraction methods on polysaccharide of clitocybe maxima stipe," *Advance Journal of Food Science and Technology*, vol. 5, pp. 370–373, 2013.

[22] H. C. Srivastava and P. P. Singh, "Structure of the polysaccharide from tamarind kernel," *Carbohydrate Research*, vol. 4, no. 4, pp. 326–342, 1967.

[23] A. M. Deters, K. R. Schröder, T. Smiatek, and A. Hensel, "Ispaghula (*Plantago ovata*) seed husk polysaccharides promote proliferation of human epithelial cells (skin keratinocytes and fibroblasts) via enhanced growth factor receptors and energy production," *Planta Medica*, vol. 71, no. 1, pp. 33–39, 2005.

[24] M. Monsigny, C. Petit, and A.-C. Roche, "Colorimetric determination of neutral sugars by a resorcinol sulfuric acid micro-method," *Analytical Biochemistry*, vol. 175, no. 2, pp. 525–530, 1988.

[25] M. M. Bradford, "A rapid and sensitive method for the quantitation of microgram quantities of protein utilizing the principle of protein dye binding," *Analytical Biochemistry*, vol. 72, no. 1-2, pp. 248–254, 1976.

[26] S. Abakuks and A. M. Deters, "Polysaccharides of St. John's Wort herb stimulate NHDF proliferation and NEHK differentiation via influence on extracellular structures and signal pathways," *Advances in Pharmacology Science*, vol. 2012, Article ID 304317, 11 pages, 2012.

[27] A. N. de Belder and K. Granath, "Preparation and properties of fluorescein-labelled dextrans," *Carbohydrate Research*, vol. 30, no. 2, pp. 375–378, 1973.

[28] K. Gescher and A. M. Deters, "*Typha latifolia* L. fruit polysaccharides induce the differentiation and stimulate the proliferation of human keratinocytes *in vitro*," *Journal of Ethnopharmacology*, vol. 137, no. 1, pp. 352–358, 2011.

[29] T. Mosmann, "Rapid colorimetric assay for cellular growth and survival: application to proliferation and cytotoxicity assays,"

Journal of Immunological Methods, vol. 65, no. 1-2, pp. 55–63, 1983.

[30] T. Schreier, E. Degen, and W. Baschong, "Fibroblast migration and proliferation during *in vitro* wound healing. A quantitative comparison between various growth factors and a low molecular weight blood dialyzate used in the clinic to normalize impaired wound healing," *Research in Experimental Medicine*, vol. 193, no. 4, pp. 195–205, 1993.

[31] M. Maas, A. M. Deters, and A. Hensel, "Anti-inflammatory activity of *Eupatorium perfoliatum* L. extracts, eupafolin, and dimeric guaianolide via iNOS inhibitory activity and modulation of inflammation-related cytokines and chemokines," *Journal of Ethnopharmacology*, vol. 137, no. 1, pp. 371–381, 2011.

[32] The GeneCards Human, Crown Human Genome Center, Department of Molecular Genetics, Weizmann Institute of Science, "hostname: 356977-web1.xennexinc.com db genecards_309_100 index build: 100 solr: 1.4".

[33] I. V. Yang, E. Chen, J. P. Hasseman et al., "Within the fold: assessing differential expression measures and reproducibility in microarray assays," *Genome Biology*, vol. 3, no. 11, Article ID research0062, 2002.

[34] M. V. Berridge, P. M. Herst, and A. S. Tan, "Tetrazolium dyes as tools in cell biology: new insights into their cellular reduction," *Biotechnology Annual Review*, vol. 11, pp. 127–152, 2005.

[35] P. Lang and K. Kajiwara, "Investigations of the architecture of tamarind seed polysaccharide in aqueous solution by different scattering techniques," *Journal of Biomaterials Science. Polymer Edition*, vol. 4, no. 5, pp. 517–528, 1993.

[36] M. J. Gidley, P. J. Lillford, D. W. Rowlands et al., "Structure and solution properties of tamarind-seed polysaccharide," *Carbohydrate Research*, vol. 214, no. 2, pp. 299–314, 1991.

[37] Y. Li, M. N. Corradetti, K. Inoki, and K.-L. Guan, "TSC2: filling the GAP in the mTOR signaling pathway," *Trends in Biochemical Sciences*, vol. 29, no. 1, pp. 32–38, 2004.

[38] J. Zhou, J. Wulfkuhle, H. Zhang et al., "Activation of the PTEN/mTOR/STAT3 pathway in breast cancer stem-like cells is required for viability and maintenance," *Proceedings of the National Academy of Sciences of the United States of America*, vol. 104, pp. 16158–16163, 2007.

[39] R. R. Ricardo-Gonzalez, A. R. Eagle, J. I. Odegaard et al., "IL-4/STAT6 immune axis regulates peripheral nutrient metabolism and insulin sensitivity," *Proceedings of the National Academy of Sciences of the United States of America*, vol. 107, no. 52, pp. 22617–22622, 2010.

[40] P. P. Roux and J. Blenis, "ERK and p38 MAPK-activated protein kinases: a family of protein kinases with diverse biological functions," *Microbiology and Molecular Biology Reviews*, vol. 68, no. 2, pp. 320–344, 2004.

[41] K. A. Gallo and G. L. Johnson, "Mixed-lineage kinase control of JNK and p38 MAPK pathways," *Nature Reviews Molecular Cell Biology*, vol. 3, no. 9, pp. 663–672, 2002.

[42] E. R. Andersson, "The role of endocytosis in activating and regulating signal transduction," *Cellular and Molecular Life Sciences*, vol. 69, pp. 1755–1771, 2012.

[43] S. Ilangumaran, B. Borisch, and D. C. Hoessli, "Signal transduction via CD44: role of plasma membrane microdomains," *Leukemia & Lymphoma*, vol. 35, no. 5-6, pp. 455–469, 1999.

[44] M. Krauss and V. Haucke, "Shaping membranes for endocytosis," *Reviews of Physiology, Biochemistry and Pharmacology*, vol. 161, pp. 45–66, 2011.

[45] M. Bienz, "β-catenin: a pivot between cell adhesion and Wnt signalling," *Current Biology*, vol. 15, no. 2, pp. R64–R67, 2005.

[46] C. R. Weston and R. J. Davis, "The JNK signal transduction pathway," *Current Opinion in Genetics and Development*, vol. 12, no. 1, pp. 14–21, 2002.

[47] M. Sano, E. Miyata, S. Tamano, A. Hagiwara, N. Ito, and T. Shirai, "Lack of carcinogenicity of tamarind seed polysaccharide in B6C3F1 mice," *Food and Chemical Toxicology*, vol. 34, no. 5, pp. 463–467, 1996.

8

A Left-Sided Prevalence of Lentigo Maligna: A UK Based Observational Study and Review of the Evidence

Mark Gorman,[1] **Andrew Hart,**[1] **and Bipin Mathew**[2]

[1]*Canniesburn Plastic Surgery Unit, Glasgow Royal Infirmary, UK*
[2]*Hull Royal Infirmary, Hull, UK*

Correspondence should be addressed to Mark Gorman; m.gorman@me.com

Academic Editor: Iris Zalaudek

Skin cancer has been shown to present asymmetrically, prevalent on the left side of the body, more so in subtypes of cutaneous melanoma such as lentigo maligna. Biases have been linked to cumulative UV light exposure and automobile driving patterns. Though left-right ratios have previously correlated with the side men or women tend to position themselves or countries drive on, more recent trends indicate a consistent left-sided bias. To clarify reasons for changing trends, a review of the evidence base and LM's laterality in a UK cohort (99 cases 2000–2011) was conducted for the first time. The strong correlation of left-sided excess, found in both genders (ratios 1.381–1.5, $P < 0.05$ X^2 0.841), is congruent with more recent findings. Though evidence indicates that driving position is no longer a risk factor for LM, due most likely to improved car window UV protection, it remains the most commonly attributed cause. Understanding phenomena such as UV lights "scatter effect" or that cumulative exposure may not be a significant risk factor helps rationalize older conclusions that would otherwise appear contradictory. The reasons for left-sided excess remain unclear but may be due to factors requiring further research such as the body's anatomical/embryological asymmetry.

1. Introduction

Since the late 1970s, studies have shown trends in which cancer presents with a bias to one side of the body [1, 2]. This has been most commonly reported in breast cancer, where a consistent left-sided excess has been shown [3]. Over the last decade, studies have also started to evidence a consistent trend of skin cancer on the left side of the body [4–6]. This work has focused more on invasive melanoma and nonmelanoma skin cancer (NMSC) than melanoma in situ (MIS) or lentigo maligna (LM). When data relating to LM has been reviewed, not only do the biases in laterality remain, but interestingly, the proportional shift seems to be more profound [7, 8]. These findings have been most commonly attributed to environmental factors such as sun damage, where it is speculated that patterns observed may relate to driving behaviors, such as positioning in a car and the resulting ultraviolet (UV) light exposure [5]. Laterality biases on the left and right sides of the body have therefore been previously linked to which side of the road individuals drive on [8–10], but more recent work indicates a left-sided

bias irrespective of such variables [4, 7]. Despite changing trends, there has been little critique of this body of work thus far. This study investigates LM's laterality in a UK cohort and reviews the evidence base to date.

As highlighted in our previous work [11], LM presents a challenge to pathologists in terms of its histological diagnosis as it can be difficult to confidently decide whether excision margins are clear. This is especially important when making management decision, such as whether to further excise lesions that present predominantly on cosmetically sensitive areas in the head and neck region [12]. Given that this is a difficult pathology to manage, it is important to identify factors that may reduce LM's risk.

Driving pattern's association with sidedness of LM at diagnosis has been found to vary based upon gender. In an Australian cohort of patients (1984–1990), the prevalence of LM was higher on the right side for men and left-side for women, explained by driving habits: men more commonly situated in the driving seat (right side) and women on the opposite passenger side [8]. However, more recent epidemiological work, with data from six different populations (including the UK), has found a consistent excess of left-sided cutaneous melanomas, irrespective of gender and driver side [4]. This has been supported by data related to MIS [7] and LM within US populations [6]. To date there have been no UK based studies investigating LM's intersex or anatomical left to right ratio.

Cumulative sunlight has been long assumed to increase melanoma risk, with a stronger association demonstrated in LM, based upon its higher preponderance in the elderly and presentation on areas of direct exposure [12]. However, case control studies over the last two decades challenge this assumption, showing that risk is increased by intermittent periods of UV exposure resulting in skin sun damage, as opposed to the total hours of sunlight [13–15]. Despite such findings, the importance of intermittent exposure has to date received little research focus, and the "cumulative hypothesis" persists in most causative explanations.

Intermittent, as opposed to cumulative, UV light would seem to explain why LM has previously been shown to present more prevalently on the side of maximum exposure whilst in a car. It does not explain why this pattern has changed, such that, irrespective of individuals positioning within a car or which side of the road they drive on, trends now indicate a consistent left-sided excess. In light of these findings, we have revisited the question of LM laterality within a UK cohort of drivers seated on the right side (affording comparison with Foley et al.'s previous cohort).

2. Methods

Patient consent was not required and the experimental methods observed the ethical principles of the Declaration of Helsinki.

2.1. Laterality Study. As a retrospective review (as part of the aforementioned wider trial), 99 cases of LM (2000–2011) were identified from a UK histopathology department (Hull and East Yorkshire NHS Trust) [11]. Cases were excluded if reports indicated invasive melanoma (LMM) or required information was omitted. The anatomical site, side, and patient demographics (gender and age) were all recorded from individual's histopathology reports.

2.2. Review of the Laterality Evidence Base. A review of the laterality evidence base to date was conducted within "Papers 2" (search engine and reference managing software available for mac and pc) [16]. "Papers 2" allows the user to define the domains (single or multiple, such as "title," "abstract," "general," "year," and "author") and portals (we selected PubMed and Google scholar), to better stratify how the chosen search terms identify relevant articles/sources of evidence. Searches were thus conducted looking within "titles" and "general," using the search terms "*melanoma, lentigo, cutaneous, skin, laterality, side, left, right and cancer.*" Abstracts were screened and articles relating to cutaneous melanoma/NMSC and LM laterality were selected for review (13 in all, five with data pertaining to MIS/LM laterality and one study exclusively focused on LM). Articles were then

TABLE 1: Variance in LM lesions anatomical site presentation for side and gender distribution.

Anatomical & intersex variation	Site distribution	
	Left side	Right side
Head & neck	56 (58%)	39 (42%)
Men	29 (58%)	21 (42%)
Women	27 (60%)	18 (40%)
Limbs	2 (50%)	2 (50%)
Total	58 (59 %)	41 (41%)

selected regarding the relationship between laterality, cancer in general, and embryology/epidemiological risk factors (15 articles). Due to the small pool of relevant papers, though higher levels of evidence were sought, no exclusion criteria were required.

2.3. Statistics. The majority of previous laterality studies had employed X^2 and odds ratio in their analysis. For direct comparison, we have employed the same statistical tests.

Pearson's X^2 test was used to analyze the probability of independence ($P < 0.05$) regarding the pattern of laterality observed between genders in the presentation of LM in the head and neck region (as in Foley et al.'s previous study) [8]. If the X^2 value was found to be less than 3.841 [17], the null hypothesis should be rejected, and males and females would be considered to follow the same pattern of laterality (df = 1) [18]. The left-right laterality odds ratio (or strictly just the ratio) was then calculated for both genders.

3. Results

LM was more common on the left side of the body (59%, $n = 58$) than on the right one (42%, $n = 41$, Table 1). This was true for both genders, the left-sided male prevalence being 58% and the female one being 60%. The left-right ratios for men, 1.381, and women, 1.5, both indicate a very strong association of left-sided excess.

The odds ratio (0.9206) and X^2 (0.841 = reject null hypothesis $P < 0.05$) indicate that there was no significant difference in laterality patterns between genders.

Of the 99 cases, the majority of lesions presented in the head and neck region ($n = 95/>95\%$, Table 1) and in the elderly, in those over 55 years of age (97%, Table 2).

4. Discussion

The strong correlation (1.381 and 1.5, resp.) in men and women towards a left-sided excess (~60%) and significant homogeneity ($P < 0.05$ X^2 0.841) between genders indicate a different pattern of LM distribution than was found in older studies [8–10]. Foley et al. found both an intersex variability and a preponderance of a right-sided prevalence in those more commonly positioned on the right side of the car. Our findings are congruent with more recent trends that indicate a consistent left-sided bias [19]. In our UK cohort,

TABLE 2: Demographics of patients presenting with LM.

Gender	
N (total)	99
Male	52 (52%)
Female	47 (47%)
Age (years)	
Median (IQR)	72 (64, 79)
[Range]	[35, 100]
<55	12 (12%)
55–74	45 (45%)
75+	42 (42%)

the proportional shift in laterality bias seems to be more profound than when compared with cutaneous melanoma in general, supporting previous data from the US and Australia [7, 8].

Returning first to the issue of gender based laterality variation, Foley et al. demonstrated a female left-sided and male a right-sided bias [20]. This was attributed to women more commonly occupying the passengers' seat. Foley et al. explained that their findings occurred in the pre-air conditioning era, leading to driving with windows down. Thus, the protection that may be afforded by glass (filtering 90% of the UV-B sunlight) was lost. Accepting this causation, our findings may, in a historical sense, follow those of Foley et al. in that our UK cohort drove approximately 20 years later, when air conditioning had become the norm and the speculated preponderance of men more commonly being on the driver's side had all but disappeared [21]. On further scrutiny, however, though Foley et al.'s conclusions may be partly valid, they are contradicted by some of their own later work and cannot be used to explain why cutaneous melanoma now seems to have a consistent left-sided bias irrespective of the causations they cite.

Continuing associative links between asymmetrical presentation and driving habits have persisted mainly in US based studies involving left-seated drivers [5, 7]. Such assertions are contradicted by both the findings of this study and the epidemiological analysis of national cancer registries, including countries where drivers are positioned/seated on the right (i.e., England, Scotland, and Australia), and the left-sided excess of cutaneous melanomas remains [19]. The left-right ratio across the six counties sampled was found to be consistently greater than 1.10 (range 1.08–1.18), the collective cohort totaling just under 100,000 cases. Given the size of the overall sample and that the ratio remained very similar across countries, it is unlikely that that trend is simply due to chance. Reflecting on their work, Brewster et al. rule out more straightforward explanations, such as recording bias and handedness of sunscreen application. Unlike previous findings, no significant differences were observed between or within subgroups, based upon gender, age, or anatomical site (i.e., upper versus lower limb, not laterality).

Factors leading to greater levels of left-sided sun exposure, other than positioning in a car, would seem to offer the most obvious explanation for laterality biases, but to date, no plausible hypotheses have been suggested. Given

that countries from both the north and south hemispheres indicate the same trend, differences such as the direction of sun set/rise and sunbathing habits may be ruled out. There has been little work investigating the link between melanoma and varying sun patterns and none that relates data directly to the laterality of presentation. On review, the only related UK melanoma study to demonstrate such data includes no analysis of laterality [22]. Though driving patterns do not explain the more recent trends, Brewster and de Vries [4] believe that they may still be a risk factor for NMSC. Without plausible epidemiological links to explain a left-sided preponderance of cutaneous melanoma, alternative explanations have been sought and considered.

An interesting hypothesis is that of the body's asymmetry. In a UK study looking at cancer in five major paired organs (the breasts, lungs, kidneys, testes, and ovaries, including ~ 250,000 patients), it was found that organ asymmetries, as opposed to epidemiological factors, coincided closely with the laterality of presentation [23]. Relating more specifically to melanoma, it has been cited that asymmetry of the lymphatic and circulatory systems may influence the immune response against or patterns of melanoma spread [19]. As yet, there has been little specific research with which to support such ideas. Brewster et al. cite a recent study involving the signaling molecule "Nodal" (belonging to the TGF-b superfamily) [24, 25], which is both involved in the left-right ratio of embryogenesis and histopathologically present when melanoma tissue excisions have been examined, not seen in normal skin. Brewster et al. hypothesize a link between these findings and data trends within the national cancer registries from their epidemiological study. Further analysis of US data (SEER "White" registry 1998–2003) revealed a more profound excess of left-sided tumors with distant metastases (ratio 1.19), compared with localized/regional spread tumors (ratios 1.09/1.06, resp.), suggesting that, as "Nodal" is secreted in more aggressive melanomas, it may be influencing the left-right ratio pattern. Individuals with situs inversus may provide the perfect cohort with which to investigate anatomical/embryological asymmetry. That no research has yet been conducted will owe in part to its rare incidence (estimated at ~1 : 8000–25000) [26].

There are few other studies demonstrating the same right-sided tendency found in Foley et al.'s study, and the evidence that does exist relates to particular subgroup stratifications of older individuals. The pattern has been demonstrated in two studies of NMSC and one of melanoma. Two are US based, the first involving a cohort from Latino/Hispanic descent presenting with NMSC [27]. The second showed an increased prevalence of right-sided melanoma in women presenting on specific anatomical sites, namely, MIS of the ear/trunk and invasive melanoma of the eyelid [6]. In both studies, all other subgroups were found to have a small left-sided majority. In the first study, it was theorized that more passengers travelled on the passenger (right) side due to decreased car ownership and increased members per Latino/Hispanic household. However, this was merely an extrapolative inference from current population statistics, and it was not based upon direct observation or data from the correct era. For the second study, the same conclusions and intersex variation apply as demonstrated in Foley et al.'s 1980s Australian cohort, when women historically occupied the passenger seat more commonly.

The other study to evidence a right-sided laterality bias was also undertaken by Foley et al. Preceding their LM study, they investigated patterns of solar keratosis (SK) presentation (related again to driving), aiming to test anecdotal assertions of the time, that skin cancer was "more frequent on the right side in Australia and Britain" ([9] page 18). They found a similar general pattern of intersex variation as within their later LM study, with more right-sided male lesions and vice versa for women. Importantly, though, this time it occurred only on the right arm for men and the head and neck region for women. Subsequent papers quote Foley's studies together as evidence to support the "window down exposure theory." However, when doing so, authors have failed to address that the studies' conclusions were somewhat contradictory. It was argued that, by being taller, men had fewer head and neck SKs, protected by the shade of car roofs. This line of argument was then omitted, despite circumstances being the same, when explaining the anatomical distribution of the LM data, for which both genders had an overwhelming majority of head and neck lesions. A US study carried out during the same period with similar driving conditions found no apparent increase in photo damage with windows down (panel based assessment of photos) but still found that asymmetry correlated with time spent driving seated on the left [10].

Paulson et al. [28] highlight that if driving habit associated UV patterns do influence the left-sided excess observed with melanoma, there would seem to be a disproportionately large number of lesions presenting on areas rarely exposed whilst in a car, such as the legs. Similarly, though the vast majority of LM lesions present in the head and neck region (>95% in our study), Foley et al.'s aforementioned contradictory conclusions also indicated that men's high prevalence of head and neck lesions occurred in spite of protective shade. The often cited "window down exposure theory" would seem to require more adequate explanation and may be answered by UV radiation's "scatter effect." It is estimated that 50% of UV-A radiation is received despite shielding from direct sunlight, be it umbrella shade or car roof. Thus, areas that are not in direct line of visible light are still affected, but prevalence should increase the nearer a body part is to an unprotected portal of entry (i.e., passenger window) [29]. The historical improvement in UV protection levels afforded by car windows, previously almost nonexistent, explains why in Singer et al.'s older study it was found that having "windows down" did not increase the positive photo damage correlation observed with driving hours in general [30]. Though the degree to which modern cars guard against UV-A (as opposed to UV-B) has been questioned [31], improvements seem the most plausible explanation as to why laterality no longer matches with driving side. Follow-up studies looking at direct skin photo damage and not just skin cancer prevalence would be useful in order to clarify this point. A summarized review of the discussion's learning points and study findings are presented as follows.

Key Findings and Learning Points from This Study. This is the first study to evidence significant *left-sided excess/prevalence of LM in a UK based population.*

(i) Previous Evidence linked laterality bias to car related UV light exposure; its key examples are as follows:

(a) LM prevalence was significantly higher on the *right side for men* and left side for women (in both the head and neck region) explained by driving habits, *men more commonly situated in the driving seat (right side)* and women on the opposite passenger's side [8];

(b) SKs and NMSC most commonly presented on the arm of the driver's side [9].

(ii) Recent Trends indicate that cutaneous melanoma prevalence now has consistent *left-sided excess*, not affected by gender or which side of the road countries drive [4, 6, 7, 19]:

(a) combined with our study, findings of the last decade indicate driving habits are no longer a risk factor for LM/melanoma (see below points);

(b) a shift to left-sided excess is explained by (a) *the previous lack of UV protection afforded by car windows +/− (b) driving with windows down* (which stopped post the advent of air conditioning).

(iii) Attribution Error. Despite evidence indicating that driving position is no longer an associated risk factor, authors still commonly cite it as the most plausible cause. Such causation error/prior assumptions may be refined with the knowledge of the following.

(a) UV radiation's "Scatter Effect": 50% of UV-A radiation is received despite shielding from direct sunlight, for example, a car roof or umbrella shade. Thus, areas not in the direct line of visible light are still affected and it is the relationship of UV intensity versus filtration, not shade, which is key [29].

(b) The evidence points to the dose of UV radiation passing through newer car windows as posing no risk, and though counterintuitive, such chronic low grade UV exposure may even be protective against melanoma (and LM) [14, 15, 32].

(iv) Moving Forward

(a) Research trends indicate that that there is no evidence justifying the need for additional sun cream protection whilst in a car (due to improved UV window protection) cited by many recent studies.

(b) The left-sided excess of cutaneous melanoma requires further research, which may, for example, include study of the body's anatomical asymmetry or epidemiological factors other than driving.

(c) Identifying risk factors/causation in LM/LMM is even more important as compared with other subtypes of melanoma; it is on the rise and demonstrates a more profound shift towards left-sided excess.

A point more widely discussed, but not within previous laterality studies, is that while LM occurs over severely sun damaged skin (part of its diagnostic histopathological criteria) [32, 33], it should not be confused with the potentiating effects of chronic sun exposure, which, without resultant "damage" per se, has been shown to reduce melanoma risk, assessed through occupational exposure groups that work outdoors [13–15, 32]. Though counterintuitive, low dose UV radiation passing through newer car windows may have very little, no, or even mildly protective effect regarding LM's prevalence and laterality of presentation. The conclusions of many recent studies that people should be more vigilant regarding sun protection whilst in cars may thus be overstated [27, 28].

5. Conclusion

This is first UK based study investigating LM's laterality, where the left-sided excess found was the same for both sexes, contrasting with older findings. Changing trends in cutaneous melanoma's laterality may be explained by factors such as the lack of protection previously afforded by car windows. Despite evidence indicating that driving position is no longer an associated risk factor for LM or cutaneous melanoma, it remains the most commonly attributed cause: an "attribution error." It is important to scrutinize the causation of LM's left-sided excess, as found by this and more recent studies, towards the identification of more likely factors, be they epidemiological *or* based upon further study of the body's anatomical/embryological asymmetry. Understanding that cumulative UV exposure may not be a significant risk factor, and being aware of UV lights "scatter effect" phenomena, may help direct future research efforts and rationalize older findings.

Conflict of Interests

The authors declare that there is no conflict of interests regarding the publication of this paper.

References

[1] Y. Melnik, P. E. Slater, R. Steinitz, and A. M. Davies, "Breast cancer in Israel: laterality and survival," *Journal of Cancer Research and Clinical Oncology*, vol. 95, no. 3, pp. 291–293, 1979.

[2] N. S. Weiss and D. T. Silverman, "Laterality and prognosis in ovarian cancer," *Obstetrics and Gynecology*, vol. 49, no. 4, pp. 421–423, 1977.

[3] M. H. Amer, "Genetic factors and breast cancer laterality," *Cancer Management and Research*, vol. 6, no. 1, pp. 191–203, 2014.

[4] D. H. Brewster and E. de Vries, "Left-sided excess of invasive cutaneous melanoma," *Journal of the American Academy of Dermatology*, vol. 65, no. 1, pp. 207–210, 2011.

[5] S. W. Fosko, S. T. Butler, and E. S. Armbrecht, "Left-sided skin cancer: importance of age, gender, body site, and tumor subtype in studying skin cancer laterality and implications for future research and public health interventions," *Journal of*

[6] G. M. Dores, M. M. Huycke, and S. S. Devesa, "Melanoma of the skin and laterality," *Journal of the American Academy of Dermatology*, vol. 64, no. 1, pp. 193–195, 2011.

[7] S. T. Butler and S. W. Fosko, "Increased prevalence of left-sided skin cancers," *Journal of the American Academy of Dermatology*, vol. 63, no. 6, pp. 1006–1010, 2010.

[8] P. A. Foley, R. Marks, and A. P. Dorevitch, "Lentigo maligna is more common on the driver's side," *Archives of Dermatology*, vol. 129, no. 9, pp. 1211–1212, 1993.

[9] P. Foley, D. Lanzer, and R. Marks, "Are solar keratoses more common on the driver's side?" *British Medical Journal*, vol. 293, no. 6538, p. 18, 1986.

[10] R. S. Singer, T. A. Hamilton, J. J. Voorhees, and C. E. M. Griffiths, "Association of asymmetrical facial photodamage with automobile driving," *Archives of Dermatology*, vol. 130, no. 1, pp. 121–123, 1994.

[11] M. Gorman, M. A. A. Khan, P. C. D. Johnson, A. Hart, and B. Mathew, "A model for lentigo maligna recurrence using melanocyte count as a predictive marker based upon logistic regression analysis of a blinded retrospective review," *Journal of Plastic, Reconstructive & Aesthetic Surgery*, vol. 67, no. 10, pp. 1322–1332, 2014.

[12] S. M. Swetter, J. C. Boldrick, S. Y. Jung, B. M. Egbert, and J. D. Harvell, "Increasing incidence of lentigo maligna melanoma subtypes: Northern California and national trends 1990–2000," *Journal of Investigative Dermatology*, vol. 125, no. 4, pp. 685–691, 2005.

[13] C. D. J. Holman, C. D. Mulroney, and B. K. Armstrong, "Epidemiology of pre-invasive and invasive malignant melanoma in Western Australia," *International Journal of Cancer*, vol. 25, no. 3, pp. 317–323, 1980.

[14] S. D. Walter, W. D. King, and L. D. Marrett, "Association of cutaneous malignant melanoma with intermittent exposure to ultraviolet radiation: results of a case-control study in Ontario, Canada," *International Journal of Epidemiology*, vol. 28, no. 3, pp. 418–427, 1999.

[15] C. Gaudy-Marqueste, N. Madjlessi, B. Guillot, M.-F. Avril, and J.-J. Grob, "Risk factors in elderly people for lentigo maligna compared with other melanomas: a double case-control study," *Archives of Dermatology*, vol. 145, no. 4, pp. 418–423, 2009.

[16] Papers, papersapp.com, your personal library of Research, 2014, http://www.papersapp.com.

[17] S. H. Online, Critical Values of the Chi-Square Distribution, 2014, http://www.itl.nist.gov/div898/handbook/eda/section3/eda3674.htm.

[18] Vassarstats. 2x2 Contingency Table, 2014, http://vassarstats.net/, http://vassarstats.net/tab2x2.html.

[19] D. H. Brewster, M.-J. D. Horner, S. Rowan, P. Jelfs, E. de Vries, and E. Pukkala, "Left-sided excess of invasive cutaneous melanoma in six countries," *European Journal of Cancer*, vol. 43, no. 18, pp. 2634–2637, 2007.

[20] R. Marks, "Prevention of skin cancer: being sunsmart in the 1990s," *Journal of Dermatological Treatment*, vol. 1, no. 5, pp. 271–274, 1990.

[21] Transport DO, *National Travel Survey 2010*, gov.uk, 2011, https://www.gov.uk/government/uploads/system/uploads/attachment_data/file/8932/nts2010-01.pdf.

[22] A. Armstrong, C. Powell, R. Powell et al., "Are we seeing the effects of public awareness campaigns? A 10-year analysis of

Breslow thickness at presentation of malignant melanoma in the South West of England," *Journal of Plastic, Reconstructive and Aesthetic Surgery*, vol. 67, no. 3, pp. 324–330, 2014.

[23] R. Roychoudhuri, V. Putcha, and H. Møller, "Cancer and laterality: a study of the five major paired organs (UK)," *Cancer Causes and Control*, vol. 17, no. 5, pp. 655–662, 2006.

[24] A. F. Schier, "Nodal signaling in vertebrate development," *Annual Review of Cell and Developmental Biology*, vol. 19, pp. 589–621, 2003.

[25] J. M. Topczewska, L.-M. Postovit, N. V. Margaryan et al., "Embryonic and tumorigenic pathways converge via Nodal signaling: role in melanoma aggressiveness," *Nature Medicine*, vol. 12, no. 8, pp. 925–932, 2006.

[26] B. A. Afzelius and B. Mossberg, *The Metabolic and Molecular Bases of Inherited Disease*, edited by C. R. Scriver, McGraw-Hill, New York, NY, USA, 1995.

[27] M. P. McLeod, K. M. Ferris, S. Choudhary et al., "Contralateral distribution of nonmelanoma skin cancer between older Hispanic/Latino and non-Hispanic/non-Latino individuals," *British Journal of Dermatology*, vol. 168, no. 1, pp. 65–73, 2013.

[28] K. G. Paulson, J. G. Iyer, and P. Nghiem, "Asymmetric lateral distribution of melanoma and Merkel cell carcinoma in the United States," *Journal of the American Academy of Dermatology*, vol. 65, no. 1, pp. 35–39, 2011.

[29] H. Schaefer, D. Moyal, and A. Fourtanier, "Recent advances in sun protection," *Seminars in Cutaneous Medicine and Surgery*, vol. 17, no. 4, pp. 266–275, 1998.

[30] E. F. Bernstein, M. Schwartz, R. Viehmeyer, M. S. Arocena, C. P. Sambuco, and S. M. Ksenzenko, "Measurement of protection afforded by ultraviolet-absorbing window film using an in vitro model of photodamage," *Lasers in Surgery and Medicine*, vol. 38, no. 4, pp. 337–342, 2006.

[31] C. Weller, Glass in Car Windows Doesn't Fully Protect from Sun's UV Rays, Could Explain Left-Side Skin Cancer, 2013, http://www.medicaldaily.com/glass-car-windows-doesnt-fully-protect-suns-uv-rays-could-explain-left-side-skin-255398.

[32] D. M. Parkin, D. Mesher, and P. Sasieni, "Cancers attributable to solar (ultraviolet) radiation exposure in the UK in 2010," *British Journal of Cancer*, vol. 105, supplement 2, pp. S66–S69, 2011.

[33] N. Agarwal-Antal, G. M. Bowen, and J. W. Gerwels, "Histologic evaluation of lentigo maligna with permanent sections: implications regarding current guidelines," *Journal of the American Academy of Dermatology*, vol. 47, no. 5, pp. 743–748, 2002.

9

Sun Protection Behaviors Associated with Self-Efficacy, Susceptibility, and Awareness among Uninsured Primary Care Patients Utilizing a Free Clinic

Akiko Kamimura,[1] Maziar M. Nourian,[2] Jeanie Ashby,[3] Ha Ngoc Trinh,[1,4] Jennifer Tabler,[1] Nushean Assasnik,[5] and Bethany K. H. Lewis[6]

[1]Department of Sociology, University of Utah, Salt Lake City, UT 84112, USA
[2]School of Medicine, University of Utah, Salt Lake City, UT 84132, USA
[3]Maliheh Free Clinic, Salt Lake City, UT 84107, USA
[4]Department of Sociology, Vietnam National University, Hanoi, Vietnam
[5]Health Society and Policy, University of Utah, Salt Lake City, UT 84112, USA
[6]Department of Dermatology, University of Utah, Salt Lake City, UT 84132, USA

Correspondence should be addressed to Akiko Kamimura; akiko.kamimura@utah.edu

Academic Editor: Iris Zalaudek

Background. Skin cancer is the most commonly diagnosed form of cancer in the United States (US). However, knowledge, behaviors, and attitudes regarding sun protection vary among the general population. The purpose of this study is to examine sun protection behaviors of low-income primary care patients and assess the association between these health behaviors and the self-efficacy, susceptibility, and skin cancer awareness. *Methods.* Uninsured primary care patients utilizing a free clinic ($N = 551$) completed a self-administered survey in May and June 2015. *Results.* Using sunscreen was the least common tactic among the participants of this study. Skin cancer awareness and self-efficacy are important to improve sun protection behaviors. Spanish speakers may have lower levels of skin care awareness compared to US born and non-US born English speakers. Male and female participants use different sun protection methods. *Conclusion.* It is important to increase skin cancer awareness with self-efficacy interventions as well as education on low-cost sun protection methods. Spanish speaking patients would be a target population for promoting awareness. Male and female patients would need separate gender-specific sun protection education. Future studies should implement educational programs and assess the effectiveness of the programs to further promote skin cancer prevention among underserved populations.

1. Introduction

Skin cancer is the most commonly diagnosed form of cancer in the United States (US) [1]. The incident rate of cancer is known to vary by race and ethnicity: non-Hispanic whites are most susceptible to skin cancer (25 per 100,000), followed by Hispanics (4 per 100,000), while blacks are least likely to be diagnosed with skin cancer (1 per 100,000) [1]. Yet, racial or ethnic minority groups tend to have higher mortality and morbidity risks from skin cancer compared to majority groups [2]. Decreasing unprotected ultraviolet

exposure is effective in preventing skin cancer [3]; thus, wearing sunscreen and wearing sun protective clothing are common recommendations for sun protection [4]. However, knowledge, behaviors, and attitudes regarding sun protection vary among the general population [5].

Variation in the knowledge, behaviors, and attitudes toward sun protection may be related to group differences in self-efficacy, perceived susceptibility, and skin cancer awareness; it is well established that individual level self-efficacy, perceived susceptibility, and awareness are important constructs influencing health behaviors [6], including sun protection behaviors and beliefs. Self-efficacy refers to confidence in one's ability to change behaviors [7] and affects sun protection intention and behavior [8–10]. Higher levels of self-efficacy are related to higher levels of desire to improve sun protection [11]. In addition, one's belief about the chance to get a disease, that is, perceived "susceptibility," is related to higher levels of motivation for sun protection behaviors [12]. Higher levels of perceived susceptibility are associated with higher levels of desire to get assistance to improve sun protection [11]. However, perceived susceptibility of skin cancer is low in general [13]. Awareness is an application for a cue to action to change health behaviors [6]. Yet skin cancer awareness is low overall, especially among minority patients [14].

Sociodemographic risk factors for reduced practice of sun protection include younger age, male gender, non-Hispanic white, Hispanic ethnicity, and low education level [5, 15, 16]. While previous studies have focused on some of the sociodemographically high risk groups, few studies examined sun protection behaviors among low-income primary care patients. In general, primary care patients are less likely to receive skin cancer screening compared to screening of other cancers [17]. Low-income primary care patients may be particularly at risk for poor skin cancer awareness and use of sun protection due to the limited access to resources. Thus, the purpose of this study is to examine sun protection behaviors of low-income primary care patients and assess the association between these health behaviors and the self-efficacy, susceptibility, and skin cancer awareness. This study increases knowledge about sun protection behaviors and influencing factors in order to develop effective intervention strategies to promote skin cancer prevention among low-income patients in a primary care setting.

In particular, this study focuses on low-income and uninsured patients who are utilizing a free clinic providing primary care for the underserved. Free clinics provide free or reduced fee healthcare to individuals who lack access to primary care and are socioeconomically disadvantaged in the US [18, 19]. Most free clinics rely on volunteer providers and staff and limited financial resources [20]. Approximately 40% of free clinic patients are immigrants [21]. Patients who utilize free clinics suffer from a wide variety of medical conditions such as respiratory diseases, circulatory diseases, and mental disorders, [22] and tend to experience poor physical and mental health and low levels of health-related quality of life [23, 24]. To the best of our knowledge, there are no previous studies that examine skin cancer risk, sun protection, and related dermatological health issues of free clinic patients.

2. Methods

2.1. Overview.
The current community-based research project was conducted at a free clinic in the Intermountain West. The clinic staff collaborated with this research team to develop the survey instrument, study protocol, participant recruitment strategies, and interpretation of study results. The clinic provides free healthcare services, mostly routine health maintenance and preventative care, for uninsured individuals who live below the 150th percentile federal poverty level and do not have access to employer-provided or government-funded health insurance. The primary focus of the clinic is routine health maintenance and preventative care for chronic conditions such as diabetes and cardiovascular diseases. The clinic is staffed by six full-time paid personnel and over 300 active volunteers, including approximately 60 volunteer interpreters. The clinic, which has been in operation since 2005, has no affiliation with religious organizations and is funded by nongovernmental grants and donations. The clinic is open five days a week. The number of patient visits was 18,967 in 2013. The clinic does not ask patients to provide documentation of legal residency or citizenship and serves undocumented immigrants as well as US citizens and documented immigrants.

2.2. Study Participants and Data Collection.
Participants were aged 18 years or older, spoke and read English or Spanish, and were patients of the clinic. A bilingual translator translated English materials into Spanish. Another bilingual translator conducted back-translation from Spanish to English. The third bilingual translator checked accuracy of the translation. Participants were divided into three groups, namely, US born English speakers, non-US born English speakers, and Spanish speakers, because previous studies on free clinic patients have indicated that these three populations have different sociodemographic characteristics, physical and mental health status, and healthcare needs [23–25].

Prior to data collection, the Institutional Review Board (IRB) approved this study. The data were collected for two months, in May and June 2015. Recruitment occurred at the free clinic by distributing flyers to patients in the waiting room. If a potential participant expressed interest in participating in the study, he or she received a consent cover letter and a self-administered paper and pencil survey. Members of the study team were available to answer any questions while participants were taking the survey. Participants received sample sunscreen or hand sanitizer (US $1 or less value) at the completion of the survey. The research assistants who collected surveys checked item nonresponses immediately after submission and asked the participant to fill in missing parts if there were any, whenever it was possible. Only completed surveys were included in the analysis.

2.3. Measures

2.3.1. Sun Protection Behaviors.
Five sun protection related questions were extracted from the Health Information National Trends Survey, the National Cancer Institute (http://hints.cancer.gov/default.aspx): (1) "When you go outside for more than 1 hour on a warm sunny day, how often do you wear long pants?"; (2) "When you go outside for more than 1 hour on a warm sunny day, how often do you wear sunscreen?"; (3) "How often do you stay in the shade or under an umbrella?"; (4) "How often do you wear a hat?"; and (5) "How often do you wear a shirt with sleeves that cover your shoulders?" The questionnaire uses a five-point Likert scale (0 = never to 4 = always) to determine the levels of sun protection behaviors.

2.3.2. Self-Efficacy. Self-efficacy was measured by the General Self-Efficacy Scale [26]. The scale has 10 items and uses a 4-point Likert scale (1 = not at all true, 4 = exactly true). The examples of the items include "I can always manage to solve difficult problems if I try hard enough" and "I can usually handle whatever comes my way." The scoring is based on a sum of all items (score range: 0–40). While there is no specific cutoff point to identify high or low levels of self-efficacy, the mean score of US-American adults is 29.48 [27]. This scale has been used in many countries and languages and its validity and reliability have been tested [27]. Cronbach's alpha for this study population was 0.905.

2.3.3. Skin Cancer Susceptibility and Awareness. Skin cancer susceptibility and awareness were measured by the scale based on the Health Belief Model [28]. There are six items for the susceptibility subscale (e.g., "My chances for getting skin cancer are high") and six items for the awareness subscale (e.g., "It's important for me to wear a hat when outside in the sun"). The mean score for each subscale was used for analysis. The scale uses a 5-point Likert scale (5 = strongly agree, 1 = strongly disagree). Higher scores indicate higher levels of perceived susceptibility or awareness. Cronbach's alpha for this study population was 0.825 for the susceptibility subscale and 0.921 for the awareness subscale.

2.3.4. Demographic Information. Demographic questions included age, gender, race/ethnicity, education level, employment status, marital status, US born or not, country of origin, length of years living in the US (non-US born participants only), and length of years as a patient of the free clinic (2+ years or less).

2.4. Data Analysis. Data were analyzed using SPSS (version 22). The participants were divided into three groups for comparison: US born English speakers, non-US born English speakers, and Spanish speakers. Descriptive statistics were used to capture the distribution of the outcome and independent variables. The three groups of the participants were compared using Pearson's Chi-square tests for categorical variables and analysis of variance (ANOVA) for continuous variables. General linear model multivariate regression analysis was conducted to assess predictors of sun protection behaviors, including self-efficacy, susceptibility, awareness, and sociodemographic factors. Sociodemographic factors for the regression analysis were selected based on previous studies on free clinic populations [23, 24].

3. Results

Table 1 describes sociodemographic characteristics of 551 participants of a convenience sample (164 US born English speakers, 129 non-US born English speakers, and 258 Spanish speakers) and descriptive statistics of sun protection behaviors, self-efficacy, susceptibility, and awareness. Based on the average number of patient visits per day (75 visits/day) and the duration of the survey collection (40 days), the estimated participation rate was 58.8%. The average age of the participants was 44.37 (SD = 13.66). More than 65% of the participants were women ($n = 365$, 66.2%). Approximately 60% of the participants ($n = 343$, 62.3%) self-identified as Hispanic, Latino, or Latina. One-quarter of the participants ($n = 138$, 25%) were white. Nearly 45% of the participants ($n = 243$, 44.1%) reported having some college or higher levels of education. US born English speakers had much higher percentage of those with some college or higher levels of education ($n = 103$, 62.8%) than non-US born English speakers ($n = 64$, 49.6%) and Spanish speakers ($n = 76$, 29.5%) ($p < 0.01$). Likewise approximately 45% of the participants ($n = 244$, 44.3%) were currently employed. Non-US born English speakers ($n = 73$, 56.6%) and Spanish speakers ($n = 147$, 57%) were more likely to be married compared to US born English speakers ($p < 0.01$). One-third of the participants ($n = 176$, 31.9%) were US born. Among those who are not US born, the average length of living in the US was 16.2 (SD = 11.92) among non-US born English speakers and 13.98 (SD = 8.1) among Spanish speakers. The participants were from 40 countries (not shown in the table). Besides the US, Mexico had the largest number of participants ($n = 192$, 34.8%) followed by Tonga ($n = 19$, 3.4%) and Peru ($n = 18$, 3.3%). Half of the participants ($n = 284$, 51.5%) had been a patient of the free clinic for two years or longer.

The common sun protection behaviors among all groups were wearing long pants (mean = 2.70, SD = 1.17) and shirts with sleeves (mean = 2.74, SD = 1.20). Using sunscreen was the least common (mean = 1.33, SD = 1.28). Spanish speakers were more likely to wear a hat but were less likely to wear shirts with sleeves compared to US born and non-US born English speakers. The overall levels of self-efficacy were very similar to that among the US general population [27]. Spanish speakers had the highest levels of self-efficacy. Spanish speakers also reported higher levels of susceptibility but lower levels of awareness than US born and non-US born English speakers.

Table 2 presents the predictors of sun protection behavior. Higher levels of self-efficacy were associated with higher levels of sunscreen use. Higher levels of awareness were associated with higher levels of using sunscreen and shade/umbrella and of wearing a hat and shirts with sleeves. Female participants were more likely to use sunscreen and shade/umbrella but were less likely to wear a hat and shirts with sleeves compared to male participants. Lastly, Spanish speakers were less likely to wear a hat compared to the other two groups.

4. Discussion

This study examined sun protection behaviors associated with self-efficacy, perceived susceptibility, and awareness among low-income primary care patients utilizing a free clinic for the uninsured. While using sunscreen is the common sun protection practice compared to wearing a hat or sleeves and/or using a shade among the general US public [29], using sunscreen was the least common tactic among the participants of this study. These results suggest that low-income primary care patients tend to use different sun protection methods from the general public. This study

TABLE 1: Sociodemographic characteristics of participants.

	Total (N = 551)	US born English speakers (n = 164)	Non-US born English speakers (n = 129)	Spanish speakers (n = 258)	p value[a]
Mean age, years	44.37 (13.66)	43.07 (14.19)	43.90 (16.38)	45.46 (11.64)	N.S.
Female	365 (66.2)	103 (62.8)	78 (60.5)	184 (71.3)	N.S.
Race/ethnicity					
White	138 (25.0)	115 (70.1)	12 (9.3)	10 (3.9)	<0.01
Hispanic/Latino/Latina	343 (62.3)	33 (20.1)	62 (48.1)	248 (96.1)	<0.01
Asian or Pacific Islander	49 (8.9)	5 (3.0)	44 (34.1)	0	
Some college or higher	243 (44.1)	103 (62.8)	64 (49.6)	76 (29.5)	<0.01
Currently employed	244 (44.3)	68 (41.5)	54 (41.9)	122 (47.3)	N.S.
Currently married	252 (45.7)	32 (19.5)	73 (56.6)	147 (57.0)	<0.01
US born	176 (31.9)	164 (100)	0	12 (4.7)	
Years in the US (non-US born only)			16.20 (11.92)	13.98 (8.10)	
Patient of the clinic (2 years or longer)	284 (51.5)	103 (62.8)	71 (55.0)	110 (42.6)	<0.01
Sun protection behavior					
Long pants	2.70 (1.17)	2.62 (1.21)	2.57 (1.14)	2.81 (1.14)	N.S.
Sunscreen	1.33 (1.28)	1.40 (1.21)	1.29 (1.36)	1.30 (1.29)	N.S.
Shade or umbrella	1.95 (1.14)	1.97 (1.13)	1.96 (1.23)	1.93 (1.11)	N.S.
Hat	1.51 (1.34)	1.36 (1.30)	1.39 (1.32)	1.66 (1.36)	<0.05
Shirts with sleeves	2.74 (1.20)	2.93 (1.15)	2.84 (1.22)	2.56 (1.19)	<0.01
Self-efficacy	30.85 (5.64)	31.03 (5.07)	29.48 (5.59)	31.48 (5.94)	<0.01
Skin cancer susceptibility	2.72 (0.90)	2.73 (0.82)	2.20 (0.82)	3.00 (0.88)	<0.01
Skin cancer awareness	2.75 (1.16)	3.45 (0.76)	3.46 (0.96)	1.88 (0.87)	<0.01

Number (%) or mean (SD). N.S.: not significant.

[a]p value denotes significance from Pearson's Chi-square tests between categorical variables (for cell size $\geq$5 only) and ANOVA tests for continuous variables comparing US born English speakers, non-US born English speakers, and Spanish speakers.

has three main findings which may provide useful information for improving or facilitating sun protection behaviors among this population. First, skin cancer awareness and self-efficacy are important to improve sun protection behaviors. Second, Spanish speakers may have lower levels of skin care awareness compared to US born and non-US born English speakers. Third, male and female participants use different sun protection methods.

The results of this study suggest that awareness and self-efficacy, especially awareness, are important to promote sun protection behavior among low-income primary care patients. The mean score of skin cancer awareness among this study population (2.75) was lower than that of general public (3.6) [28]. Promoting skin cancer awareness may not necessarily be the main focus for free clinics given that free clinics tend to target treating patients' chronic conditions such as diabetes, hypertension, and heart disease [22]. However, because skin cancer is a common cancer, sun protection needs to be promoted among low-income patients utilizing a free clinic. Since free clinics are mostly volunteer-based [21], it may be challenging for volunteer physicians to provide skin cancer interventions. Using nonphysician providers potentially increases skin cancer screening [30] and may be feasible for free clinics to implement skin cancer prevention education. Since individuals who received

self-efficacy interventions are more likely to accept sun protection messages than those without interventions [31], self-efficacy interventions should be included in skin cancer prevention education to make the educational programs effective. At the same time, the low use of sunscreens among the participants may be clearly associated with the cost of these products. Thus, interventions in skin awareness or self-efficacy may not achieve positive results because of cost of sunscreens. In this scenario other measures of sun protection such as clothes and hats may be more efficient.

While previous studies suggest that Hispanics have low levels of skin cancer susceptibility [32], the results of the current study indicate that Spanish speakers may be at greater risk for skin cancer given that Spanish speakers reported lower levels of skin cancer awareness compared to US born or non-US born English speakers. There are some barriers to engaging sun protection behaviors; for example, wearing sunscreen or protective clothing is "not part of my daily routine" was a common statement in a study analyzing barriers to sun protection in Hispanics [33]. Given this, sun protection behaviors practiced by Hispanics need to be improved [34]. However, individuals of Hispanic origin are not homogeneous and there are differences in sun protection behaviors across Hispanic subgroups: for example, Mexican heritage Hispanics are more likely to perform sun protection

TABLE 2: Predictors of sun protection behavior ($N = 551$).

Dependent variables	Long pants β	p value	Sunscreen β	p value	Shade/umbrella β	p value	Hat β	p value	Sleeves β	p value
Independent variables										
Age	0.01	N.S.	−0.003	N.S.	0.01	<0.05	0.02	<0.01	0.004	N.S.
Female	0.01	N.S.	0.58	<0.01	0.29	<0.05	−0.48	<0.01	−0.26	<0.05
Some college or higher	−0.15	N.S.	0.03	N.S.	0.06	N.S.	0.02	N.S.	−0.07	N.S.
Employed	0.07	N.S.	−0.02	N.S.	−0.12	N.S.	−0.07	N.S.	0.09	N.S.
Married	0.15	N.S.	0.15	N.S.	0.05	N.S.	0.16	N.S.	0.15	N.S.
Clinic patient, 2+ years	0.03	N.S.	−0.07	N.S.	0.13	N.S.	−0.002	N.S.	0.16	N.S.
Self-efficacy	−0.003	N.S.	0.03	<0.05	0.00	N.S.	0.02	N.S.	−0.004	N.S.
Susceptibility	0.03	N.S.	0.03	N.S.	−0.10	N.S.	−0.03	N.S.	0.00	N.S.
Awareness	0.04	N.S.	0.25	<0.01	0.22	<0.01	0.24	<0.01	0.16	<0.05
US born English speakers[#]	−0.09	N.S.	−0.16	N.S.	−0.30	N.S.	−0.70	<0.01	0.11	N.S.
Non-US born English speakers[#]	−0.22	N.S.	−0.31	N.S.	−0.37	N.S.	−0.72	<0.01	−0.07	N.S.
(Intercept)	2.33	<0.01	−0.45	N.S.	1.10	<0.05	0.25	N.S.	2.22	<0.01
Multivariate tests										
Effect size	0.02									
F	1.85									
p value	<0.05									

Multivariate regression analysis (general linear model). p values are based on parameter estimates. N.S.: not significant.
Multivariate tests based on Wilks' lambda.
[#]Reference variable (reference = Spanish speakers).

behavior but also experience more sunburns more often compared to other Hispanic subgroups [15]. It is therefore important to develop sun protection educational programs for Spanish speaking patients that consider within group differences in sun protection behaviors.

The results of this study also indicate that female participants are more likely to use sunscreen and shade/umbrella but are less likely to wear hat and shirts with sleeves for sun protection compared to men. Previous studies show that men are less likely to practice sun protection than women [5, 35]. Based on the results of this study, men and women use different methods for sun protection. Gender differences in clothing preference or the use of lotion may affect the choice of sun protection methods. Gender-specific sun protection interventions are necessary so that male and female patients can choose the methods with which they are familiar and may potentially implement.

This study has limitations. The cross-sectional design of this study examines associations but does not assess causal relationships among variables. Patients who were not literate in either English or Spanish were not included in this study. Non-US born English speakers have very diverse backgrounds but did not have a sample size large enough to divide them into subgroups. While participants were not selected based on specific skin types, there is a possibility that the high percentage of the minority groups (Hispanic or Asian/Pacific Islander) could affect the results of this study,

which were very different from the US national average. In addition, the participants were not asked about their reasons for visiting the clinic or their health status. Because the clinic provides services primarily for chronic or comorbid conditions such as diabetes and cardiovascular diseases, patient health status could have affected the results of low interest in sun protection. While this study is based on one free clinic, the results of this study can be valuable to other free clinic populations and increase knowledge about free clinic patients who are significantly understudied because the free clinic that carried out this study shares common characteristics with other free clinics such as uninsured patients only, income requirements, 0% revenue from government, no affiliation with other organizations (an independent organization), and volunteer providers [21]. The low-income primary care patient population has not been well studied in sun protection behaviors before. This study provides new knowledge about sun protection and skin cancer prevention among the population who have been understudied.

5. Conclusion

Sun protection education and skin cancer prevention strategies among low-income primary care patients have not been well examined. This study contributes to the increased knowledge about the understudied population related to sun protection behaviors and skin cancer preventions. It is important to increase skin cancer awareness with self-efficacy interventions as well as education on low-cost sun protection methods. Spanish speaking patients would be a target population for promoting awareness. Male and female patients would need separate gender-specific sun protection education. Future studies should implement educational programs and assess the effectiveness of the programs to further promote skin cancer prevention among underserved populations.

Ethical Approval

The University of Utah Institutional Review Board (IRB) approved this study.

Conflict of Interests

The authors have no financial interest with regard to the paper.

Acknowledgments

This project was funded by the Public Service Professorship, Lowell Bennion Community Service Center at the University of Utah. The authors want to thank the patients who participated in this study and acknowledge the contribution of the staff and volunteers of the Maliheh Free Clinic. In addition, they thank Guadalupe Aguilera, Alla Chernenko, Travis Dixon, Anthony Mills, Molly Pace, Liana Prudencio, Naveen Rathi, Monica Scott, Emily Stephens, Tamara Stephens, and Lindsey Wright for their help in data collection, data entry, and translation related to this study.

References

[1] American Cancer Society, *Cancer Facts & Figures 2015*, American Cancer Society, Atlanta, Ga, USA, 2015.

[2] P. T. Bradford, "Skin cancer in skin of color," *Dermatology Nurse*, vol. 21, no. 4, pp. 170–177, 2009.

[3] Center for Disease Control and Prevention, "Preventing skin cancer: findings of the Tasks Force on Community Preventive Services on reducing exposure to ultraviolet light and counseling to prevent skin cancer: recommendations and rationale of the U.S. Preventive Task Force," *Morbidity and Mortality Weekly Report*, vol. 52, no. 15, pp. 1–12, 2003.

[4] J. H. Cooley and L. M. Quale, "Skin cancer preventive behavior and sun protection recommendations," *Seminars in Oncology Nursing*, vol. 29, no. 3, pp. 223–226, 2013.

[5] A. Lee, K. B. Garbutcheon-Singh, S. Dixit, P. Brown, and S. D. Smith, "The influence of age and gender in knowledge, behaviors and attitudes towards sun protection: a cross-sectional survey of Australian outpatient clinic attendees," *The American Journal of Clinical Dermatology*, vol. 16, no. 1, pp. 47–54, 2014.

[6] V. L. Champion and C. S. Skinner, "The health belief model," in *Health Behavior and Health Education: Theory, Research, and Practice*, K. Glanz, B. K. Rimer, and K. Viswanath, Eds., Jossey-Bass, San Francisco, Calif, USA, 4th edition, 2008.

[7] I. M. Rosenstock, V. J. Strecher, and M. H. Becker, "Social learning theory and the Health Belief Model," *Health Education Quarterly*, vol. 15, no. 2, pp. 175–183, 1988.

[8] C. Craciun, N. Schüz, S. Lippke, and R. Schwarzer, "A mediator model of sunscreen use: a longitudinal analysis of social-cognitive predictors and mediators," *International Journal of Behavioral Medicine*, vol. 19, no. 1, pp. 65–72, 2012.

[9] D. Hedeker, R. J. Mermelstein, and K. A. Weeks, "The thresholds of change model: an approach to analyzing stages of change data," *Annals of Behavioral Medicine*, vol. 21, no. 1, pp. 61–70, 1999.

[10] L. B. Myers and M. S. Horswill, "Social cognitive predictors of sun protection intention and behavior," *Behavioral Medicine*, vol. 32, no. 2, pp. 57–63, 2006.

[11] T. D. Street and D. L. Thomas, "Employee factors associated with interest in improving sun protection in an Australian mining workforce," *Health Promotion Journal of Australia*, vol. 26, no. 1, pp. 33–38, 2015.

[12] J. W. M. Ch'ng and A. I. Glendon, "Predicting sun protection behaviors using protection motivation variables," *Journal of Behavioral Medicine*, vol. 37, no. 2, pp. 245–256, 2014.

[13] R. Garside, M. Pearson, and T. Moxham, "What influences the uptake of information to prevent skin cancer? A systematic review and synthesis of qualitative research," *Health Education Research*, vol. 25, no. 1, pp. 162–182, 2010.

[14] D. Z. Korta, V. Saggar, T. P. Wu, and M. Sanchez, "Racial differences in skin cancer awareness and surveillance practices at a public hospital dermatology clinic," *Journal of the American Academy of Dermatology*, vol. 70, no. 2, pp. 312–317, 2014.

[15] E. J. Coups, J. L. Stapleton, S. V. Hudson, A. Medina-Forrester, A. Natale-Pereira, and J. S. Goydos, "Sun protection and exposure behaviors among Hispanic adults in the United States: differences according to acculturation and among Hispanic subgroups," *BMC Public Health*, vol. 12, no. 1, article 985, 2012.

[16] M. Falk and C. D. Anderson, "Influence of age, gender, educational level and self-estimation of skin type on sun exposure habits and readiness to increase sun protection," *Cancer Epidemiology*, vol. 37, no. 2, pp. 127–132, 2013.

[17] G. L. Rodriguez, F. Ma, D. G. Federman et al., "Predictors of skin cancer screening practice and attitudes in primary care," *Journal of the American Academy of Dermatology*, vol. 57, no. 5, pp. 775–781, 2007.

[18] M. M. Nadkarni and J. T. Philbrick, "Free clinics and the uninsured: the increasing demands of chronic illness," *Journal of Health Care for the Poor and Underserved*, vol. 14, no. 2, pp. 165–174, 2003.

[19] M. M. Nadkarni and J. T. Philbrick, "Free clinics: a national survey," *American Journal of the Medical Sciences*, vol. 330, no. 1, pp. 25–31, 2005.

[20] S. L. Isaacs and P. Jellinek, "Is there a (volunteer) doctor in the house? Free clinics and volunteer physician referral networks in the United States—what was learned from a W.K. Kellogg Foundation-funded effort to understand the role of volunteerism in health care for the underserved," *Health Affairs*, vol. 26, no. 3, pp. 871–876, 2007.

[21] J. S. Darnell, "Free clinics in the United States. A nationwide survey," *Archives of Internal Medicine*, vol. 170, no. 11, pp. 946–953, 2010.

[22] S. J. Notaro, M. Khan, N. Bryan et al., "Analysis of the demographic characteristics and medical conditions of the uninsured utilizing a free clinic," *Journal of Community Health*, vol. 37, no. 2, pp. 501–506, 2012.

[23] A. Kamimura, N. Christensen, J. Tabler, J. Ashby, and L. M. Olson, "Patients utilizing a free clinic: physical and mental

health, health literacy, and social support," *Journal of Community Health*, vol. 38, no. 4, pp. 716–723, 2013.

[24] A. Kamimura, N. Christensen, J. Tabler et al., "Depression, somatic symptoms, and perceived neighborhood environments among US-born and non-US-born free clinic patients," *Southern Medical Journal*, vol. 107, no. 9, pp. 591–596, 2014.

[25] A. Kamimura, J. Ashby, K. Myers, M. M. Nourian, and N. Christensen, "Satisfaction with healthcare services among free clinic patients," *Journal of Community Health*, vol. 40, no. 1, pp. 62–72, 2015.

[26] R. Schwarzer and M. Jerusalem, "Generalized self-efficacy scale," in *Measures in Health Psychology: A User's Portfolio. Causal and Control Beliefs*, J. Weinman, S. Wright, and M. Johnston, Eds., pp. 35–37, NFER-NELSON, Windsor, UK, 1995.

[27] R. Schwarzer, "Everything you want to know about the general Self-Efficacy Scale but were afraid to ask," 2014, http://userpage .fu-berlin.de/~health/faq_gse.pdf.

[28] D. Shelestak and K. Lindow, "Beliefs and practices regarding skin cancer prevention," *Journal of the Dermatology Nurses' Association*, vol. 3, no. 3, pp. 150–155, 2011.

[29] E. Linos, E. Keiser, T. Fu, G. Colditz, S. Chen, and J. Y. Tang, "Hat, shade, long sleeves, or sunscreen? Rethinking US sun protection messages based on their relative effectiveness," *Cancer Causes & Control*, vol. 22, no. 7, pp. 1067–1071, 2011.

[30] S. A. Oliveria, J. F. Altman, P. J. Christos, and A. C. Halpern, "Use of nonphysician health care providers for skin cancer screening in the primary care setting," *Preventive Medicine*, vol. 34, no. 3, pp. 374–379, 2002.

[31] A. Good and C. Abraham, "Can the effectiveness of health promotion campaigns be improved using self-efficacy and self-affirmation interventions? an analysis of sun protection messages," *Psychology & Health*, vol. 26, no. 7, pp. 799–818, 2011.

[32] M. Santiago-Rivas, C. Wang, and L. Jandorf, "Sun protection beliefs among hispanics in the US," *Journal of Skin Cancer*, vol. 2014, Article ID 161960, 10 pages, 2014.

[33] E. J. Coups, J. L. Stapleton, S. L. Manne et al., "Psychosocial correlates of sun protection behaviors among U.S. Hispanic adults," *Journal of Behavioral Medicine*, vol. 37, no. 6, pp. 1082–1090, 2014.

[34] J. Weiss, R. S. Kirsner, and S. Hu, "Trends in primary skin cancer prevention among US hispanics: a systematic review," *Journal of Drugs in Dermatology*, vol. 11, no. 5, pp. 580–586, 2012.

[35] M. A. Katz, C. D. Delnevo, D. A. Gundersen, and D. Q. Rich, "Methodologic artifacts in adult sun-protection trends," *American Journal of Preventive Medicine*, vol. 40, no. 1, pp. 72–75, 2011.

10

Collagen and Elastic Fiber Content Correlation Analysis between Horizontal and Vertical Orientations of Skin Samples of Human Body

Naveen Kumar,[1] Pramod Kumar,[2] Satheesha Nayak Badagabettu,[1] Ranjini Kudva,[3] Sudarshan Surendran,[1] and Murali Adiga[4]

[1]*Department of Anatomy, Melaka Manipal Medical College, Manipal University, Manipal Campus, Manipal 576104, India*
[2]*King Abdul Aziz Hospital, Al Jouf 42421, Saudi Arabia*
[3]*Department of Pathology, Kasturba Medical College, Manipal, Manipal University, Manipal 576104, India*
[4]*Department of Physiology, Kasturba Medical College, Manipal, Manipal University, Manipal 576104, India*

Correspondence should be addressed to Pramod Kumar; pkumar86@hotmail.com

Academic Editor: Bruno A. Bernard

Background. Unequal distribution of dermal collagen and elastic fibers in different orientations of skin is reported to be one of the multifocal causes of scar related complications. Present study is to understand the correlation pattern between collagen in horizontal (C_H) and in vertical (C_V) directions as well as that of elastic in horizontal (E_H) and vertical (E_V) directions. *Materials and Method*. A total of 320 skin samples were collected in two orientations from suprascapular, anterior chest, lateral chest, anterior abdominal wall, and inguinal regions of 32 human cadavers. Spearman correlation coefficient (r) was calculated between the variables (C_H, C_V, E_H, and E_V). *Results*. Significant positive correlation between C_H and C_V, and between E_H and E_V observed in all 5 areas tested. A negative correlation between C_V and E_V at suprascapular, lateral chest, and inguinal regions and negative correlation between C_H and E_H at anterior chest and anterior abdominal wall have been identified. *Conclusion*. Knowledge of asymmetric content of dermal collagen and elastic fibers together with the varied strength and degree of association in the given area provides guidelines to the dermatologists and aesthetic surgeons in placing elective incisions in the direction maximally utilizing the anatomical facts for aesthetically pleasing result.

1. Introduction

The dermis of the skin has two parts that are accountable for sustaining the epidermis. The papillary part of the dermis is a thin sheet located just below the epidermis. It contains a small number of collagen and elastic fibers. The reticular layer of dermis lies deep into it, which contains larger bundles of collagen and elastic fibers that usually run parallel to surface of the skin.

Skin incisions or injury to the skin is known to produce scar. Hence, appearance of a scar, following wound repair, is a natural process. Intercomplimentary functions of collagen and elastic fibers play a key role in the wound healing and its subsequent consequences resulting in the formation of the scar. Sherratt reported that the types of collagen present

in the scar tissue and the normal skin are similar, but with the diverged pattern of arrangement and distribution as compared to normal [1]. Similarly, Rnjak et al. reported the useful role of dermal elastic fibers in the process of wound healing and improvement of scar appearance [2].

Hypertrophic scars more commonly affect young individuals. Females are more prone to hypertrophic scars when compared to males for unknown etiology. The anterior chest, presternal region, shoulders, and deltoid regions are predisposed to hypertrophic scars [3–7]. Anterior chest area is also vulnerable for keloid formation [8]. Nevertheless, scar stretching occurs most frequently in the lower third of the scar overlying the xiphisternum and it may extend onto the abdomen [3].

In this study, we aimed to analyze the possible correlation between collagen and elastic fiber content in dermis of skin samples obtained from horizontal and vertical directions from selected areas of body and its possible effect in scar related complications.

2. Materials and Method

Three hundred and twenty (320) skin samples (160 each in horizontal and vertical orientations) at 5 different areas of human body were obtained from 32 formalin embalmed adult cadavers of either gender, aged between 50–70 years. Before obtaining the samples, the gross appearance of the skin quality of the cadaver was examined thoroughly to ensure its healthy appearance. The samples were obtained in two different orientations (horizontal and vertical) at randomly selected areas with the following descriptions:

(1) Suprascapular area: skin samples were obtained along the superior border of trapezius muscle overlying the scapula.

(2) Anterior chest area: skin overlying body of the sternum (at the level of 3rd costal cartilage) along its midline was taken. The vertical section was obtained along the vertical axis of the sternum, while horizontal section was across the former.

(3) Lateral chest area: samples from skin covering 8th rib at anterior axillary line were collected in both the directions.

(4) Anterior abdominal wall: samples of skin were taken at infraumbilical part (1 cm below the umbilicus) of anterior abdominal wall, overlying midline of linea alba.

(5) Inguinal region: skin casing the inguinal ligament was collected. Skin along the direction of the ligament (horizontal) and perpendicular to it (vertical) was collected.

2.1. Tissue Processing. All the skin samples were processed for the histological preparation and employed with a special stain known as Verhoeff-van Gieson stain. While picrofuchsin solution of van Gieson selectively stains the collagen fibers, the elastic tissue is readily penetrated by the Verhoeff's stain by the multipurpose role of iodine in the solution [9].

2.2. Image Procurement and Image Analysis. From the special stained sections, photomicrographs were taken from entire thickness of dermis (involving both papillary and reticular parts) in 3 different fields of vision using Progress capture Pro 2.1 Jenoptic microscopic camera under 20x magnification. A total of 960 images were collected and subjected to image analysis by "Tissue-Quant" software version 1.0. Semiquantitative measure of dermal collagen and elastic fibers was performed in terms of percentage area occupied by these tissue structures [10, 11].

2.3. Statistical Analysis. Spearman correlation coefficient (r) was computed using SPSS package (version 15.0) to determine

TABLE 1: Comparative description of correlation coefficient (r) and strength of association.

Correlation coefficient (r)	Strength of association
0.7 to 1 (positive) −0.7 to −1 (negative)	Strong
0.5 to 0.7 (positive) −0.5 to −0.7 (negative)	Moderate
0.3 to 0.5 (positive) −0.3 to −0.5 (negative)	Low

the linear association between the variables. Correlation coefficient (r) values were obtained in accordance with the following combined variables:

(i) C_H and C_V (collagen content between horizontal and vertical directions).

(ii) C_H and E_H (between collagen and elastic fibers in horizontal direction).

(iii) C_V and E_V (between collagen and elastic fibers in vertical direction).

(iv) E_H and E_V (elastic fiber content between horizontal and vertical directions).

The results obtained by these calculations were interpreted according to the strength of association (strong, moderate, and low) and degree of correlation (positive or negative) according to reference table (Table 1) after taking into consideration the significant correlation ($p < 0.01$ or $p < 0.05$).

3. Results

Descriptive statistics of Spearman's rho correlation coefficient (r) and the level of significance (p) as computed from the selected areas of body are presented in Table 2 and corresponding scatter plots of significant (two-tailed) correlations are depicted in Figures 1–5. Comprehensive data with statistically significant ($p < 0.01$ or $p < 0.05$) correlation coefficient with the pattern of strength of association in each area are given in Table 3.

Spearman's correlation revealed a statistically significant positive correlation between C_H and C_V in all areas: suprascapular area ($r = 0.75$, $p < 0.01$), anterior chest area ($r = 0.56$, $p < 0.01$), lateral chest area ($r = 0.55$, $p < 0.01$), anterior abdominal wall ($r = 0.57$, $p < 0.01$), and inguinal region ($r = 0.77$, $p < 0.01$).

Similar to C_H and C_V, statistically significant positive correlation was also noticed between E_H and E_V in all areas: suprascapular area ($r = 0.77$, $p < 0.01$), anterior chest area ($r = 0.62$, $p < 0.01$), lateral chest area ($r = 0.43$, $p < 0.05$), anterior abdominal wall ($r = 0.69$, $p < 0.01$), and inguinal region ($r = 0.62$, $p < 0.01$).

Significant negative correlations between C_H and E_H were seen only at anterior chest area ($r = -0.55$, $p < 0.01$) and in anterior abdominal wall ($r = -0.57$, $p < 0.01$).

Statistically significant negative correlation between C_V and E_V was also seen at suprascapular ($r = -0.37$, $p < 0.05$),

(a)

(b)

(c)

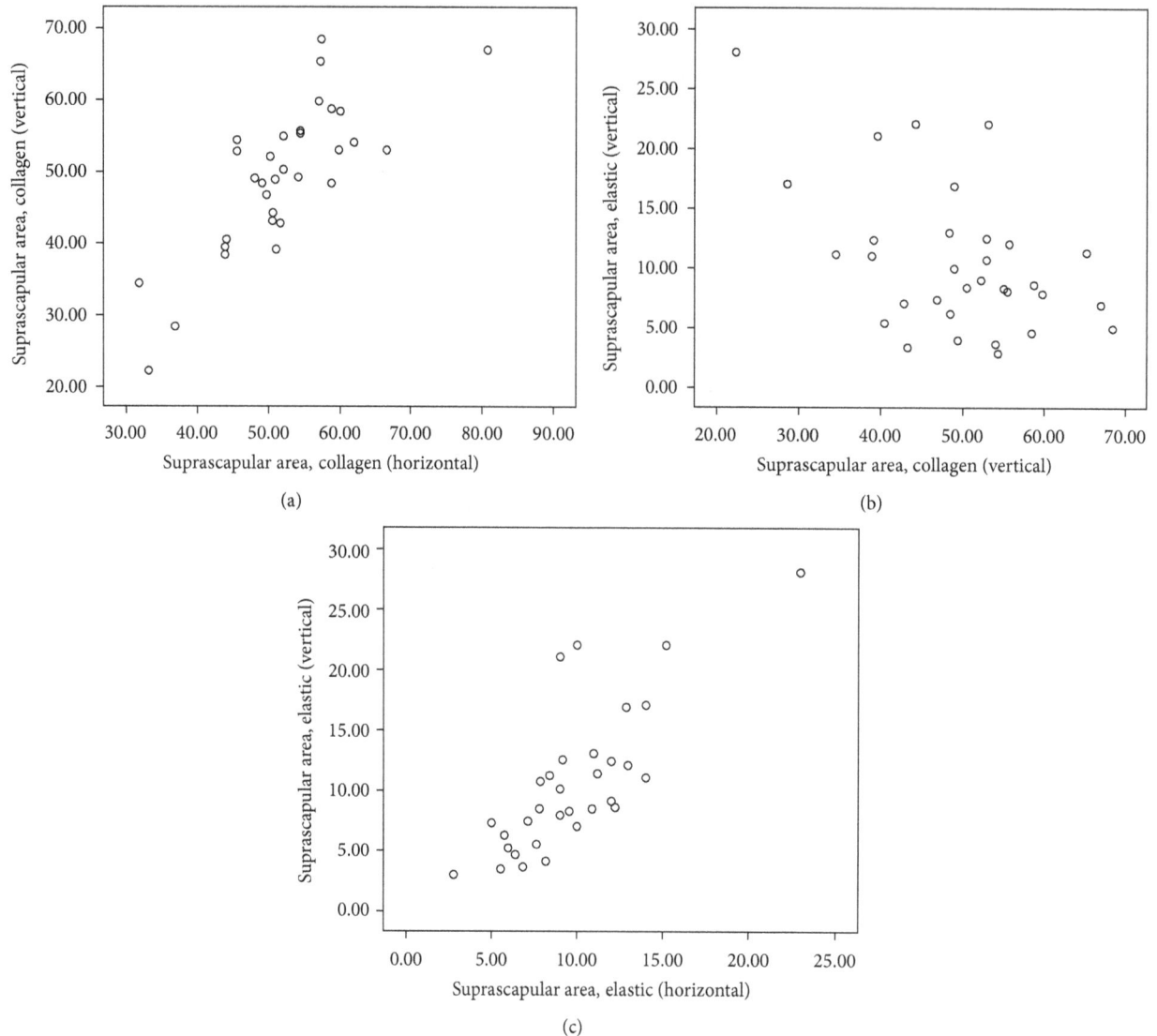

FIGURE 1: Scatter plot of significant Spearman correlation pattern at suprascapular area. (a) Strong positive correlation between C_H and C_V, (b) low negative correlation between C_V and E_V, and (c) strong positive correlation between E_H and E_V (C_H: collagen in horizontal, C_V: collagen in vertical, E_H: elastic in horizontal, and E_V: elastic in vertical direction).

TABLE 2: Spearman's correlation coefficient (r) and its level of significance (p).

Variables between	Suprascapular area		Anterior chest area		Lateral chest area		Anterior abdominal wall		Inguinal region	
	r	p	r	p	r	p	r	p	r	p
C_H & C_V	0.75	**0.000**[#]	0.56	**0.001**[#]	0.55	**0.001**[#]	0.57	**0.001**[#]	0.77	**0.000**[#]
C_H & E_H	−0.08	**0.62**	−0.55	**0.001**[#]	−0.14	**0.41**	−0.57	**0.001**[#]	−0.25	**0.15**
C_V & E_V	−0.37	**0.03**[*]	−0.22	**0.21**	−0.43	**0.01**[*]	−0.33	**0.059**	−0.42	**0.01**[*]
E_H & E_V	0.77	**0.000**[#]	0.62	**0.000**[#]	0.43	**0.01**[*]	0.69	**0.000**[#]	0.62	**0.000**[#]

[#]Correlation is significant at $p < 0.01$; [*]correlation is significant at $p < 0.05$.
(C_H: collagen in horizontal, C_V: collagen in vertical, E_H: elastic in horizontal, and E_V: elastic in vertical direction).

lateral chest ($r = −0.043$, $p < 0.05$), and inguinal areas ($r = −0.42$, $p < 0.05$).

4. Discussion

The management of scar in the clinical setup is one of the most challenging tasks for aesthetic surgeons. This has not been resolved even after the incisions had been made on the skin in accordance with the standard lines of choice. The varied quantity and asymmetric content of dermal collagen and elastic fibers in different orientations of skin plane affecting the formation of scar remain a possibility [12].

Asymmetric distribution of dermal collagen and elastic fibers in different regions of human body is said to have

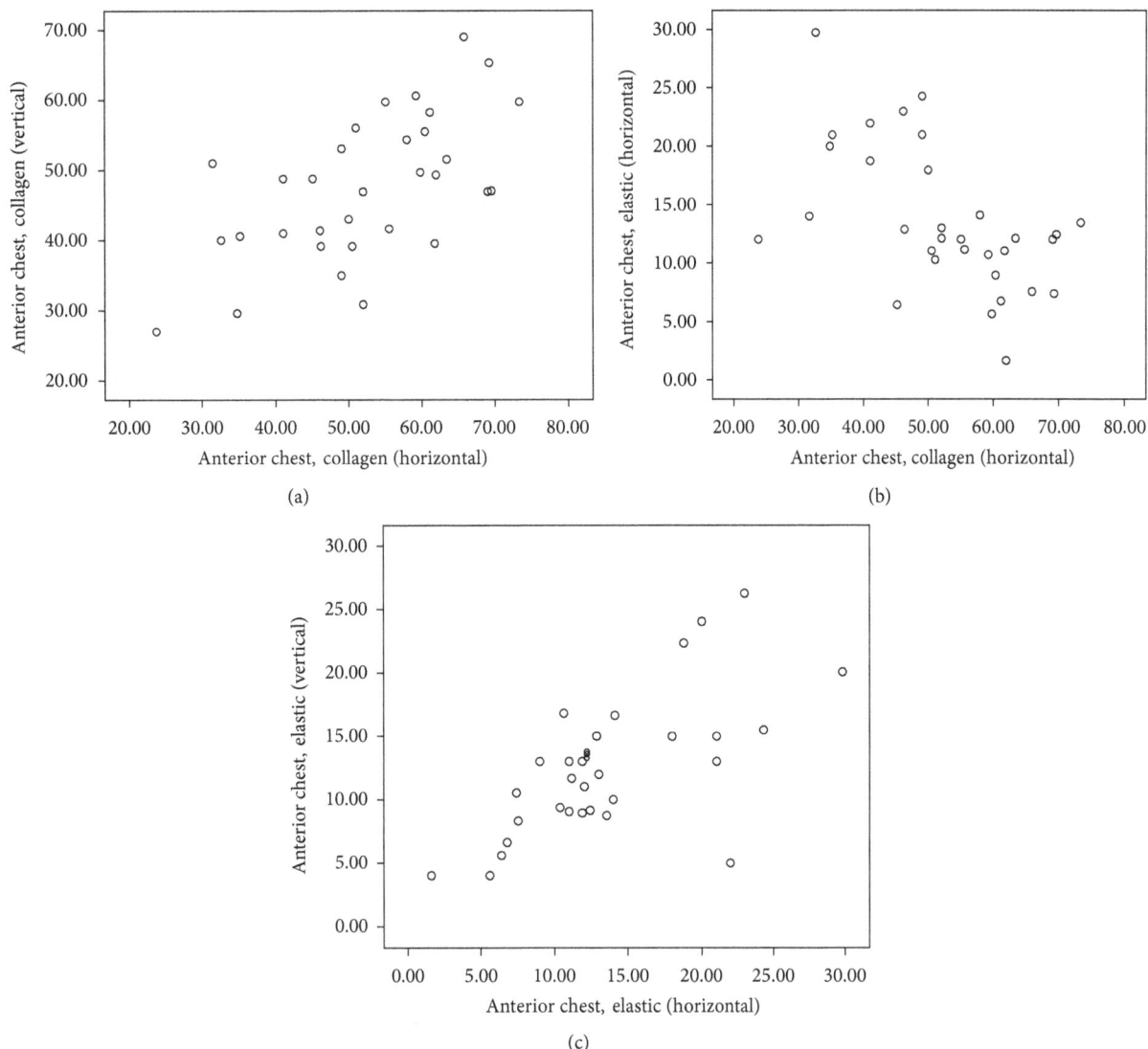

FIGURE 2: Scatter plot of significant Spearman correlation pattern at anterior chest area. (a) Moderate positive correlation between C_H and C_V. (b) Moderate negative correlation between C_H and E_H. (c) Moderate positive correlation between E_H and E_V (C_H: collagen in horizontal, C_V: collagen in vertical, E_H: elastic in horizontal, and E_V: elastic in vertical direction).

TABLE 3: Significant Spearman coefficient (r) and pattern of correlation trend profile.

	Between C_H and C_V	Between E_H and E_V	Between C_V and E_V	Between C_H and E_H
Suprascapular area	0.75 Strong +ve	0.77 Strong +ve	−0.37 Low −ve	—
Anterior chest	0.56 Moderate +ve	0.62 Moderate +ve	—	−0.55 Moderate −ve
Lateral chest	0.55 Moderate +ve	0.43 Low +ve	−0.43 Low −ve	—
Anterior abdominal wall	0.57 Moderate +ve	0.69 Moderate +ve	—	−0.57 Moderate −ve
Inguinal region	0.77 Strong +ve	0.62 Moderate +ve	−0.42 Low −ve	—

r = Spearman's correlation coefficient; +ve: positive correlation; −ve: negative correlation.
(C_H: collagen in horizontal, C_V: collagen in vertical, E_H: elastic in horizontal, and E_V: elastic in vertical direction).

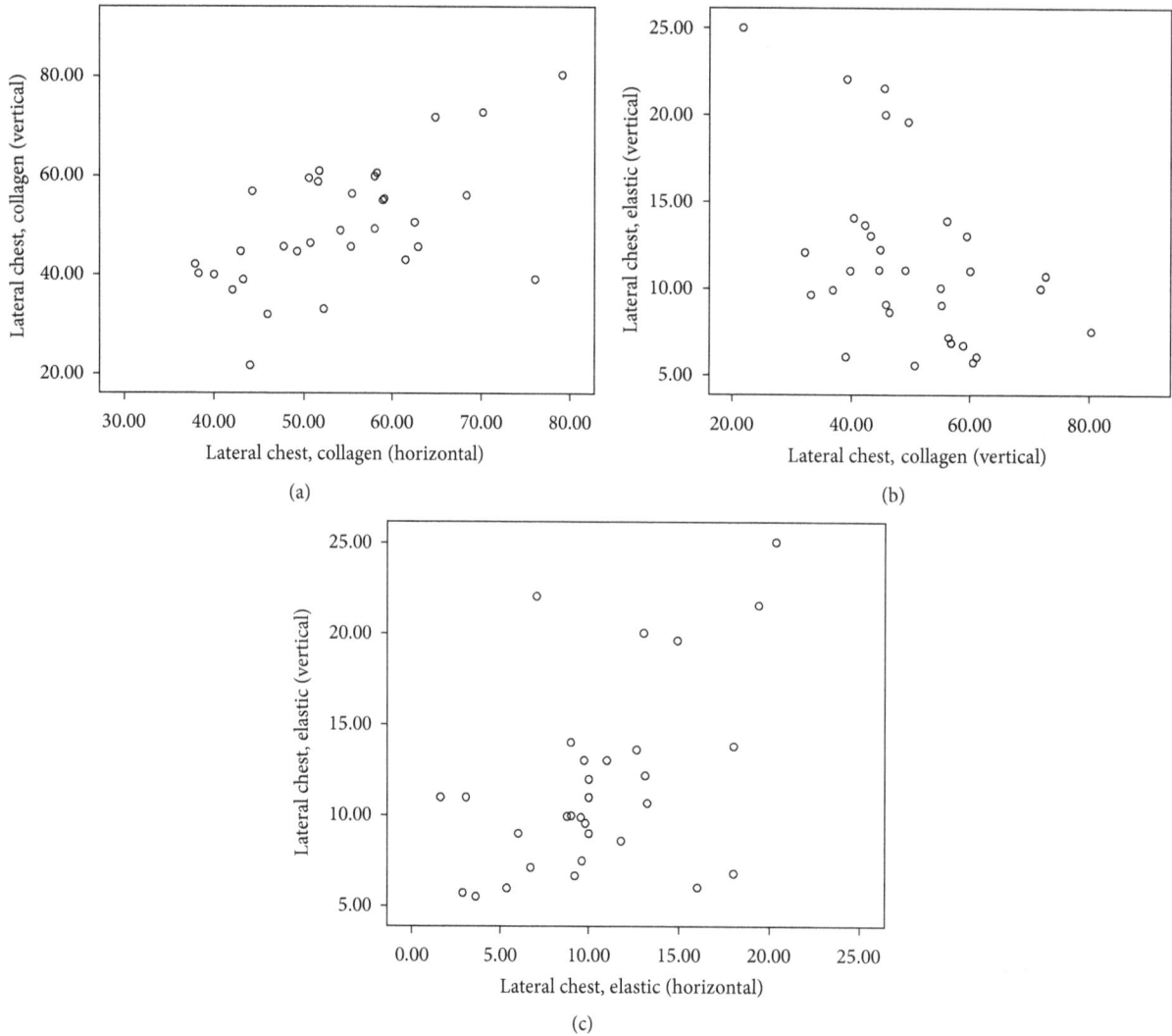

FIGURE 3: Scatter plot of significant Spearman correlation pattern at lateral chest area. (a) Moderate positive correlation between C_H and C_V. (b) Low negative correlation between C_V and E_V. (c) Low positive correlation between E_H and E_V (C_H: collagen in horizontal, C_V: collagen in vertical, E_H: elastic in horizontal, and E_V: elastic in vertical direction).

regional discrepancies. It may be depending on the texture of the skin, as in head and neck region [13], anatomic, functional, or physical cause of skin tension as applicable in trunk region [10], and may be due to effect of various forces like burst force and stretch force exerted at joints [14]. These factors are found to be applicable in the management of wound healing consequences and scar management.

Selective incision on the skin was preferred to be line of Langer's. However, in some topographic sites of human body these lines are obscure and poorly differentiated. Conversely, role of an unequal distribution of dermal collagen and elastic fibers, as observable in two different orientations of the skin, is worth noticeable. Understanding the possible correlation between the collagen and elastic fibers between two different skin planes serves a valuable basis in the management of aesthetic procedures.

The correlation pattern analysis revealed that skin over the suprascapular area had strong positive correlation between C_H and C_V and between E_H and E_V. Lateral chest showed moderate positive correlation between C_H and C_V and low positive correlation between E_H and E_V. Inguinal region also showed strong positive correlation between C_H and C_V and moderate positive correlation between E_H and E_V contents. But all three areas exhibited low negative correlation between C_V and E_V.

This indicates that the content of collagen and elastic fibers in these areas changes in accordance with their positive manner of correlation across two directions (horizontal and vertical), while, in the vertical direction, the content change between collagen and elastic fibers would be in reversed manner due to negative correlation between them.

In the remaining two areas, that is, anterior chest area and anterior abdominal wall, moderate positive correlation was observed between C_H and C_V, and between E_H and E_V. And in both areas, moderate negative correlation between C_H and E_H was observed. Therefore, in these areas, both

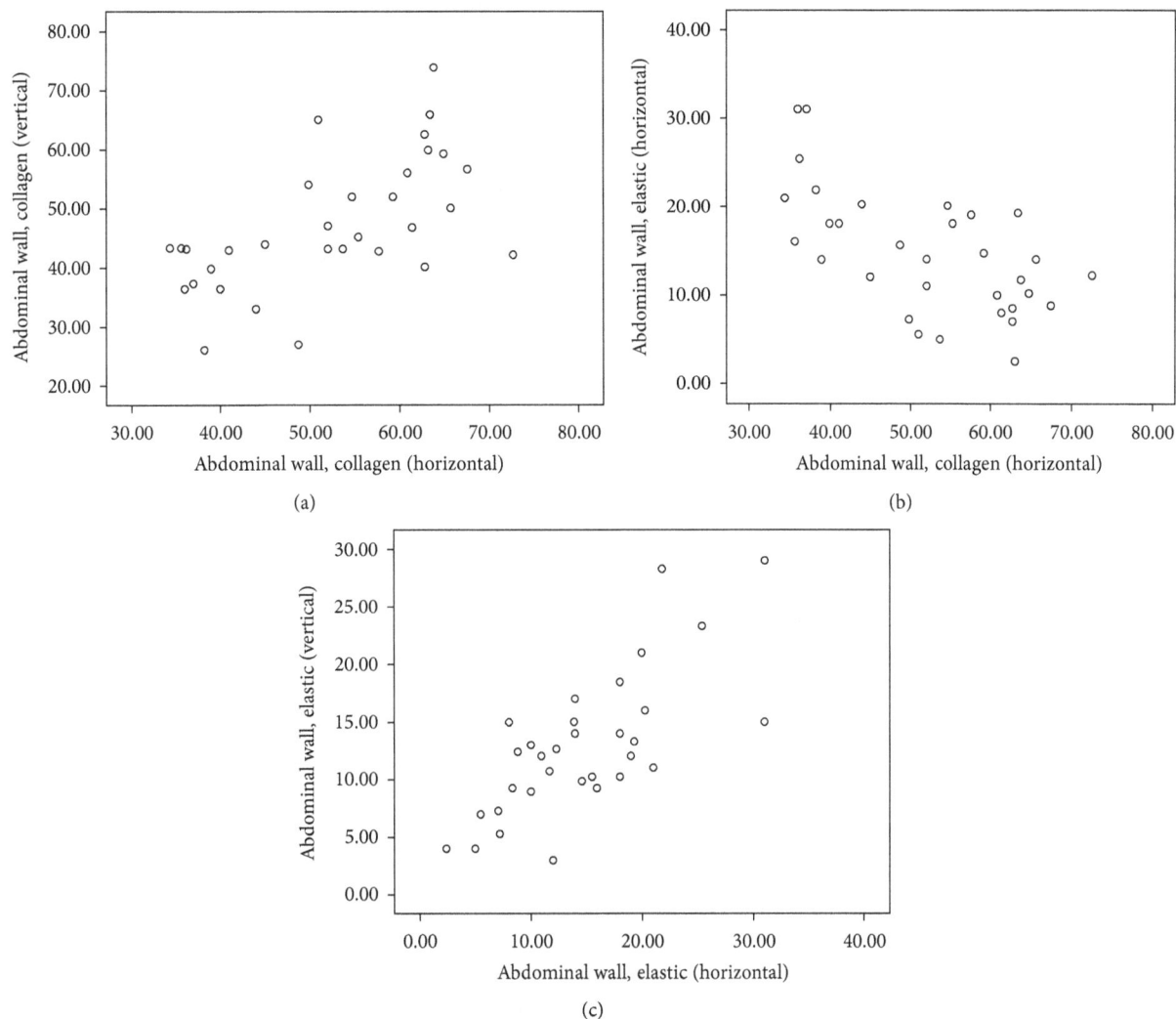

Figure 4: Scatter plot of significant Spearman correlation pattern at anterior abdominal wall. (a) Moderate positive correlation between C_H and C_V. (b) Moderate negative correlation between C_H and E_H. (c) Moderate positive correlation between E_H and E_V (C_H: collagen in horizontal, C_V: collagen in vertical, E_H: elastic in horizontal, and E_V: elastic in vertical direction).

the collagen and elastic fibers content between horizontal and vertical directions change in positive manner, but along the horizontal direction when collagen is increased corresponding elastic fiber content will be decreased and vice versa occurring consequently due to negative correlation effect.

Previous research study analyzing the unequal distribution of dermal collagen and elastic fibers across two directions in these areas reported that the abdomen area with higher content of both collagen and elastic fibers in horizontal direction accomplishes the functional cause factor together with Langer's line concept. Whereas the suprascapular, presternal, and lateral chest areas fulfill the dominance of functional cause factor over anatomical cause. Thus, in these areas, the collagen content in horizontal direction is significantly higher than vertical direction without any similar changes in their elastic fiber content between two directions. The groin area, on the other hand, witnesses the nullified effect of elastic fibers that necessitates its increased content in vertical direction without the changes of collagen content [10].

To summarize, significant positive correlation between C_H and C_V and between E_H and E_V as observed in all areas tested is dependent on the functional reason due to local stretch force effect rather than the anatomical cause factor as reported earlier [10]. This correlation pattern in these areas is in accordance with the collagen content pattern in two different directions as the collagen content is more in horizontal direction than in their vertical direction ($C_H > C_V$).

On the other hand, negative correlation between C_H and E_H at anterior chest and anterior abdominal wall and negative correlation between C_V and E_V at suprascapular, lateral chest, and inguinal regions have been observed. This may be due to the fact that, in certain areas, constant active or passive stretch force works for the movements and gravity (as weight of upper limb which constantly produces rotation force on scapula/pulls the shoulder downward direction). The effect of these forces may be more in one or more directions which necessitates the requirement of increased elastic fiber content

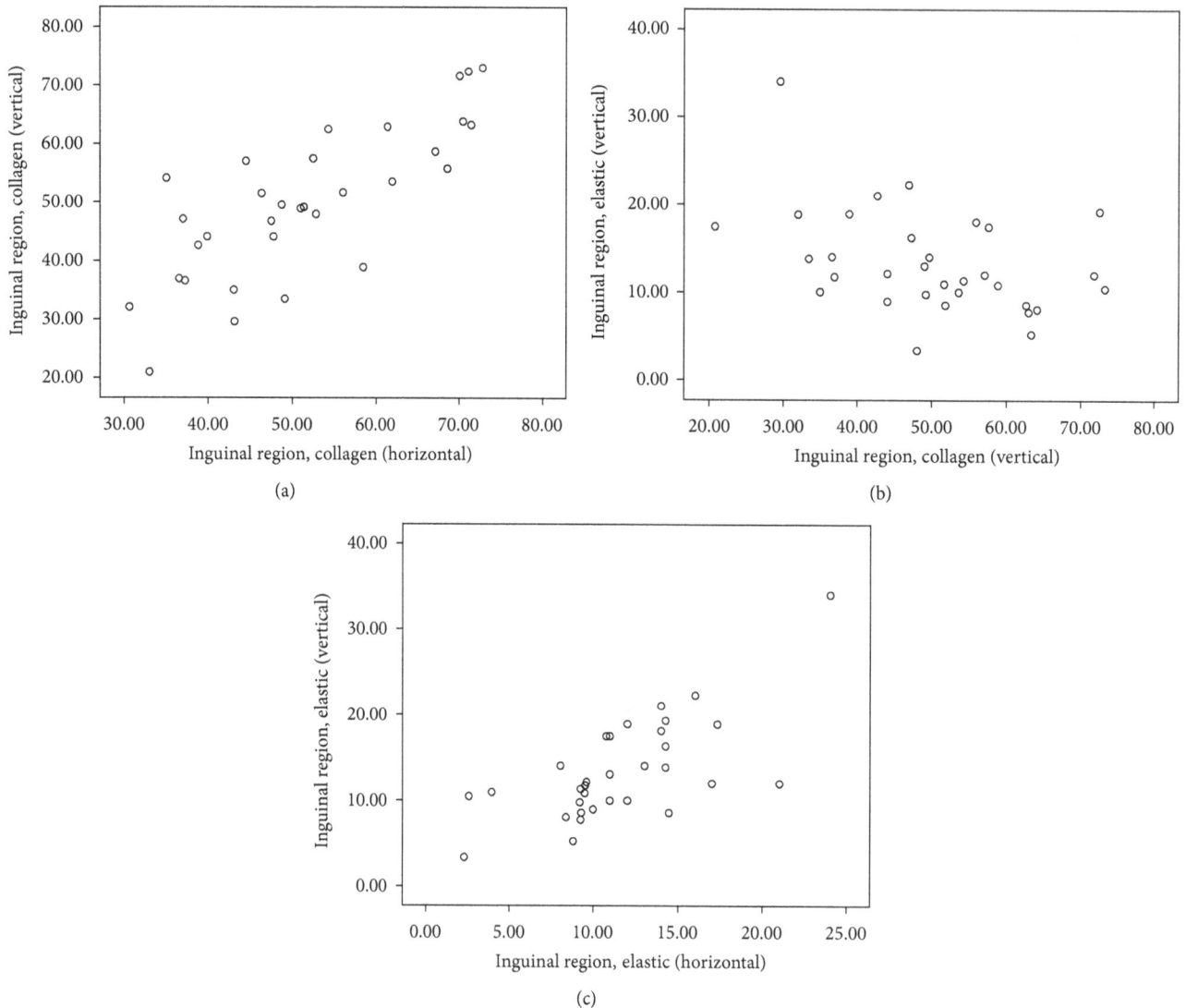

FIGURE 5: Scatter plot of significant Spearman correlation pattern at inguinal area. (a) Strong positive correlation between C_H and C_V. (b) Low negative correlation between C_V and E_V. (c) Moderate positive correlation between E_H and E_V (C_H: collagen in horizontal, C_V: collagen in vertical, E_H: elastic in horizontal, and E_V: elastic in vertical direction).

in that specific direction. Accordingly, the higher allotment of elastic fibers in horizontal direction than in the vertical direction ($E_H > E_V$) was attributed to the areas where the negative correlation between C_H and E_H was noted, while reversal of this was seen in the remaining areas where the negative correlation between C_V and E_V exists.

5. Conclusion

Understanding the pattern of asymmetric content of dermal collagen and elastic fibers in a given area together with the stress on proposed incision in that area and degree of association between them in two different planes provides a valuable guideline to the dermatologists and surgeons in elective incisions that necessitates providing aesthetically pleasing results and in the management of scar related complications.

Conflict of Interests

The authors declare that there is no conflict of interests regarding the publication of this paper.

Authors' Contribution

Naveen Kumar is responsible for integrity and accuracy of the data analysis, Pramod Kumar and Satheesha Nayak Badagabettu are responsible for study concept and design, Murali Adiga is responsible for histological technique and data analysis, Ranjini Kudva and Sudarshan Surendran are responsible for critical revision of the paper, and Pramod Kumar and Satheesha Nayak Badagabettu are responsible for study supervision.

References

[1] J. A. Sherratt, *Mathematical Modelling of Scar Tissue Formation*, Department of Mathematics, Heriot-Watt University, Edinburgh. UK, 2010, http://www.ma.hw.ac.uk/~jas/research-interests/scartissueformation.html.

[2] J. Rnjak, S. G. Wise, S. M. Mithieux, and A. S. Weiss, "Severe burn injuries and the role of elastin in the design of dermal substitutes," *Tissue Engineering Part B: Reviews*, vol. 17, no. 2, pp. 81–91, 2011.

[3] D. Elliot, R. Cory-Pearce, and G. M. Rees, "The behaviour of pre-sternal scars in a fair-skinned population," *Annals of the Royal College of Surgeons of England*, vol. 67, no. 4, pp. 238–240, 1985.

[4] I. F. K. Muir, "On the nature of keloid and hypertrophic scars," *British Journal of Plastic Surgery*, vol. 43, no. 1, pp. 61–69, 1990.

[5] L. From and D. Assad, "Neoplasms, pseudo-neoplasms and hyperplasia of supporting tissue origin," in *Dermatology in General Medicine*, J. D. Jeffers and M. R. Englis, Eds., pp. 1198–1199, McGraw-Hill, New York, NY, USA, 1993.

[6] H. K. Hawkins, "Pathophysiology of the burn scar," in *Total Burn Care*, D. N. Herndon, Ed., pp. 608–619, Saunders Elsevier, Philadelphia, Pa, USA, 2007.

[7] S. W. Norman, J. K. B. Christopher, and P. R. O'Connel, "Abnormal scars inflammation and abnormal wounds after healing," in *Bailey and Love's Short Practice of Surgery*, pp. 598–599, Hodder Arnold, 25th edition, 2008.

[8] F. B. Niessen, P. H. M. Spauwen, J. Schalkwijk, and M. Kon, "On the nature of hypertrophic scars and keloids: a review," *Plastic and Reconstructive Surgery*, vol. 104, no. 5, pp. 1435–1458, 1999.

[9] J. D. Bancroft and M. Gamble, *Theory and Practice of Histological Techniques*, edited by: M. Gamble, Churchill Livingstone, 5th edition, 2002.

[10] K. Naveen, K. Pramod, N. B. Satheesha, P. Keerthana, K. Ranjini, and C. V. Raghuveer, "Quantitative fraction evaluation of dermal collagen and elastic fibres in the skin samples obtained in two orientations from the trunk region," *Dermatology Research and Practice*, vol. 2014, Article ID 251254, 7 pages, 2014.

[11] K. Prasad, P. B. Kumar, M. Chakravarthy, and G. Prabhu, "Applications of 'TissueQuant'—a color intensity quantification tool for medical research," *Computer Methods and Programs in Biomedicine*, vol. 106, no. 1, pp. 27–36, 2012.

[12] K. Naveen, K. Pramod, P. Keerthana, and N. B. Satheesha, "A histological study on the distribution of dermal collagen and elastic fibers in different regions of the body," *International Journal of Medicine and Medical Sciences*, vol. 4, no. 8, pp. 171–176, 2012.

[13] K. Naveen, K. Pramod, N. B. Satheesha, P. Keerthana, K. Ranjini, and C. V. Raghuveer, "Histomorphometric analysis of dermal collagen and elastic fibers in skin tissues taken perpendicular to each other from Head and Neck region," *Journal of Surgical Academia*, vol. 4, no. 1, pp. 30–36, 2014.

[14] K. Naveen, N. B. Pramod, P. Satheesha, K. Keerthana, and R. C. Vasudevarao, "Surgical implications of asymmetric distribution of dermal collagen and elastic fibres in two orientations of skin samples from extremities," *Plastic Surgery International*, vol. 2014, Article ID 364573, 7 pages, 2014.

11

Some Epidemiological Aspects of Cutaneous Leishmaniasis in a New Focus, Central Iran

M. R. Yaghoobi-Ershadi,[1] **N. Marvi-Moghadam,**[1] **R. Jafari,**[2] **A. A. Akhavan,**[1] **H. Solimani,**[3] **A. R. Zahrai-Ramazani,**[1] **M. H. Arandian,**[2] **and A. R. Dehghan-Dehnavi**[4]

[1]*Department of Medical Entomology and Vector Control, School of Public Health, Tehran University of Medical Sciences, Tehran, Iran*
[2]*Isfahan Research Station, National Institute of Health Research, Isfahan, Iran*
[3]*Yazd Health Research Station, National Institute of Health Research, Yazd, Iran*
[4]*School of Public Health, Yazd University of Medical Sciences, Yazd, Iran*

Correspondence should be addressed to N. Marvi-Moghadam; nr_moghadam@yahoo.com

Academic Editor: Iris Zalaudek

Following the epidemic of cutaneous leishmaniasis in Khatam County, Yazd Province, this study was carried out to determine vector, and animal reservoir host(s) and investigate the human infection during 2005-2006. Four rural districts where the disease had higher prevalence were selected. Sticky paper traps were used to collect sand flies during April to November, biweekly. Meanwhile rodents were captured using Sherman traps from August to November. Households and primary schools were visited and examined for human infection in February 2006. The parasite was detected by RAPD-PCR method. The rate of ulcers and scars among the inhabitants was 4.8% and 9.8%, respectively. Three rodent species were captured during the study: *Meriones libycus*, *Rhombomys opimus*, and *Tatera indica*. Six sand fly species were also collected and identified; among them *Phlebotomus papatasi* had the highest frequency. *Leishmania major* was detected as the agent of the disease in the area. It was detected from *R. opimus* and native people.

1. Introduction

In the old world, cutaneous leishmaniasis (CL) is a major public health problem in the Eastern Mediterranean Region of World Health Organization (WHO), with more than reported cases [1]. In this region, Iran is known as one of the high risk countries for the disease with more than 20000 annual cases. The endemic foci of CL are reported in 17 out of 31 provinces of the country while foci of Isfahan, Yazd, Khorasan-e-Razavi, Golestan, and Fars Province are more important [2–11].

Previous studies in Iran indicated *Phlebotomus papatasi* as the main vector among 45 reported sand fly species [12, 13]. *Rhombomys opimus* and *Meriones libycus* are the main and secondary reservoir hosts and *Leishmania major* is the agent of zoonotic cutaneous leishmaniasis (ZCL) [2–11].

In recent years, CL cases have been reported increasingly from different areas of Yazd Province, central Iran, including Khatam County. Due to lake of data in this area, current study was designed and conducted to determine some epidemiological aspects of the statistical evaluation of patients with cutaneous in Health Center of Yazd during 2000–2004 that shows that most of cases exist in Khatam city, the southernmost province of Yazd There were 1509 cases recorded during these years. Most cases are in Herat (Fathabad Village) and Marvast (village of Harabarjan), and it has become a common disease in the last four years.

2. Objects and Methods

2.1. Study Area. Khatam County with 7931 km^2 area and total population of about 35000 is located in the southeast of Yazd Province, central Iran. The elevation of the county ranges between 1500 and 3005 m above the sea level. The climate is hot and dry. Khatam County has two towns of Marvast and Harat as well as four rural districts of Fathabad, Harabarjan, Chahak, and Isar. Agriculture, animal husbandry, service affairs, office affairs, and trading are the main occupations

TABLE 1: Prevalence of acute lesion and scar in the studied families, Khatam County, Yazd Province, central Iran, 2006.

Age	Males					Females					Total				
	Visited	Scar		Acute lesion		Visited	Scar		Acute lesion		Visited	Scar		Acute lesion	
		Number	%	Number	%		Number	%	Number	%		Number	%	Number	%
0–4	25	1	4	1	4	28	0	0	1	3.57	53	1	1.88	2	3.7
5–9	45	1	2.22	2	4.44	40	2	5	4	10	85	3	3.52	6	7.05
10–14	72	6	8.33	8	11.11	76	10	1.31	4	5.26	148	16	10.81	12	8.10
15–19	124	16	12.9	5	4.03	134	6	4.47	6	4.47	259	22	8.49	11	4.24
20–24	98	6	6.12	1	1.02	76	7	9.21	2	2.63	174	13	7.47	3	1.72
+25	332	41	17.67	16	4.81	314	37	11.78	15	4.77	645	78	12.09	30	4.65
Total	696	71	10.20	33	4.74	668	62	9.28	32	4.79	1364	133	9.75	65	4.76

in the county (Yazd Province statistics 2005). The study was carried out in Fathabad, Harabarjan, and Marvast areas.

2.2. Study of Human Infection. Prevalence of cutaneous leishmaniasis was studied during February and 300 households were visited and interviewed. Family size, infected members, age, gender, disease condition (acute wound or scar), place or number of wounds, and time and place of infection were considered in the questionnaires. Smears were prepared and examined from the acute lesions of native people who had no history of travel to other endemic foci of the disease during past year. All students of the primary schools were also visited. The serosity of lesions was inoculated to the tail base of Balb/C mice in the field. After infection of the mice and wound formation, the serosity of their wounds was cultivated in the Schneider-RPMI media. After one week, promastigote stage of the parasite was developed and used for species identification using RAPD-PCR [14].

2.3. Study of Rodents. For this purpose wild rodents were captured around the study area during September to November biweekly using Sherman traps. Traps were installed before sunset and collected next early morning. Trapped rodents were identified using morphological and morphometric characteristics [15] and after anaesthesia two slides were prepared from each ear of the rodents [16]. Species recognition results and direct examination of parasitology were recorded by number, date, and trapping location.

2.4. Study of Sand Flies. Sand flies were collected biweekly from indoor (bedrooms, toilets, hall, etc.) and outdoor (rodent burrows) resting places using 30 sticky traps (castor oil coated on A_5 white papers) from the beginning to the end of the active season. The traps were placed before sunset and collected next early morning. For species identification, sand flies were mounted in Puri's medium and identified using the relevant keys [17]. Sex ratio was calculated as the number of males/females × 100. Study on sand fly infection was performed during August-September using dissection method and direct observation of head and gut under the light microscope. Susceptibility of sand flies to Deltamethrin was evaluated using WHO test kits in the diagnostic dose [1].

2.5. Parasite Detection. Schneider medium was used to transfer and culture the parasite in the field. The parasites then were transferred to RPMI medium in the laboratory and, after sufficient amplification, the species was identified using RAPD-PCR method [14].

2.6. Statistical Analysis. SPSS version 11.5 and χ^2 test were used to analyse data.

3. Results

3.1. Human Infection. During February 2006 a total of 300 families with a population of 1364 (696 males and 668 females) were visited and their demographic as well as the disease data was recorded. Out of them, 4.64% had acute lesions (Table 1). χ^2 analysis showed no significant difference between males and females ($\alpha = 5\%$). Most of the wounds were found in 10–14 years age group (8.1%), while the lowest rate was found in 20–24 years age group (1.72%). All students of primary schools of the area were also visited. The active lesions were found in 4.94% of them (Table 2). There was no significant difference between boys and girls ($P > 0.05$).

The isolated parasite from the local patients with no history of travel was detected as *L. major.*

3.2. Rodents. During this study 15 rodents were trapped and identified as follows: *Meriones libycus* (66.7%), *Rhombomys opimus* (20%), and *Tatera indica* (13.3%). One *M. libycus,* one *T. indica,* and all *R. opimus* specimens were found to be infected with the amastigotes of *Leishmania* parasite (Figure 1). The isolated parasites were identified as *L. major.*

3.3. Sand Flies. A total of 5571 sand flies (772 indoors and 4999 outdoors) were collected and identified as *Phlebotomus papatasi* (85.35%), *Ph. mongoliensis* (0.03%), *Ph. kazeruni* (0.03%), *Ph. sergenti* (0.03%), *Sergentomyia baghdadis* (0.3%), and *Se. sintoni* (14.28%). The dominant species were found to be *Ph. papatasi* and *Se. sintoni,* respectively. *Phlebotomus mongoliensis* and *Ph. sergenti* were collected only indoors, while *Se. baghdadis* was found only outdoors (Table 3).

TABLE 2: Prevalence of acute lesion and scar in primary schools of the studied area, Khatam County, Yazd Province, central Iran, 2006.

| | | Boys | | | | | Girls | | | | | Total | | | |
| | | Scar | | Acute lesion | | | Scar | | Lesion | | | Scar | | Acute lesion | |
Age	Visited	Number	%	Number	%	Visited	Number	%	Number	%	Visited	Number	%	Number	%
7	77	3	3.89	2	2.59	71	4	5.63	4	5.63	148	7	9.52	6	8.22
8	72	3	4.16	2	2.77	75	5	6.66	2	2.66	147	8	10.82	4	5.43
9	59	4	6.77	2	3.38	52	3	5.76	1	1.92	111	7	12.53	3	5.3
10	82	16	19.51	6	7.31	75	6	8	6	8	157	22	27.51	12	15.31
11	70	17	10	5	7.14	63	7	11.11	4	6.34	134	14	21.11	9	13.48
12	18	2	11.11	1	5.55	12	1	0.82	0	0	30	13	11.93	1	5.55
Total	379	36	9.94	18	4.74	348	26	7.47	17	4.88	727	62	8.29	36	4.95

TABLE 3: Fauna, density, and sex ratio of sand flies in Khatam County, Yazd Province, 2006.

| | Indoors | | Outdoors | | Total | | Sex ratio | |
Species	Number	%	Number	%	Number	%	Indoors	Outdoors
Ph. papatasi	735	95.08	4190	83.82	4925	85.33	383.5	159.76
Ph. mongoliensis	2	0.26	0	0	2	0.03	—	—
Ph. kazeruni	1	0.13	1	0.02	2	0.03	—	—
Ph. sergenti	2	0.26	0	0	2	0.03	—	—
Se. baghdadis	0	0	17	0.34	17	0.3	—	—
Se. sintoni	33	4.27	791	15.82	824	14.28	106.25	239.48
Total	773	13.39	4999	86.61	5772	100	—	—

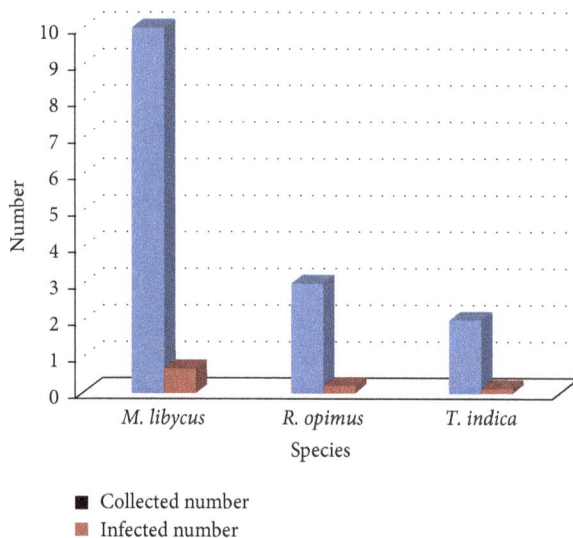

FIGURE 1: Trapped rodents and their infection to *Leishmania* parasite, Khatam County, Yazd Province, 2006.

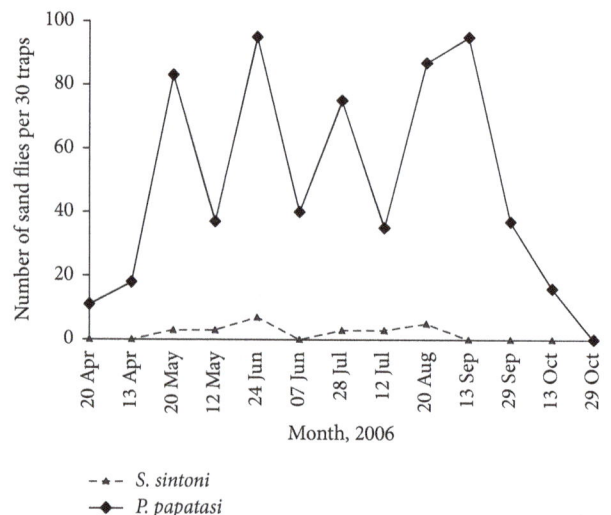

FIGURE 2: Monthly prevalence of *Se. sintoni*, *Ph. papatasi* indoors of Khatam County, Yazd Province, central Iran, 2006.

The monthly activity of two main species, that is, *Ph. papatasi* and *Se. sintoni* both indoors and outdoors, was studied. Both species were collected in all sampling months, from May to October with 2 peaks of activity (Figures 2 and 3).

Sex ratio for *Ph. papatasi* was calculated as 383.55 indoors and 159.76 outdoors. This ratio for *Se. sintoni* was found to be 106.25 and 239.48 in indoor and outdoor resting places, respectively.

During August and September a total of 295 female sand flies were dissected for the parasitic infection, but finding the promastigote was failed.

Susceptibility test with Deltamethrin 0.025% resulted in 100% mortality in tested *Ph. papatasi*.

4. Discussion

This is the first time that an epidemiological study was conducted in Khatam County. In this survey six sand fly species

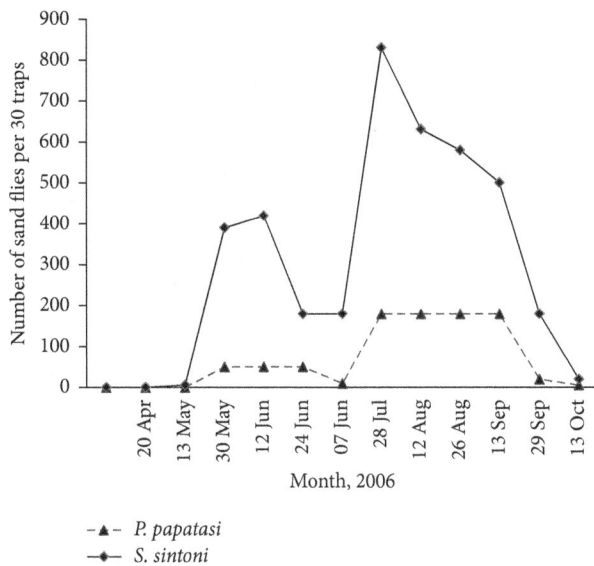

FIGURE 3: Monthly activity of *Se. sintoni*, *Ph. papatasi* outdoors of Khatam County, Yazd Province, central Iran, 2006.

were collected and identified; among them *Ph. papatasi* was the dominant species indoors (95.2%). This high indoor density confirms the endophilicity behavior of this sand fly and proves its domestic comparing other collected species. It is also found that because of neighborhood of rodent burrows and villages *Se. sintoni* had a relative high density indoors. This is the same as some other parts of Iran [7, 18].

Although the promastigotes of *Leishmania* parasite were not found in dissected *Ph. papatasi* specimens, high density of this species in both indoor and outdoor resting places, as well as isolation of *L. major* from this sand fly in close foci, that is, Ardakan, seems to be the main vectors of cutaneous leishmaniasis in the study area and has a critical role in the disease transmission from rodents to human [19, 20]. Test of *Ph. papatasi* against Deltamethrin 0.05 showed it is susceptible. Although there is a report of tolerance to DDT 4% in this species [21], it is now susceptible to all tested insecticides. Therefore, these insecticides can be used in epidemics of zoonotic cutaneous leishmaniasis for sand fly control [22, 23].

With due attention to leptomonad infection of all three captured rodents, detection of *L. major* from *R. opimus*, and history of studies in Iran, *R. opimus* and *M. libycus* are introduced as reservoir hosts of ZCL in Khatam County. These gerbils have been found to be infected in central and northeastern foci of the disease in Iran [2, 3, 6, 7, 9, 20, 21, 24–27].

Study on prevalence of the disease in the inhabitant population of Khatam County showed the acute lesions existed in all age groups and both genders ($\alpha = 0.05$). This means we encounter a new focus of cutaneous leishmaniasis. As *L. major* was isolated from native people without history of travel, it can be concluded that ZCL has prevalence in the

county. This parasite is the causative agent of ZCL in other foci of the disease in Iran [7]. So, new focus of ZCL has been established in Khatam County with *L. major* as agent, *Ph. papatasi* as suspected vector, and *R. opimus* as the main reservoir host. It also seems that *M. libycus* and *T. indica* play a role in preserving this focus with *R. opimus*.

It is conjectured that development of agriculture in the area, especially cultivating crops like sugar beet and vegetables, and construction of numerous water wells for the agricultural purposes have increased the soil moisture and resulted in the colonization of gerbils and increasing the population of sand flies.

Outdoor sleeping behavior of people during the disease transmission months in summer and close contact of farmers with the infected sand flies in farms have resulted in increasing the rate of human infection.

For control of the disease it is suggested to start a rodent control program within a radius of 500 m around the infected/at risk villages prior to starting the active season of sand flies. Health education and improving the knowledge of people regarding ZCL can help to prevent the disease transmission. Self-protection using long-lasting insecticide treated net as well as repellents can also decrease the human-vector contact and therefore collapse the disease prevalence in the area.

5. Conclusion

In this study, *P. papatasi and S. sintoni were, respectively, predominant species* both indoors and outdoors. *T. indica, M. libycus, and R. opimus* were found to be infected with amastigotes of *Leishmania* parasite. Study of prevalence among 1364 inhabitants of Marvast and Harat district showed rate of 4.95% for active lesions and the scar rate was 9.75% but our studies showed that the majority of scars were due to the treatment of ulcers in the same year. Based on the findings of this study, zoonotic cycle of the disease exists in the area. Therefore planning for the disease control should be based on this form.

Conflict of Interests

The authors declare that there is no conflict of interests regarding the publication of this paper.

Acknowledgments

Authors wish to thank and appreciate Dr. Salari honorable Director of Yazd Health Research Station, Dr. Nouri Shadkam honorable Health Deputy of Yazd Province, Dr. Jafari Health Network Director of Khatam Township, and Dr. Forghani and Mr. Ezzat, experts of Yazd Province Health Center, for their sincere cooperation for better accomplishment of this project. They thank Mr. Kafi, Mr. Noroozi, and Mr. Mousavi who are experts of health network for their cooperation in field operations. This research has been done with support of scientific pole of Health Research Institute, Tehran University of Medical Sciences (Project no. t-241/68/).

References

[1] WHO, "Report of the consultative meeting on cutaneous leishmaniasis," March 2010, http://www.who.int/leishmaniasis/resources/Cutaneous_leish_cm_2008.pdf.

[2] R. Jafari, *Study of cutaneous leishmaniasis in Nikabad town [M.S. thesis of Health Sciences in Medical Insectology and Fighting with Vectors Course]*, Tehran University of Medical Sciences, Tehran, Iran, 1997.

[3] E. Javadian, A. Nadim, G. H. Tahvildare-Bidruni, and V. Assefi, "Epidemiology of cutaneous leishmaniasis in Iran: B. Khorassan. Part V: report on a focus of zoonotic cutaneous leishmaniasis in Esferayen," *Bulletin de la Societe de Pathologie Exotique et de ses Filiales*, vol. 69, no. 2, p. 140, 1976.

[4] H. Kasiri, E. Javadian, and M. A. Seyedi-Rashti, "Liste des phlebotominae (Diptera: Psychodidae) d'Iran," *Bulletin de la Société de Pathologie Exotique*, vol. 93, no. 2, pp. 129–130, 2000.

[5] R. P. Lane and R. W. Crosskey, *Medical Insects and Arachnids*, Springer, 1993.

[6] M. R. Yaghoobi-Ershadi, A. A. Akhavan, and M. Mohebali, "Meriones libycus and *Rhombomys opimus* (Rodentia: Gerbillidae) are the main reservoir hosts in a new focus of zoonotic cutaneous leishmaniasis in Iran," *Transactions of the Royal Society of Tropical Medicine and Hygiene*, vol. 90, no. 5, pp. 503–504, 1996.

[7] M. R. Yaghoobi-Ershadi, A. A. Akhavan, A. V. Zahraei-Ramazani et al., "Epidemiological study in a new focus of cutaneous leishmaniasis in the Islamic Republic of Iran," *Eastern Mediterranean Health Journal*, vol. 9, no. 4, pp. 816–826, 2003.

[8] M. R. Yaghoobi-Ershadi, A. A. Hanafi-Bojd, A. A. Akhavan, R. Jafari, and M. Mohebali, "Study of animal sources of cutaneous leishmaniasis in two epidemic focuses in Yazd province," *Scientific Research Magazine of Yazd University of Medical Sciences*, vol. 2, pp. 38–43, 2001.

[9] M. R. Yaghoobi-Ershadi, A. A. Hanafi-Bojd, A. A. Akhavan, A. R. Zahrai-Ramazani, and M. Mohebali, "Epidemiological study in a new focus of cutaneous leishmaniosis due to Leishmania major in Ardestan town, central Iran," *Acta Tropica*, vol. 79, no. 2, pp. 115–121, 2001.

[10] M. R. Yaghoobi-Ershadi and E. Javadian, "Epidemiological study of reservoir hosts in an endemic area of zoonotic cutaneous leishmaniasis in Iran," *Bulletin of the World Health Organization*, vol. 74, no. 6, pp. 587–590, 1996.

[11] M.-R. Yaghoobi-Ershadi, A.-R. Zahraei-Ramazani, A.-A. Akhavan, A.-R. Jalali-Zand, H. Abdoli, and A. Nadim, "Rodent control operations against zoonotic cutaneous leishmaniasis in rural Iran," *Annals of Saudi Medicine*, vol. 25, no. 4, pp. 309–312, 2005.

[12] A. Karimi, A. A. Hanafi-Bojd, M. R. Yaghoobi-Ershadi, A. A. Akhavan, and Z. Ghezelbash, "Spatial and temporal distributions of phlebotomine sand flies (Diptera: Psychodidae), vectors of leishmaniasis, in Iran," *Acta Tropica*, vol. 132, no. 1, pp. 131–139, 2014.

[13] M. Yaghoobi-Ershadi, "Phlebotomine sand flies (Diptera: Psychodidae) in Iran and their role on leishmania transmission," *Journal of Arthropod-Borne Diseases*, vol. 6, no. 1, pp. 1–17, 2012.

[14] S. Ardehali, H. V. Rezaie, and A. Nadim, *Leishmaniasis Parasite an Leishmaniasis*, Publication Center of Tehran University, Tehran, Iran, 2nd edition, 1998.

[15] A. Etemad, "Rodents and their detection key," in *Iran Mammals*, vol. 1, pp. 288–298, National Institute of Natural Resources and Human Environment Preservation, Tehran, Iran, 1978.

[16] G. H. Edrissian, Z. Zovein, and A. Nadim, "A simple technique for preparation of smears from the ear of *Rhombomys opimus* for the detection of leishmanial infection," *Transactions of the Royal Society of Tropical Medicine and Hygiene*, vol. 76, no. 5, pp. 706–707, 1982.

[17] O. Theodor, *Revue de la Faculté des Sciences de l'Université d'Istanbul Série B*, vol. 17, p. 107, 1952.

[18] A. A. Akhavan, M. R. Yaghoobi-Ershadi, and M. Mohebali, "Epidemiology of dermal leishmaniasis (human infection) in the region of badrood, natanz township," in *Proceedings of the 1st Congress and Reeducation of Iran Medical Insectology*, Tehran, Iran, 2005.

[19] M. A. Seyedi-Rashti and A. Nadim, "Cutaneous leishmaniasis in Baluchistan, Iran," in *Proceedings of the 11th International Congress for Tropical Medicine and Malaria*, Abstract and Poster, Calgary, Canada, September 1984.

[20] M. A. Seyedi-Rashti and A. Salehzadeh, "A new focus of zoonotic cutaneous leishmaniasis near Tehran, Iran," *Bulletin de la Société Française de Parasitologie*, vol. 8, 1990.

[21] M. R. Yaghoob-Ershadi and E. Javadian, "Susceptibility of *Phlebotomus papatasi* to DDT in the most important focus of zoonotic cutaneous leishmaniasis, Isfahan province, Iran," *Journal of Entomological Society of Iran*, vol. 12, no. 13, pp. 27–37, 1993.

[22] A. A. Afshar, Y. Rassi, I. Sharifi et al., "Susceptibility status of *Phlebotomus papatasi* and *P. sergenti* (Diptera: Psychodidae) to DDT and deltamethrin in a focus of cutaneous leishmaniasis after earthquake strike in Bam, Iran," *Iranian Journal of Arthropod-Borne Diseases*, vol. 5, no. 2, pp. 32–14, 2011.

[23] M. A. Seyedi-Rashti, H. Yazdan-panah, H. Shah-Mohammadi, and M. Jedari, "Susceptibilityof *Phlebotomus papatasi* (Diptera: Psychodidae) to D.D.T. in some foci of cutaneous leishmaniasis in Iran," *Journal of the American Mosquito Control Association*, vol. 8, no. 1, pp. 99–100, 1992.

[24] E. Javadian, "Reservoir host of cutaneous leishmaniasis in Iran," in *Proceedings of the 12th International Congress for Tropical Medicine and Malaria*, Amsterdam, The Netherlands, September 1988.

[25] E. Javadian, M. Dehestani, N. Nadim et al., "Confirmation of *Tatera indica* (Rodentia: Gerbilldae) as the main reservoir host of zoonotic cutaneous leishmaniasis in the west of Iran," *Iranian Journal of Public Health*, vol. 27, no. 1-2, 1998.

[26] A. Nadim, M. A. Seyedi-Rashti, and A. Mesghali, "Epidemiology of cutaneous leishmaniasis in Turkemen Sahara, Iran," *The Journal of Tropical Medicine and Hygiene*, vol. 71, no. 9, pp. 238–239, 1968.

[27] M. R. Yaghoobi-Ershadi, R. Jafari, and A. A. Hanafi-Bojd, "A new epidemic focus of zoonotic cutaneous leishmaniasis in central Iran," *Annals of Saudi Medicine*, vol. 24, no. 2, pp. 98–101, 2004.

12

The Importance of Trichoscopy in Clinical Practice

Ana Filipa Pedrosa,[1] Paulo Morais,[1,2] Carmen Lisboa,[1,2] and Filomena Azevedo[1]

[1] *Department of Dermatology and Venereology, Centro Hospitalar São João EPE Porto, Alameda Prof. Hernani Monteiro, 4200-319 Porto, Portugal*
[2] *Faculty of Medicine, University of Porto, Alameda Prof. Hernani Monteiro, 4200-319 Porto, Portugal*

Correspondence should be addressed to Ana Filipa Pedrosa; anabastospedrosa@gmail.com

Academic Editor: Craig G. Burkhart

Trichoscopy corresponds to scalp and hair dermoscopy and has been increasingly used as an aid in the diagnosis, follow-up, and prognosis of hair disorders. Herein, we report selected cases harbouring scalp or hair diseases, in whom trichoscopy proved to be a valuable tool in their management. A review of the recent literature on this hot topic was performed comparing the described patterns with our findings in clinically common conditions, as well as in rare hair shaft abnormalities, where trichoscopy may display pathognomonic features. In our view, trichoscopy represents a valuable link between clinical and histological diagnosis. We detailed some trichoscopic patterns, complemented with our original photographs and our insights into nondescribed patterns.

1. Introduction

Trichoscopy (scalp and hair dermoscopy) represents a valuable noninvasive and low-cost technique, still underutilized, to rapidly differentiate clinically frequent hair disorders [1]. In their revision, Miteva and Tosti give a comprehensive and a thorough description of the usefulness of this technique in the diagnosis and follow-up of most common hair and scalp disorders, based on updated data from the literature and their personal experience [1]. We, herein, describe its application in randomly selected patients harbouring miscellaneous hair disorders, not only as a diagnostic tool, but also in monitoring treatment response or giving an insight of prognosis.

Trichoscopy may help to distinguish scarring versus nonscarring alopecia, early androgenetic alopecia (AGA) versus telogen effluvium, and it also supports the diagnosis and predicts the prognosis of alopecia areata (AA) [1].

2. Materials and Methods

From our clinical practice, we randomly selected patients harbouring hair or scalp complaints in whom trichoscopy assumed particular importance in clarifying the diagnosis, differential diagnosis, and prognosis and/or in monitoring the treatment response. The trichoscopic features were compared with data from the literature, when available.

3. Results and Discussion

Considering the conditions causing scarring alopecia, the key point seems to be the reduction or the absence of follicular orifices and the presence of peripilar casts or erythema (Figure 1(a)) [2]. Hair tufting can be seen in cases of lichen planopilaris [3]. In addition to dermoscopy, clinical presentation and physician's expertise are crucial for the diagnosis of such condition, subsequently confirmed by histopathology. There has been an effort to recognize specific features to distinguish the causes of scarring alopecia by trichoscopy. Tosti et al. [4] reported that follicular red dots seem to be a specific finding of scalp discoid lupus erythematosus (DLE), and their presence may denote disease activity, as we found in some patients with active biopsy-proven DLE (Figure 1(b)).

Regarding nonscarring alopecia, hair diameter diversity greater than 20% remains the most consistent finding in AGA in addition to perifollicular pigmentation (Figure 1(c)), whereas in telogen effluvium, there may be noticeable empty follicles and short regrowing normal thickness hairs [1].

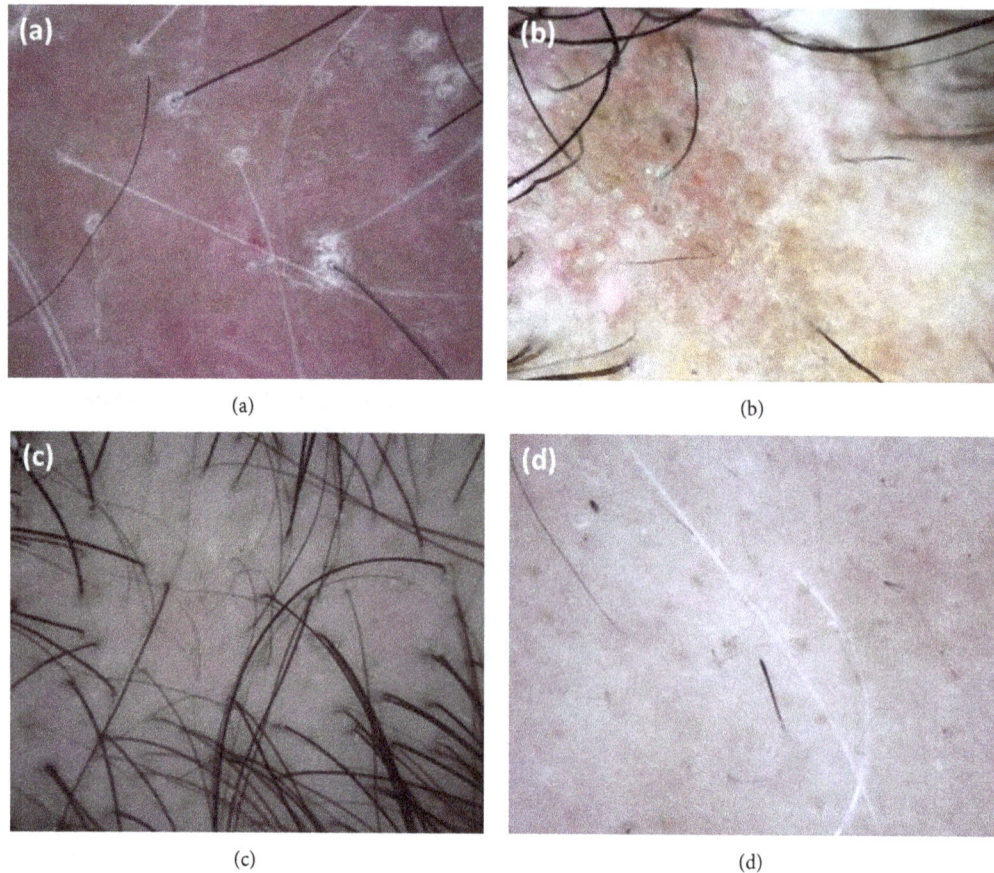

FIGURE 1: Clinically frequent hair disorders. Examples of scarring and nonscarring alopecia: (a) lichen planopilaris; (b) active scalp discoid lupus erythematosus with red follicular dots interspersed with scar areas; (c) androgenetic alopecia; (d) active alopecia areata. (a), (c), and (d) were captured with DermLite II PRO (3 Gen, San Juan Capistrano, CA, USA); (b) was captured with FotoFinder systems (Handyscope, Bad Birnbach, Germany) attached to the iPhone 4S (Apple, Cupertino, CA, USA).

In contrast, trichoscopy in AA may reveal uniform miniaturization of hair shafts which is most common in the remitting disease. According to other authors [1, 3], we frequently found yellow dots in both AGA and AA, although in the latter they are usually present in a greater number and may be associated with more specific markers, namely, black dots and broken and exclamation mark hairs (Figure 1(d)), which are predictors of disease activity [1, 3, 5].

Recently, we have emphasized the role of trichoscopy in the diagnosis of congenital atrichia and its distinction from other forms of childhood hair loss, especially AA universalis [6]. Trichotillomania (TTM), the compulsive desire to pull the hair, is another common cause of childhood alopecia, difficult to differentiate from AA, even with the aid of trichoscopy as both display broken hairs and black and yellow dots [5]. Some clues to TTM include the presence of scalp hemorrhages, different shaft lengths and the absence of exclamation mark hairs [7].

We had the opportunity to diagnose hair infestations with the aid of the handheld dermatoscope. Pediculosis capitis is reliably diagnosed unveiling the presence of lice nits (empty or full of nymphs) [8], and the iconographic proof of the infestation can be provided to the sceptic patients or their parents.

Genetic hair shaft abnormalities may be visualized by trichoscopy avoiding the need to pluck or cut hairs to perform light microscopy [9]. We display an example of trichorrhexis invaginata in a patient with Comèl-Netherton syndrome, highlighting the multiple nodes along the hair shafts, giving the appearance of "bamboo hair" (Figure 2(a)), which is considered pathognomonic for the disease [9].

Additionally, a case of nevoid pili multigemini in a patient complaining of skin roughness of the back was diagnosed with trichoscopy that enabled the recognition of multiple hair shafts emerging from the same follicle. After plucking the hairs, dermatoscopy suggested their true multigeminate nature coming from a single papilla and looking identical in a brush-like pattern (Figure 2(b)), different from the more commonly found compound follicles [10, 11].

4. Conclusions

In conclusion, we aimed to have briefly presented our experience in the daily clinical practice using a handheld dermatoscope coupled with a digital camera (or a smartphone) in the study of hair and scalp disorders. Trichoscopy represents a valuable link between clinical and histologic diagnoses.

(a)

(b)

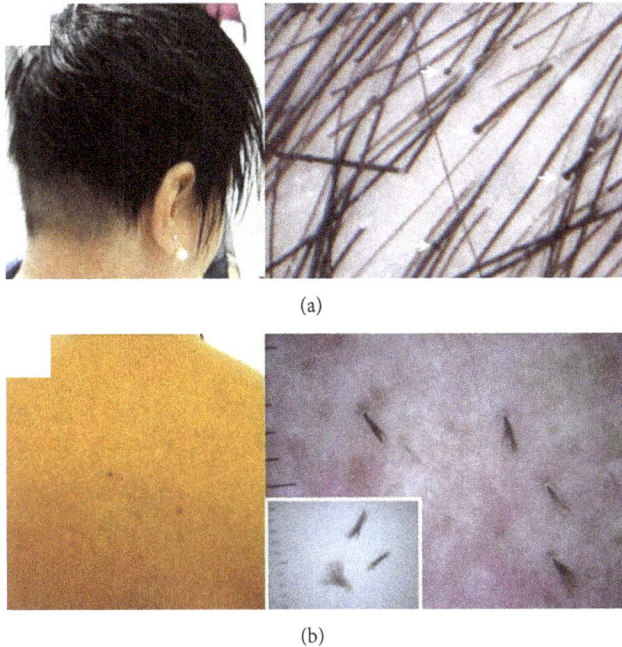

FIGURE 2: Rare hair shaft abnormalities. (a) Trichorhexis invaginata in a patient with Comèl-Netherton syndrome. Clinically hair appears sparse, brittle, and short; trichoscopy shows nodes along the hair shafts (white arrows). (b) Pili multigemini on the back. Dermoscopy highlighting the multiple hair shafts emerging from the same follicular ostia. Dermlite II Pro (3 Gen, San Juan Capistrano, CA, USA).

We have found reproducibility of many trichoscopic patterns complemented with our dies and original photographs.

References

[1] M. Miteva and A. Tosti, "Hair and scalp dermatoscopy," *Journal of the American Academy of Dermatology*, vol. 67, no. 5, pp. 1040–1048, 2012.

[2] L. Rudnicka, M. Olszewska, A. Rakowska, E. Kowalska-Oledzka, and M. Slowinska, "Trichoscopy: a new method for diagnosing hair loss," *Journal of Drugs in Dermatology*, vol. 7, no. 7, pp. 651–654, 2008.

[3] S. Inui, "Trichoscopy for common hair loss diseases: algorithmic method for diagnosis," *Journal of Dermatology*, vol. 38, no. 1, pp. 71–75, 2011.

[4] A. Tosti, F. Torres, C. Misciali et al., "Follicular red dots: a novel dermoscopic pattern observed in scalp discoid lupus erythematosus," *Archives of Dermatology*, vol. 145, no. 12, pp. 1406–1409, 2009.

[5] S. Inui, T. Nakajima, and S. Itami, "Coudability hairs: a revisited sign of alopecia areata assessed by trichoscopy," *Clinical and Experimental Dermatology*, vol. 35, no. 4, pp. 361–365, 2010.

[6] A. Pedrosa, A. Nogueira, P. Morais et al., "Photoletter to the editor: congenital atrichia associated with an uncommon mutation of HR gene," *Journal of Dermatological Case Reports*, vol. 7, no. 1, pp. 18–19, 2013.

[7] L. Peralta and P. Morais, "Photoletter to the editor: the friar tuck sign in trichotillomania," *Journal of Dermatological Case Reports*, vol. 6, no. 2, pp. 63–64, 2012.

[8] R. M. Bakos and L. Bakos, "Dermoscopy for diagnosis of pediculosis capitis," *Journal of the American Academy of Dermatology*, vol. 57, no. 4, pp. 727–728, 2007.

[9] A. Rakowska, M. Slowinska, E. Kowalska-Oledzka, and L. Rudnicka, "Trichoscopy in genetic hair shaft abnormalities," *Journal of Dermatological Case Reports*, vol. 2, no. 2, pp. 14–20, 2008.

[10] L. Lester and C. Venditti, "The prevalence of pili multigemini," *The British Journal of Dermatology*, vol. 156, no. 6, pp. 1362–1363, 2007.

[11] J. S. Lee, Y. C. Kim, and H. Y. Kang, "The nevoid pili multigemini over the back," *European Journal of Dermatology*, vol. 15, no. 2, pp. 99–101, 2005.

13

Is There Really Relationship between Androgenetic Alopecia and Metabolic Syndrome?

Seyran Ozbas Gok,[1] **Asli Akin Belli,**[2] **and Emine Dervis**[1]

[1]*Department of Dermatology, Haseki Training and Research Hospital, 34080 Istanbul, Turkey*
[2]*Department of Dermatology, Mugla Sitki Kocman University Training and Research Hospital, 48000 Mugla, Turkey*

Correspondence should be addressed to Asli Akin Belli; dr_asliakin@hotmail.com

Academic Editor: Craig G. Burkhart

Background. There are several studies investigating the relationship between androgenetic alopecia (AGA) and metabolic syndrome (MS) with conflicting results. *Objective.* We sought to investigate whether there is a relationship between AGA and MS. *Methods.* A case-control study including 74 male patients with AGA and 42 male controls was conducted. Age, duration of AGA, AGA onset age, anthropometric measures, body mass index, lipid parameters, fasting blood glucose, blood pressure, and presence of MS were recorded. *Results.* Of the 74 male AGA patients (age range 20–50 years, mean 32.14), 24 were in stage 2, 26 were in stage 3, 17 were in stage 3V, 1 was in stage 5, and 6 were in stage 7. There was no significant difference in the rate of MS between AGA and control groups ($P = 0.135$). Among the evaluated parameters, only systolic blood pressure in AGA group was significantly higher than control group. *Conclusion.* In contrast to the most of the previous studies, our study does not support the link between AGA and MS. To exclude confounding factors such as advanced age and therefore metabolic disturbances, further studies are needed with large group of AGA patients including different age groups and varying severity.

1. Introduction

Androgenetic alopecia (AGA) is a hair loss in specific patterns depending on circulating androgens in genetically predisposed men and women. Androgenetic alopecia affects 80% of men by the age of 70 years. In women, the incidence of AGA is 2–5% by the age of 50 and the ratio rises to 40% at age of 70. Although the main etiological factors are the same, phenotypic manifestations are different in men and women. Men usually have bitemporal and vertex hair loss leading to the complete baldness. In women, frontal hairline is usually preserved and complete baldness does not occur [1].

Metabolic syndrome (MS) is a group of metabolic disorders such as glucose intolerance, insulin resistance (IR), central obesity, dyslipidemia, and hypertension associated with increased risk of cardiovascular disease [2]. There are several studies investigating the relationship between AGA and MS, as well as IR with conflicting results [3–8]. In this study, we aimed to investigate whether there is a relationship between AGA and MS.

2. Patients and Methods

Between August 2012 and January 2013, a case-control study including 74 patients with AGA and 42 male controls was conducted in the Dermatology Outpatient Clinic of Haseki Training and Research Hospital, Istanbul. Ethic committee approval was obtained prior to the study. Inclusion criteria for patients with AGA were as follows:

(1) Being between 20 and 50 years of age.

(2) Absence of a known glucose metabolism disease.

(3) Absence of a known coronary artery disease.

(4) No history of drug use that affects carbohydrates metabolism (especially glucocorticoids).

The control group included age- and gender-matched male patients who have the inclusion criteria and admitted to the outpatient clinic with various dermatological complaints except alopecia.

AGA group included the patients who admitted to our outpatient clinic for alopecia or any dermatological problems that meet the inclusion criteria. Diagnosis of AGA was based on characteristic clinical findings. For grading AGA; Hamilton-Norwood classification was used in the patient group [1, 9].

Age, anthropometric measures (weight, height, and waist circumference), body mass index (BMI), lipid parameters (triglyceride, total cholesterol, high density lipoprotein, and low density lipoprotein), fasting blood glucose (FBG), blood pressure values of the participants' were evaluated. Waist circumference (WC) levels of >94 cm were recommended as cutoff point for abdominal obesity. BMI was calculated using the formula weight (kg)/height (m^2). Lipid parameters and FBG levels were studied after a 12-hour fasting period. Triglyceride level >150 mg/dL and HDL level <40 mg/dL were recommended as cutoff for dyslipidemia. FBG level ≥100 mg/dL was recommended as cutoff for impaired fasting glycemia. Systolic BP ≥135 mmHg and diastolic BP ≥85 mmHg were recommended as cutoff points for hypertension. The onset age, the duration of AGA, smoking history, and sports life were also recorded. The onset age of ≤35 years was recommended as early-onset AGA.

Based on the diagnostic criteria of International Diabetes Federation (IDF-2005), waist circumference >94 cm and at least two of the following criteria, triglyceride value >150 mg/dL or specific treatment for this lipid abnormality, high density lipoprotein <40 mg/dL or specific treatment for this lipid abnormality, blood pressure ≥130/85 mmHg or antihypertensive treatment, and fasting blood glucose ≥100 mg/dL or diagnosed diabetes mellitus, were accepted as MS [10].

In all patients, complete blood count, serum iron, total iron binding capacity, serum ferritin, free T3, free T4, and thyroid stimulating hormone (TSH) were performed to determine possible iron deficiency anemia and thyroid disorders.

For the data analysis, the statistical program "SPSS for windows 21.0" was employed. Mean, standard deviation, ratio, and frequency were used for descriptive statistics of the data. The distribution of variables was checked with Kolmogorov-Smirnov test. Independent samples t-test and Mann-Whitney u test were used for the analysis of quantitative data. The chi-square test was used for the analysis of categorical data. $P < 0.05$ was assessed as significant.

3. Results

Seventy four male AGA patients (age range 20–50 years, mean 32.14) and 42 controls (age range 20–50 years, mean 34.40) were investigated. Of 74 AGA patients 24 (32.4%) were in stage 2, 26 (35.1%) were in stage 3, 17 (23%) were in stage 3V, 1 (1.4%) was in stage 5, and 6 (8.1%) were in stage 7 according to Hamilton-Norwood classification.

In AGA group, there were no significant differences in the participants' age, weight, height, BMI, sport life, TG, total cholesterol, HDL, LDL, and diastolic pressure values

TABLE 1: Comparison of MS parameters and BMI in AGA and control groups.

	Patients ($n = 74$) n (%)	Controls ($n = 42$) n (%)	P
BMI ≥25 kg/m^2	35 (47.2)	26 (61.9)	0.130
FBG ≥100 mg/dL	1 (1.3)	9 (21.4)	**<0.001**
TG ≥150 mg/dL	23 (31)	17 (40.4)	0.306
HDL <40 mg/dL	28 (37.8)	17 (40.4)	0.779
Systolic BP ≥135 mmHg	16 (21.6)	3 (7.1)	**0.043**
Diastolic BP ≥85 mmHg	5 (6.7)	1 (2.3)	0.415
Waist C >94 cm	23 (31.1)	21 (50)	**0.044**

Chi-square test. MS: metabolic syndrome; AGA: androgenetic alopecia; BMI: body mass index; FBG: fasting blood glucose; TG: triglyceride; HDL: high density lipoprotein; BP: blood pressure; Waist C: waist circumference.

TABLE 2: The rate of metabolic syndrome in AGA and control groups.

	AGA group		Control group		P
	n	%	n	%	
Metabolic syndrome					
Present	11	14.9%	11	26.2%	0.135
Absent	63	85.1%	31	73.8%	

Chi-square test. AGA: androgenetic alopecia.

$(P > 0.05)$. AGA group had significantly high systolic blood pressure levels and control group had significantly high FBG and waist circumference levels $(P < 0.05)$ (Table 1). There was no significant difference in the rate of MS between AGA and control groups (Table 2) $(P > 0.135)$.

In AGA group, the onset age of AGA and the duration of AGA were not significantly different in the patients with or without MS $(P > 0.05)$.

When patients with stages I–IV were assessed as mild-moderate and patients with stages V–VII were assessed as severe, there was no significant difference between the patients with or without MS $(P < 0.05)$.

4. Discussion

There are several studies investigating AGA and metabolic disorders related to MS with conflicting results [3–8]. Although some studies have reported a relationship between AGA and MS, pathophysiological connection between these two diseases has not been completely elucidated [11].

Metabolic syndrome is a group of metabolic disorders associated with increased risk of cardiovascular disease [2]. In the pathogenesis of MS, several factors such as genetic predisposition, insulin resistance (IR), obesity, hypertension, dyslipidemia, vascular abnormalities, inflammation, hyperandrogenism, uric acid deficiency, and vitamin D deficiency are considered to be responsible. In a study performed by Acibucu et al., the rate of IR and MS was significantly high in 80 early AGA patients [3]. The link between AGA and

MS has not been clarified yet. However, two hypotheses have been proposed that, firstly, both of AGA and cardiovascular diseases are related to excess of androgens and secondly, hormonal changes such as hyperandrogenism may play a role in the development of AGA and hypertension [12]. Mumcuoglu et al. found a relationship between AGA and IR but not with MS in 50 male patients with grade ≥3 AGA [4]. The action mechanism of insulin on the AGA is not clear. It has been suggested that insulin may be an important factor in the pathogenesis of AGA by causing vasoconstriction and nutrient deficiency. It may also be effective by enhancing the effects of testosterone [5]. Insulin and insulin-like growth factor-1 may enhance DHT levels by inducing 5-α-reductase activity in obese patients [13]. Matilainen et al. noted that IR may be a pathophysiological mechanism or enhancing factor in early AGA [6]. In another study performed by Matilainen et al., some parameters associated with IR were significantly high in 342 female AGA patients [7]. In our study, insulin levels and insulin resistance were not evaluated.

In contrast to the other studies, Nabaie et al. did not find a relationship between AGA and the parameters, FBG, serum fasting insulin levels, total cholesterol, TG, HDL, and IR in 97 male AGA patients [8]. Similarly, we did not find a positive correlation between AGA and MS. Only systolic blood pressure levels were significantly higher than control group. Although controls were selected metabolically normal subjects, FBG and mean waist circumference levels were significantly higher in the control group. These unexpected results were attributed to be incidental. Additionally, there was no relationship between the AGA onset age and the duration of AGA and MS. Positive relation of AGA with MS and IR reported in the previous studies may be due to the confounding factors that the patients had advanced age and thus metabolic abnormalities could be plausible. The study reported by Giltay et al. also supports our results. In this study, 81 female-to-male transsexuals treated with testosterone esters had male-pattern baldness without any cardiovascular disease risk factors such as increased blood pressure, levels of lipid, and insulin. It was noted that male-pattern alopecia does not indicate increased cardiovascular disease risk [14]. In another study involving 60 AGA patients with or without MS, the patients with MS were likely to have IR rather than the patients without MS, and true association between AGA and IR has been denied [5].

The relationship between early AGA and serious cardiovascular events such as myocardial infarction (MI) and fatal ischemic heart disease has been shown, but explaining mechanisms are not clear [6]. Androgen receptors have been found in the arterial wall endothelium but have not clarified whether there are direct effects [15]. Lesko et al. investigated 665 male AGA patients and 772 control patients who had acute myocardial infarction under 55 years of age; they found higher rates of AGA on the vertex [16]. In terms of cardiovascular risk factors, systolic blood pressure levels were significantly higher in our AGA group. There are some studies reporting an association between hypertension, as well as aldosterone levels and AGA. It has been proposed that specific mineralocorticoid receptor antagonists could be used in the treatment of AGA [17, 18].

5. Conclusions

Even though some studies undetected a relationship between AGA and MS, it has been found in many and has emphasized the importance of early diagnosis. In contrast to previous reports, we did not find a relationship between AGA and MS. Although there was no correlation between AGA and MS, to detect an increase in systolic blood pressure levels may be remarkable in terms of being a cardiovascular disease risk factor. Moreover, this low rate of MS may be related to the fact that our study did not include elderly patients and majority of our patients had mild alopecia compared to the other studies. On this topic, there is a need of large group of AGA patients including different age groups and varying severity.

Conflict of Interests

The authors declare that there is no conflict of interests regarding the publication of this paper.

References

[1] R. Paus, E. A. Olsen, and A. G. Messenger, "Hair growth disorders," in *Fitzpatrick's Dermatology in General Medicine*, K. Wolff, L. A. Goldsmith, S. I. Katz, B. A. Gilchrest, A. S. Paller, and D. J. Leffell, Eds., pp. 753–777, McGraw-Hill, New York, NY, USA, 7th edition, 2008.

[2] T. Fulop, D. Tessier, and A. Carpentier, "The metabolic syndrome," *Pathologie Biologie*, vol. 54, no. 7, pp. 375–386, 2006.

[3] F. Acibucu, M. Kayatas, and F. Candan, "The association of insulin resistance and metabolic syndrome in early androgenetic alopecia," *Singapore Medical Journal*, vol. 51, no. 12, pp. 931–936, 2010.

[4] C. Mumcuoglu, T. R. Ekmekci, and S. Ucak, "The investigation of insulin resistance and metabolic syndrome in male patients with early-onset androgenetic alopecia," *European Journal of Dermatology*, vol. 21, no. 1, pp. 79–82, 2011.

[5] N. S. A. Abdel Fattah and Y. W. Darwish, "Androgenetic alopecia and insulin resistance: are they truly associated?" *International Journal of Dermatology*, vol. 50, no. 4, pp. 417–422, 2011.

[6] V. Matilainen, P. Koskela, and S. Keinänen-Kiukaanniemi, "Early androgenetic alopecia as a marker of insulin resistance," *The Lancet*, vol. 356, no. 9236, pp. 1165–1166, 2000.

[7] V. Matilainen, M. Laakso, P. Hirsso, P. Koskela, U. Rajala, and S. Keinänen-Kiukaanniemi, "Hair loss, insulin resistance, and heredity in middle-aged women. A population-based study," *Journal of Cardiovascular Risk*, vol. 10, no. 3, pp. 227–231, 2003.

[8] L. Nabaie, S. Kavand, R. M. Robati et al., "Androgenic alopecia and insulin resistance: are they really related?" *Clinical and Experimental Dermatology*, vol. 34, no. 6, pp. 694–697, 2009.

[9] E. A. Olsen, "Female pattern hair loss," *Journal of the American Academy of Dermatology*, vol. 45, no. 3, supplement, pp. S70–S80, 2001.

[10] K. G. Alberti, P. Zimmet, and J. Shaw, "The metabolic syndrome—a new worldwide definition," *The Lancet*, vol. 366, no. 9491, pp. 1059–1062, 2005.

[11] M. Arslan, "Metabolik sendrom: tanımı, patogenezi, tanı kriterleri ve bileşenleri," *Turkiye Klinikleri Journal of Internal Medical Sciences*, vol. 2, no. 3, pp. 1–7, 2006.

[12] N. Trieu and G. D. Eslick, "Alopecia and its association with coronary heart disease and cardiovascular risk factors: a meta-analysis," *International Journal of Cardiology*, vol. 176, no. 3, pp. 687–695, 2014.

[13] C.-C. Yang, F.-N. Hsieh, L.-Y. Lin, C.-K. Hsu, H.-M. Sheu, and W. Chen, "Higher body mass index is associated with greater severity of alopecia in men with male-pattern androgenetic alopecia in Taiwan: a cross-sectional study," *Journal of the American Academy of Dermatology*, vol. 70, no. 2, pp. 297–302, 2014.

[14] E. J. Giltay, A. W. F. T. Toorians, A. R. Sarabjitsingh, N. A. de Vries, and L. J. G. Gooren, "Established risk factors for coronary heart disease are unrelated to androgen-induced baldness in female-to-male transsexuals," *Journal of Endocrinology*, vol. 180, no. 1, pp. 107–112, 2004.

[15] J. H. Pinkney, C. D. A. Stehouwer, S. W. Coppack, and J. S. Yudkin, "Endothelial dysfunction: cause of the insulin resistance syndrome," *Diabetes*, vol. 46, no. 2, pp. 9–13, 1997.

[16] S. M. Lesko, L. Rosenberg, and S. Shapiro, "A case-control study of baldness in relation to myocardial infarction in men," *The Journal of the American Medical Association*, vol. 269, no. 8, pp. 998–1003, 1993.

[17] S. Ahouansou, P. Le Toumelin, B. Crickx, and V. Descamps, "Association of androgenetic alopecia and hypertension," *European Journal of Dermatology*, vol. 17, no. 3, pp. 220–222, 2007.

[18] S. Arias-Santiago, M. T. Gutiérrez-Salmerón, A. Buendía-Eisman, M. S. Girón-Prieto, and R. Naranjo-Sintes, "Hypertension and aldosterone levels in women with early-onset androgenetic alopecia," *British Journal of Dermatology*, vol. 162, no. 4, pp. 786–789, 2010.

14

Dermatological Diseases Associated with Pregnancy: Pemphigoid Gestationis, Polymorphic Eruption of Pregnancy, Intrahepatic Cholestasis of Pregnancy, and Atopic Eruption of Pregnancy

Christine Sävervall,[1] Freja Lærke Sand,[1] and Simon Francis Thomsen[1,2]

[1]Department of Dermatology, Bispebjerg Hospital, 2400 Copenhagen NV, Denmark
[2]Center for Medical Research Methodology, Department of Biomedical Sciences, University of Copenhagen, 2200 Copenhagen N, Denmark

Correspondence should be addressed to Simon Francis Thomsen; simonfrancisthomsen@gmail.com

Academic Editor: Lajos Kemény

Dermatoses unique to pregnancy are important to recognize for the clinician as they carry considerable morbidity for pregnant mothers and in some instances constitute a risk to the fetus. These diseases include pemphigoid gestationis, polymorphic eruption of pregnancy, intrahepatic cholestasis of pregnancy, and atopic eruption of pregnancy. This review discusses the pathogenesis, clinical importance, and management of the dermatoses of pregnancy.

1. Introduction

Three general categories of skin conditions occur during pregnancy. First, a number of benign skin conditions can occur because of normal physiological/hormonal changes during pregnancy; second, preexisting skin conditions can show signs of flare (or quiescence) during pregnancy due to immune-hormonal alterations, and third, several pregnancy-specific dermatoses can occur [1].

Pregnancy-specific dermatoses represent a group of pruritic skin diseases unique to pregnancy. Due to the not fully elucidated etiopathogenesis, the rarity of these diseases, and the clinical overlap between them, there is an ongoing discussion on how to classify the specific diseases. The latest classification is proposed by Ambrus-Rudolph [2] in 2006 and includes pemphigoid gestationis (PG), polymorphic eruption of pregnancy (PEP), intrahepatic cholestasis of pregnancy (ICP), and atopic eruption of pregnancy (AEP) (Table 1).

The purpose of this review is to elucidate these four pregnancy-specific dermatoses and their clinical importance.

Some of the diseases are correlated with fetal risks, making pregnancy-specific dermatoses an important topic for the clinician. Several other dermatological diseases exist, which can be associated with pregnancy. However, these are not dealt with herein.

2. Pemphigoid Gestationis (PG)

PG is a rare and intensely pruritic autoimmune skin disorder that only occurs in association with pregnancy. In terms of clinical and immunologic features it is similar to the pemphigoid group of autoimmune blistering skin disorders.

PG was formerly termed herpes gestations, because of the similar morphology of the blisters. The name was changed as PG was shown not to be related to, or associated with, any prior or active herpes virus infection. The disease commonly presents in the second or third trimester of pregnancy [2, 3] but cases have also been reported in the first trimester and postpartum period [2, 4, 5]. The incidence is approximately 1 in 60.000 [6, 7] pregnancies and the disease shows a worldwide distribution. The pathogenesis is not yet fully

TABLE 1

Pregnancy dermatosis	Suggested pathogenesis	Clinical features	Localisation	Paraclinical diagnosis	Treatment	Fetal concerns
Pemphigoid gestationis (PG)	Complement-fixing IgG antibodies and complement C3 react with the amniotic epithelium of placental tissues and the basement membrane of the skin causing an autoimmune response resulting in tissue damage and blister formation	Pruritic urticarial papules and annular plaques followed by vesicles and finally large tense bullae on an erythematous background	Eruption site is the periumbilical area (most common), rest of the abdomen, thighs, palms, and soles	Histology: urticarial lesions with superficial and deep perivascular lymphohistiocytic eosinophil infiltration DIF: linear deposition of IgG and C3 complement at the BMZ	Oral corticosteroids at a daily dose of 0.5 mg/kg gradually tapered to a maintenance dose depending on the activity of the disease Classes III-IV topical steroids. Cyclosporine A, dapsone, azathioprine, or methotrexate (postpartum)	Passive transfer of IgG1 antibodies can cause mild urticaria-like or vesicular skin lesions in newborns Risk for premature birth and small-for-gestational-age babies Risk of small-for-gestational-age and preterm birth with cyclosporine A Drug toxicity should also be monitored in the mother
Polymorphic eruption of pregnancy (PEP)	Abdominal distension causing subsequent damage to the connective tissue triggering an inflammatory response Differences in cortisol level in patients with PEP Connection to atopy	Intensely pruritic urticarial rash with erythematous, edematous papules, and plaques, developing into polymorphic features such as papulovesicles, erythema, and annular wheals	Onset on the abdomen with sparing of the umbilical region as a characteristic finding, which later spreads to thighs, buttocks, and back	Histology: dermal edema with a superficial to mid-dermal perivascular lymphohistiocytic infiltrate composed of eosinophils, Th cells, and macrophages	Topical corticosteroids and oral antihistamines Oral corticosteroids	No adverse effects related to PEP Prednisone and prednisolone do not readily cross the placenta and can be safely used during pregnancy Drug toxicity should be monitored in the mother Only certain antihistamines approved during pregnancy
Intrahepatic cholestasis of pregnancy (ICP)	Hormonal changes Genetic predisposition Exogenous factors (seasonal variability and dietary factors)	Severe pruritus with no primary skin lesions occurring with or without jaundice	Onset on palms and soles to later become generalized Secondary lesions such as excoriations, scratch marks, and prurigo nodules might develop	Elevated serum bile acid levels (and aminotransferases)	Ursodeoxycholic acid to alleviate the severity of pruritus and to give a more favorable outcome of pregnancy and the absence of adverse events UVB Phototherapy	Premature birth Intrapartal fetal distress Stillbirth Vitamin K deficiency and coagulopathy in the mother and newborn
Atopic eruption of pregnancy (AEP)	Altered pattern of Th cells with a reduced production of Th1 cytokines (IL-2, interferon gamma, and IL-12) and an increased Th2 cytokine (IL-4 and IL-10) production	Pruritus, prurigo lesions/excoriations, and eczematous-like skin lesions Secondary infection due to excoriations	66% present with widespread eczematous changes affecting typical atopic sites 33% have small pruritic, erythematous papules on the trunk and limbs	No pathognomonic findings specific to AEP Elevated serum IgE levels in 20–70%	Topical corticosteroids classes II-IV Oral corticosteroids and antihistamines UVB phototherapy Antibiotics in cases of secondary infection	No adverse effects except the uncertain risk for the child to develop atopic dermatitis

DIF: direct immunofluorescence; BMZ: basement membrane zone; Th: T-helper.

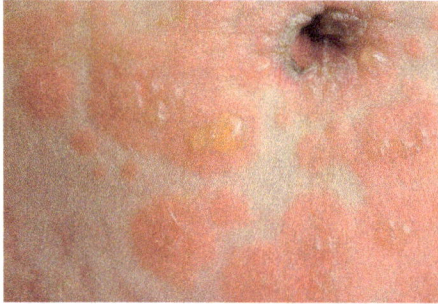

FIGURE 1: Periumbilical eruption in PG.

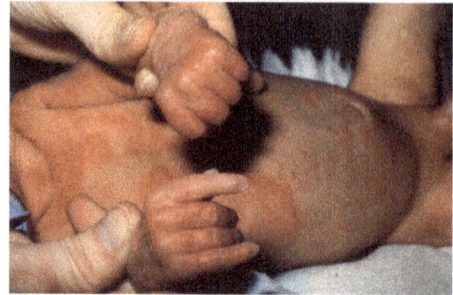

FIGURE 2: Urticaria-like and vesicular skin lesions in neonatal PG.

established but an association with the haplotypes HLA-DR3 in 61–80% of patients and HLA-DR4 in 52-53% of patients has been delineated [8].

2.1. Pathogenesis.

In PG the first immune response is located within the placenta. Circulating complement-fixing IgG antibodies develop that react with the amniotic epithelium of placental tissues and the basement membrane of the skin. The autoimmune response in the skin consists of deposition of immune complexes, complement activation, consecutive chemoattraction of eosinophils, and degranulation, resulting in tissue damage and blister formation [9]. The underlying factor that initiates the process remains unclear, but a theory proposes that an allogeneic or autoimmune response to an abnormal MHC class TI product expression in the placenta is important [10].

PG is also reported to exacerbate or flare during menstruation, or following administration of postpartum oral contraceptives. These observations suggest that changes in sex hormones might play a role in the pathogenesis of PG [6, 11, 12], although this is not congruent with some studies [13].

2.2. Clinical Features.

Initially the disease presents with pruritic urticarial papules and annular plaques, followed by vesicles and finally large tense bullae on an erythematous background. The most common eruption site is the periumbilical area (Figure 1). In 90% of the cases, it later spreads to the rest of the abdomen and, in some cases, even to thighs, palms, and soles [11]. During the last month of pregnancy the patient experiences a remission commonly followed by a flare immediately after delivery. The activity of PG decreases and often disappears during the first months after delivery but will often return in subsequent pregnancies. The disease is self-limiting and most patients exhibit a spontaneous remission in weeks to months after delivery, even without treatment.

2.3. Diagnosis.

The diagnosis of PG relies on the clinical evaluation, histological findings, and direct immunofluorescence (DIF). The classic histologic picture shows urticarial lesions with superficial and deep perivascular lymphohistiocytic eosinophil infiltration. DIF shows a linear deposition of IgG and C3 complement at the basement membrane antigenic zone [4, 11]. C3 is reported in up to 100% of cases, while IgG is seen in 25 to 50% [11].

2.4. Treatment.

The treatment is oral corticosteroids with a daily dose of 0.5 mg/kg, gradually tapered to a maintenance dose depending on the activity of the disease. For mild disease the use of class III or IV topical steroids can be sufficient. If topical and oral corticosteroid treatment is insufficient, systemic immunosuppressants such as cyclosporine A, dapsone, azathioprine, or methotrexate (postpartum) might be beneficial.

2.5. Fetal Concerns.

PG is associated with several risks for the fetus. Because of the passive transfer of IgG1 antibodies from the mother to the fetus, approximately 10% of newborns develop a mild clinical picture consisting of urticaria-like or vesicular skin lesions [9] (Figure 2). There is also a risk for premature birth and small-for-gestational-age babies. Some have theorized that systemic use of corticosteroids during pregnancy might increase the risk of developing fetal abnormities, but this is probably associated with the activity of the disease rather than the systemic use of corticosteroids. The fetal risks are especially found related to the onset of PG in the first or second trimester. The presence of blisters and/or the systemic prednisolone treatment did not appear to affect, or worsen, pregnancy outcomes in women with PG [14]. However, adverse effects of topical and systemic corticosteroids in the mother should be monitored. Also, toxicity in the mother and risk of premature birth and small-for-gestational-age babies related to cyclosporine A should be monitored closely. Azathioprine can be used during pregnancy but toxicity related to the mother should be monitored. Methotrexate is contraindicated during pregnancy.

2.6. Comorbidities.

PG is often found in association with other autoimmune diseases such as Graves' disease, thyroiditis, and pernicious anemia [5, 11]. This can be partially explained by the presence of HLA-DR3 and DR4 [15] in both PG and these autoimmune diseases.

3. Polymorphic Eruption of Pregnancy (PEP)

PEP (earlier termed pruritic urticarial papules and plaques of pregnancy, PUPPP) is a benign, self-limiting inflammatory disorder that usually affects *primigravida* in the third trimester of pregnancy or immediately in the postpartum period [9, 16, 17]. It rarely recurs in subsequent pregnancies [17]. It is the most common pregnancy-specific dermatosis

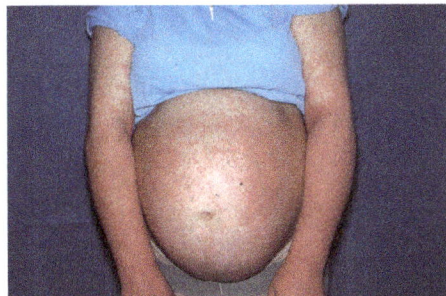

FIGURE 3: Pruritic urticarial rash in PEP.

with an incidence of 1 in 160 pregnancies [9, 18]. Despite the relatively high frequency of PEP, little is known about its etiology. It is suggested that changes in sex hormones and immunologic responses to abdominal distension may trigger PEP, but none of these theories are substantiated [3, 9, 18].

3.1. Pathogenesis. The pathogenesis is still unknown and not sufficiently elucidated. *The distension theory* suggests that an overdistension of the abdominal wall causes subsequent damage to the connective tissue triggering an inflammatory response [9, 18]. A study of 200 patients found a statistically significant reduction in serum cortisol among patients with PEP [3] compared to controls, but the relevance of this is still unclear. Another theory suggests that PEP might be connected to atopy, after a study of 181 patients with PEP revealed a frequency of atopy among 55% of the included patients [18]. So far it has not been possible to find evidence of circulating immune complexes or specific HLA associations for PEP, so the pathogenic mechanisms remain unknown.

3.2. Clinical Features. The site of onset of symptoms is usually the abdomen, often within *striae distensae* and with an intensely pruritic urticarial rash with erythematous, edematous papules, and plaques (Figure 3). Sparing of the umbilical region is a characteristic finding. The disease spreads to other body sites such as proximal thighs, buttocks, and the back. Rarely the eruption spreads ideally involving arms and legs [9]. The morphology changes while the disease advances, developing polymorphic features such as papulovesicles, erythema, and annular wheals.

3.3. Diagnosis. There are no tests that definitely can decide whether a woman has PEP. DIF and indirect immunofluorescence are negative in PEP. The histopathology varies with the stage of the disease. The diagnosis is based on the clinical picture, with the abovementioned characteristics, and a biopsy showing dermal edema, a superficial to mid-dermal perivascular lymphohistiocytic infiltrate composed of eosinophils, T-helper cells, and macrophages. At a later stage a biopsy reveals epidermal changes including hyper- and parakeratosis [9, 16].

3.4. Treatment. Treatment is symptomatic. In order to control pruritus and advancement of the skin rash it is usually sufficient to use topical corticosteroids with or without oral antihistamines, but in severe cases a short treatment burst with systemic corticosteroids may be necessary [9, 16]. The disease is self-limiting and the lesions usually resolve within weeks after birth, with no postinflammatory pigmentary change or scarring.

3.5. Fetal Concerns. PEP is not associated with cutaneous manifestations or risk to the newborn or fetus. The maternal prognosis is excellent in most cases [18]. Maternal adverse effects of systemic and topical corticosteroids should be monitored. Not all antihistamines are approved during pregnancy; cetirizine, loratadine, and fexofenadine should be preferred.

4. Intrahepatic Cholestasis of Pregnancy (ICP)

ICP, also known as pruritus gravidarum, is a liver disorder characterized by severe pruritus and secondary skin lesions in the third trimester of pregnancy. The symptoms develop from a reversible form of hormonally triggered cholestasis that typically develops in genetically predisposed individuals. ICP is not a primary dermatosis, but due to its correlation with fetal risks and skin symptoms, it is regarded as a pregnancy-specific dermatosis. The prevalence of ICP is around 1% [9, 16, 19, 20] but it shows a striking geographical pattern with a higher prevalence in Scandinavia and South Africa.

4.1. Pathogenesis. The pathogenesis is multifactorial involving an interaction between hormonal changes (being the main factor), genetic predisposition, and exogenous factors [9]. Exogenous factors include environmental factors such as seasonal variability [21] and dietary factors such as decreased selenium levels [22]. The role of the exogenous factors is still debated.

4.2. Clinical Features. ICP is characterized by severe pruritus with no primary skin lesions with or without jaundice, which is seen in 0.02–2.4% [23]. Pruritus typically starts on the palms and soles and later becomes generalized. Later secondary lesions such as excoriations, scratch marks, and prurigo nodules might develop as a result of scratching (Figure 4). This commonly involves the shins and lower arms. The symptoms usually disappear 1-2 days after delivery, but in some cases they can persist for 1-2 weeks [9]. There is a high risk of recurrence of ICP in subsequent pregnancies (50–70%) and with the use of oral contraceptives.

4.3. Diagnosis. The hallmarks for diagnosing ICP are the generalized pruritus and the elevated serum bile acid levels and aminotransferases.

4.4. Treatment. Treatment aims to lower the level of serum bile acid and to alleviate pruritus. Ursodeoxycholic acid can be used to alleviate the severity of pruritus and has shown to give a more favorable outcome of pregnancy and the absence of adverse events [24]. Treatments with cholestyramine, antihistamines, and oral corticosteroids have been tried, but none are supported by current evidence or may have

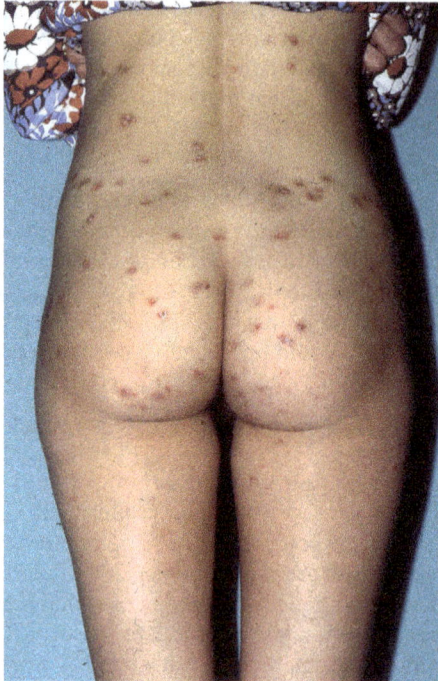

FIGURE 4: Excoriations, scratch marks, and prurigo nodules in ICP.

adverse effects [1, 24]. Phototherapy with UVB can be used in refractory cases.

4.5. Fetal Concerns. ICP is correlated with fetal risks, the most common being premature birth (20–60%) followed by intrapartal fetal distress (20–30%) and stillbirth (1-2%) [9]. In severe or prolonged ICP, cholestasis might cause vitamin K deficiency and coagulopathy in patients and their children [1]. These risks make it necessary to closely follow these during and after pregnancy.

5. Atopic Eruption of Pregnancy (AEP)

AEP is a benign pruritic condition that is characterized by eczematous or papular lesions in patients with a history of, or predisposition to, atopic dermatitis or with new onset of atopic dermatitis during pregnancy. The term AEP covers a heterogeneous group of pruritic conditions during pregnancy also known as prurigo of pregnancy, pruritic folliculitis of pregnancy, and eczema in pregnancy. AEP is the most common cause of pruritus during pregnancy [2, 16] with a prevalence of 5–20%. AEP includes two groups of patients, one who during pregnancy either experience atopic skin changes for the first time or after a long remission and, second, patients who suffer from an exacerbation of preexisting atopic dermatitis. A study of 505 women showed that 80% experienced skin changes for the first time [2]. The symptoms usually start early in the first or second trimester and typically reoccur in subsequent pregnancies due to the atopic background. Many women with AEP have elevated serum IgE, a positive allergy test for airborne allergens, and a family history of atopic diseases.

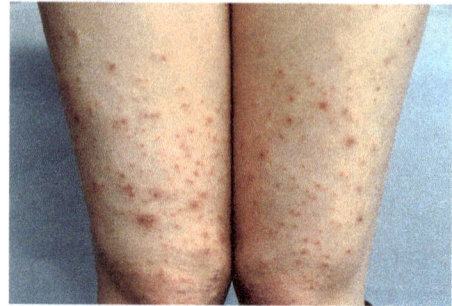

FIGURE 5: Prurigo lesions/excoriations and eczematous-like skin lesions in AEP.

5.1. Pathogenesis. The pathogenesis of AEP and the late onset of symptoms are thought to be triggered by pregnancy-specific immunological changes. During pregnancy, women have an altered pattern of T-helper (Th) cells with a reduced production of Th1 cytokines (IL-2, interferon gamma, and IL-12) and an increased Th2 cytokine (IL-4 and IL-10) production [25]. The Th2 response is thought to be responsible for the skin changes seen in pregnant women.

5.2. Clinical Features. The main clinical features are pruritus, prurigo lesions/excoriations, and eczematous-like skin lesions (Figure 5). Two-thirds present with widespread eczematous changes affecting typical atopic sites such as the face, neck, and the flexor surfaces of the extremities, while one-third have small pruritic, erythematous papules on the trunk and limbs. Scratching causes excoriations and might result in secondary skin infections. The eczema usually disappears after pregnancy.

5.3. Diagnosis. The diagnosis is mostly based on the clinical characteristics. There are no pathognomonic findings specific to AEP, but laboratory tests might reveal elevated serum IgE levels in 20–70% [2].

5.4. Treatment. Treatment strategy depends on the severity of the condition. The treatment is topical corticosteroids class III or IV. This is usually sufficient, but in severe cases systemic corticosteroids or antihistamines may be required. UVB phototherapy is used for recalcitrant cases. In case of secondary bacterial infection with hemolytic streptococci or staphylococci, treatment with antibiotics is necessary.

5.5. Fetal Concerns. AEP is not associated with fetal risks, except the uncertain risk for the child to develop atopic dermatitis.

6. Conclusion

Pruritus and skin changes are common during pregnancy and are usually benign and self-limiting. In some cases, however, they are symptoms of pregnancy-specific dermatoses. These constitute a rare group of inflammatory dermatoses specifically related to pregnancy and/or the immediate postpartum period, which can be associated with severe fetal outcomes such as fetal distress, stillbirth, and premature birth [23].

Pruritus represents the leading symptom in this group of diseases. Skin changes vary in morphology, location, and time of onset, but still there are many similarities. For the untrained eye it might be difficult to separate the different diagnoses by only using clinical characteristics. Direct immunofluorescence, histopathology, and blood analyses are used as complementary diagnostic tools for a more correct diagnosis. Only for PG and ICP laboratory tests can substantiate the clinical diagnosis. Therefore, it is important for the clinician to combine the medical history, the morphologic criteria, and the histopathology of the lesions to establish the correct diagnosis.

Fetal risks have only been associated with PG and ICP, but with the overlapping symptoms between the diseases pruritus in pregnancy should never be neglected. Interdisciplinary management involving dermatologists, pediatricians, obstetricians, and gastroenterologists is mandatory to acquire a better outcome for the mother and the fetus.

Conflict of Interests

The authors declare that there is no conflict of interests regarding the publication of this paper.

Acknowledgment

The authors are indebted to Nis Kentorp, clinical photographer, for producing the illustrations.

References

[1] M. Tunzi and G. R. Gray, "Common skin conditions during pregnancy," *American Family Physician*, vol. 75, no. 2, pp. 211–218, 2007.

[2] C. M. Ambros-Rudolph, R. R. Müllegger, S. A. Vaughan-Jones, H. Kerl, and M. M. Black, "The specific dermatoses of pregnancy revisited and reclassified: results of a retrospective two-center study on 505 pregnant patients," *Journal of the American Academy of Dermatology*, vol. 54, no. 3, pp. 395–404, 2006.

[3] S. A. Vaughan Jones, S. Hern, C. Nelson-Piercy, P. T. Seed, and M. M. Black, "A prospective study of 200 women with dermatoses of pregnancy correlating clinical findings with hormonal and immunopathological profiles," *British Journal of Dermatology*, vol. 141, no. 1, pp. 71–81, 1999.

[4] J. Lipozenčić, S. Ljubojevic, and Z. Bukvić-Mokos, "Pemphigoid gestationis," *Clinics in Dermatology*, vol. 30, no. 1, pp. 51–55, 2012.

[5] R. E. Jenkins, S. Hern, and M. M. Black, "Clinical features and management of 87 patients with pemphigoid gestationis," *Clinical and Experimental Dermatology*, vol. 24, no. 4, pp. 255–259, 1999.

[6] J. K. Shornick, J. L. Bangert, R. G. Freeman, and J. N. Gilliam, "Herpes gestationis: clinical and histologic features of twenty-eight cases," *Journal of the American Academy of Dermatology*, vol. 8, no. 2, pp. 214–224, 1983.

[7] R. C. Kolodny, "Herpes gestationis. A new assessment of incidence, diagnosis, and fetal prognosis," *American Journal of Obstetrics & Gynecology*, vol. 104, no. 1, pp. 39–45, 1969.

[8] R. E. Jenkins and J. Shornick, "Pemphigoid (herpes) gestationis," in *Obstetric and Gynecologic Dermatology*, M. Black, C. M. Ambros-Rudolph, L. Edwards, and P. J. Lynch, Eds., pp. 37–47, Mosby, 3rd edition, 2008.

[9] M.-M. Roth, "Pregnancy dermatoses: diagnosis, management, and controversies," *American Journal of Clinical Dermatology*, vol. 12, no. 1, pp. 25–41, 2011.

[10] S. E. Kelly, M. M. Black, and S. Fleming, "Pemphigoid gestationis: a unique mechanism of initiation of an autoimmune response by MHC class II molecules," *Journal of Pathology*, vol. 158, no. 1, pp. 81–82, 1989.

[11] L. R. A. Intong and D. F. Murrell, "Pemphigoid gestationis: pathogenesis and clinical features," *Dermatologic Clinics*, vol. 29, no. 3, pp. 447–452, 2011.

[12] K. Semkova and M. Black, "Pemphigoid gestationis: current insights into pathogenesis and treatment," *European Journal of Obstetrics Gynecology and Reproductive Biology*, vol. 145, no. 2, pp. 138–144, 2009.

[13] R. E. Jenkins, S. Hern, and M. M. Black, "Clinical features and management of 87 patients with pemphigoid gestationis," *Clinical & Experimental Dermatology*, vol. 24, no. 4, pp. 255–259, 1999.

[14] C.-C. Chi, S.-H. Wang, R. Charles-Holmes et al., "Pemphigoid gestationis: early onset and blister formation are associated with adverse pregnancy outcomes," *British Journal of Dermatology*, vol. 160, no. 6, pp. 1222–1228, 2009.

[15] J. K. Shornick and M. M. Black, "Secondary autoimmune diseases in herpes gestationis (pemphigoid gestationis)," *Journal of the American Academy of Dermatology*, vol. 26, no. 4, pp. 563–566, 1992.

[16] C. M. Ambros-Rudolph, "Dermatoses of pregnancy—clues to diagnosis, fetal risk and therapy," *Annals of Dermatology*, vol. 23, no. 3, pp. 265–275, 2011.

[17] C. M. Ambros-Rudolph and M. M. Black, "Polymorphic eruption of pregnancy," in *Obstetric and Gynecologic Dermatology*, M. M. Black, C. M. Ambros-Rudolph, L. Edwards, and P. J. Lynch, Eds., pp. 49–55, Mosby, 3rd edition, 2008.

[18] C. M. Rudolph, S. Al-Fares, S. A. Vaughan-Jones, R. R. Müllegger, H. Kerl, and M. M. Black, "Polymorphic eruption of pregnancy: clinicopathology and potential trigger factors in 181 patients," *British Journal of Dermatology*, vol. 154, no. 1, pp. 54–60, 2006.

[19] K. T. Ahmed, A. A. Almashhrawi, R. N. Rahman, G. M. Hammoud, and J. A. Ibdah, "Liver diseases in pregnancy: diseases unique to pregnancy," *World Journal of Gastroenterology*, vol. 19, no. 43, pp. 7639–7646, 2013.

[20] K. Turunen, M. Sumanen, R.-L. Haukilahti, P. Kirkinen, and K. Mattila, "Good pregnancy outcome despite intrahepatic cholestasis," *Scandinavian Journal of Primary Health Care*, vol. 28, no. 2, pp. 102–107, 2010.

[21] B. Berg, G. Helm, L. Petersohn, and N. Tryding, "Cholestasis of pregnancy. Clinical and laboratory studies," *Acta Obstetricia et Gynecologica Scandinavica*, vol. 65, no. 2, pp. 107–113, 1986.

[22] H. Reyes, M. E. Báez, M. C. González et al., "Selenium, zinc and copper plasma levels in intrahepatic cholestasis of pregnancy, in normal pregnancies and in healthy individuals, in Chile," *Journal of Hepatology*, vol. 32, no. 4, pp. 542–549, 2000.

[23] M. M. Păunescu, V. Feier, M. Păunescu, F. Dorneanu, A. Sisak, and C. M. Ambros-Rudolph, "Dermatoses of pregnancy," *Acta Dermatovenerologica Alpina, Pannonica et Adriatica*, vol. 17, no. 1, pp. 4–11, 2008.

[24] J. Kondrackiene, U. Beuers, and L. Kupcinskas, "Efficacy and safety of ursodeoxycholic acid versus cholestyramine in intrahepatic cholestasis of pregnancy," *Gastroenterology*, vol. 129, no. 3, pp. 894–901, 2005.

[25] R. L. Wilder, "Hormones, pregnancy, and autoimmune diseases," *Annals of the New York Academy of Sciences*, vol. 840, pp. 45–50, 1998.

15

Quality of Life in Alopecia Areata: A Sample of Tunisian Patients

Jawaher Masmoudi,[1] **Rim Sellami,**[1] **Uta Ouali,**[1] **Leila Mnif,**[1] **Ines Feki,**[1] **Mariam Amouri,**[2] **Hamida Turki,**[2] **and Abdellaziz Jaoua**[1]

[1] *Department of Psychiatry A, Hédi Chaker University Hospital, Sfax, Tunisia*
[2] *Department of Dermatology, Hédi Chaker University Hospital, Sfax, Tunisia*

Correspondence should be addressed to Jawaher Masmoudi; amirsoussi@yahoo.fr

Academic Editor: Masutaka Furue

Background. Alopecia areata (AA) has a significant impact on the quality of life and social interaction of those suffering from it. Our aim was to assess the impact of AA on the quality of life. *Methods.* Fifty patients diagnosed with AA seen in the Department of Dermatology of Hedi Chaker University Hospital, between March 2010 and July 2010, were included. Quality of life was measured by SF 36; severity of AA was measured by SALT. *Results.* Eighty percent had patchy alopecia with less than 50% involvement, 12% had patchy alopecia with 50–99% involvement, and 8% had alopecia totalis. Compared with the general population, AA patients presented a significantly altered quality of life, found in the global score and in five subscores of the SF-36: mental health, role emotional, social functioning, vitality, and general health. Gender, age, marital status, and severity of alopecia areata had a significant influence on patients' quality of life. *Conclusions.* This study indicates that patients with AA experience a poor quality of life, which impacts their overall health. We suggest screening for psychiatric distress. Studies of interventions such as counseling, psychoeducation, and psychotherapeutic interventions to reduce the impact of the disease may be warranted.

1. Introduction

Alopecia areata (AA) is a common disease with an incidence of 2-3% among the dermatoses and 0.1% in the population at large [1]. This disorder occurs in both sexes, at all ages [2], and is characterized by the sudden appearance of areas of hair loss on the scalp and other hair-bearing areas. Various factors, including immunologic and endocrine abnormalities [3], genetic factors [4], infections [5], and psychological/psychiatric disturbances, have been claimed to play a role in its etiopathogenesis [6]. Hence, it is suspected to be an autoimmune disease having a genetic predisposition and being influenced by environmental and ethnic factors. Epidemiological studies of AA are available from the USA, Japan, and European countries [7–9]. However, there is a paucity of data from Arab countries, with especially one published study from Kuwait done in the pediatric age group [10].

Hair loss significantly impacts an individual's self image, and studies indicate that patients with both clinically apparent and clinically imperceptible hair loss may have significantly decreased quality of life [11, 12]. Quality of life is defined as the subjective perception of the impact on the health status and on the physical, psychological, and social functioning and well-being of the patients [13]. Although AA is a medically benign condition, it can affect patients' quality of life [2]. Indeed, AA can have psychosocial complications, including depression, low self-esteem, altered self-image, and less frequent and enjoyable social engagements [14–16]. To assess the severity of AA, quality of life seems to be a more relevant criterion than clinical evaluation such as AA extension because the perception of patients may differ significantly from those of their health-care providers [13].

The aim of our study was to examine the impact of AA on the different dimensions of quality of life and to determine factors related to an altered quality of life.

2. Methods

All new patients diagnosed with AA seen in the Department of Dermatology of Hedi Chaker University Hospital between March 2010 and July 2010 were included in the study.

Informed consent was obtained from all subjects enrolled. The diagnosis of AA was made by a qualified dermatologist on a clinical basis. Sociodemographic and clinical data including age, sex, family history of AA, site of onset, and associated diseases were recorded for all patients. Included patients underwent full clinical examination to determine the number and extension of the sites affected by AA and the severity of the disease.

The severity of hair loss was assessed by measuring the percentage of the alopecic area on the scalp. Patients with AA were evaluated using Severity of Alopecia Tool (SALT) [17]. The SALT score is computed by measuring the percentage of hair loss in each of 4 areas of the scalp (40% vertex, 18% right profile, 18% left profile, 24% posterior) and adding the total to achieve a composite score.

Patients were divided into four groups according to disease severity: S1-S2: hair loss below 50%; S3-S4: hair loss of 50–99%; S5: total scalp hair loss.

Following examination, a health survey in its short form (SF36) was administered to all included patients. The SF36 health survey is a widely used generic, 36-item, self-reported health status questionnaire assessing eight domains of health status (1) physical functioning; (2) role physical; (3) bodily pain; (4) mental health; (5) role emotional; (6) social functioning; (7) vitality; (8) general health. A score from 0 to 100 is calculated for each subscale, with higher scores indicating better quality of life. It has been translated into Arabic and validated but not yet published [18]. Physical functioning domain addresses physical activities associated with daily life, such as bathing, walking, or carrying groceries. Role-physical domain assesses how physical health affects work. Bodily pain domain measures pain severity and how it interferes with daily activities. Mental health domain assesses the subject's mood, specifically focusing on feelings of sadness and anxiety. Role emotional domain addresses how the subject's emotional state has influenced work and other daily activities. Social functioning domain measures how much emotional or physical problems have interfered with usual social activities. Vitality domain assesses how energetic or tired the subject feels. Finally, general health domain describes how the patient perceives health status. The findings of the SF-36 were compared with those of a control group consisting of healthy volunteers, with no known chronic skin disease, of similar age, sex, and level of education. The group of patients and 50 controls did not show significant differences concerning age ($P = 1.000$), educational level ($P = 0.802$), and gender ($P = 0.987$). The control group had not any organic or psychiatric disease.

The mean total score of each domain of SF36 in patients with AA was compared with the mean score of the control group by t-test. The t-test comparisons for each subscale were evaluated with statistical significance designated as P less than 0.05. We also examined the relationship between different domains of quality of life and several independent variables, including marital status, gender, illness severity, and age. Associations with quality of life were tested using t tests and one-way ANOVAs with post hoc LSD multiple comparison tests and correlations (Spearman and Pearson). The use of parametric versus nonparametric tests was

TABLE 1: Quality of life comparisons between AA patients and controls.

Dimensions of SF-36	Patients M ± ET	Controls M ± ET	P
D1: physical functioning	93.10 ± 12.45	88.30 ± 17.57	0.118
D2: role physical	95.50 ± 10.93	90.20 ± 16.31	0.059
D3: bodily pain	95.40 ± 12.48	89.80 ± 16.22	0.056
D4: mental health	63.64 ± 16.61	77.14 ± 11.03	<0.001
D5: role emotional	33.33 ± 36.26	83.06 ± 24.40	<0.001
D6: social functioning	54.60 ± 33.75	82.20 ± 18.56	<0.001
D7: vitality	62.40 ± 21.19	77.00 ± 14.70	<0.001
D8: general health	58.17 ± 17.06	71.62 ± 13.71	<0.001
Mean score	68.95 ± 13.10	80.52 ± 9.14	<0.001

dependent on the scale of measurement and distribution of the results.

3. Results

Fifty patients were included in the study. Their mean age was 32.92 years (SD = 11.81), having a minimum of 18 years and a maximum of 60 years. There were 48% males and 52% females with a male to female ratio of 0.92. As to the level of education, 18% had elementary school education, 40% had secondary school education, and 42% had higher education level.

Fifty-two percent of patients were single, 46% were married, and 2% of them were divorced. As to occupation, most worked (52%) some were retired (2%), and whereas the others were studying (24%) or unemployed (22%).

At the time of first presentation, 80% had patchy alopecia with less than 50% involvement (S1-S2), 12% had patchy alopecia with 50–99% involvement (S3-S4), and 8% had alopecia totalis.

Patient's quality of life, demonstrated by SF-36 scores, ranged from 38.54 to 92.7 with a mean 68.95 (±13.10). Compared with the general population (Table 1), AA patients presented a significantly altered quality of life, found in the global score and in five subscores of the SF-36: mental health (D4), role emotional (D5), social functioning (D6), vitality (D7), and general health (D8) (Table 1).

Females scored lower on the SF 36 than males: this gender difference was significant for the global score ($P = 0.007$) and three subscores: physical functioning ($P = 0.028$), general health ($P = 0.012$), and role emotional ($P = 0.018$).

The correlation of Pearson indicated a significantly altered mental health domain in younger patients ($r = 0.336$, $P = 0.017$).

Furthermore, we observed a significant difference in the scores of the mental health subscale (D4) between married and unmarried patients ($P = 0.050$): unmarried patients scored lower than married patients.

In our study, we found a relationship between poorer quality of life and severity of AA. This relationship was significant in the SF-36 subscale of mental health and social functioning: patients with 51% to 75% of hair loss (S3)

TABLE 2: Correlation between quality of life and severity.

Dimensions of SF-36	S1 M ± ET	S2 M ± ET	S3 M ± ET	S5 M ± ET	ANOVA F	P
D1: physical functioning	93.87 ± 10.3	86.66 ± 21.06	99.16 ± 2.04	92.5 ± 8.66	1.347	0.271
D2: role physical	94.35 ± 10.62	100	91.66 ± 20.41	100	1.099	0.359
D3: bodily pain	92.58 ± 15.26	100	100	100	1.422	0.249
D4: mental health	66.54 ± 13.93	67 ± 15.65	56.66 ± 20.61	44 ± 21.66	2.978	0.041
D5: role emotional	40.85 ± 38.2	18.51 ± 33.79	33.33 ± 29.81	8.33 ± 16.66	1.641	0.193
D6: social functioning	64.83 ± 29.19	48.88 ± 30.18	21.66 ± 32.5	37.5 ± 43.49	3.856	0.015
D7: vitality	61.45 ± 19.67	59.62 ± 12.07	61.66 ± 32.5	72.5 ± 5	0.316	0.814
D8: general health	59.21 ± 16.65	66.37 ± 13.33	52.2 ± 26.35	55.83 ± 17.92	0.315	0.815
Mean score	71.22 ± 13.33	80.52 ± 9.14	64.54 ± 14.45	63.82 ± 12.09	0.850	0.474

showed significantly lower scores on the social functioning subscale compared to those with hair loss less than 25% (S1) (Table 2). Patients with 100% extent of hair loss (S5) showed significantly lower scores on the mental health subscale compared to those with 51% to 75% of hair loss (S3). Severity of AA was related to lower scores in the mental health domain ($r = -0.379$; $P = 0.007$) as well as lower scores in the social functioning domain ($r = -0.365$; $P = 0.009$).

4. Discussion

In our study, we observed a slight female preponderance for AA. (M/F: 0.92). This is in agreement with other studies [19–21]. However, the results of the literature are disparate. Thus, for some authors, AA affects men and women with the same proportions [2, 22, 23].

We have found that included patients had a lower quality of life compared to the control group. Dimensions of the SF36 referring to psychological and social components were particularly affected. Indeed, several studies underline that the experience of AA is psychologically damaging, causes intense emotional suffering, and leads to personal, social, and work related problems [24]. Our results are in line with authors' findings that report quality of life to be seriously impaired, mainly, by altering self-perception and self-esteem [25, 26].

This may be because of the special importance of hair in appearance [27]. Hair is a distinctive and valued facial characteristic, and the way it is styled helps to define the individual's self-concept and identity. Through hair loss, the ability to manipulate and improve appearance may become uncertain and out of one's control [28, 29]. In fact, AA might make the individual focus on the bold patches, which leads to even greater distress.

On the other hand, the alteration of psychological and relational dimensions of patients' quality of life could be dependent on the regular recurrence and unpredictable severity of AA, leaving a feeling of incomprehension and vulnerability [30]. Moreover, the unpredictable hair loss and the fact that there is currently no effective remedy could cause particular anxiety related to uncertainty about the patient's future appearance [31].

The disease not only has a severe psychological impact but also causes a marked disturbance in the social life of the patients forcing them to avoid social meetings, change their hair style, and alter the type of clothing. In Tunisia, where Islamic customs prevail, women try to cover their hair. This observation was found in Kuwaiti and Egyptian studies [32].

Our results showed that women have a more significantly altered quality of life than men. The dimensions of general health and role emotional were particularly affected. In consistency with our findings, several other studies have reported a particularly impaired quality of life for women [11, 33]. Femininity, sexuality, and personality are symbolically linked to a woman's hair, more so than for a man [34]. Indeed, a women's self-esteem is often more dependent on physical appearance compared to men [29], and hair strongly influences whether or not an individual is seen as physically attractive [35]. In line with social stereotypes, men were more likely to express concern over work interference, whereas women were more concerned with the social impact of such a visible condition. There is an important link between hair and identity, especially for women, even in Arab Muslim culture. Hair loss may be seen in terms of abnormality and as a failure to conform to the norms of physical appearance in society, which has the potential to set people apart in their own estimation and in the estimation of others. So, AA in women significantly affects self-image, and psychosocial factors often negatively impact patients' quality of life [33, 36–38].

In our study, we found that a patient's age was correlated to the SF 36 dimension of mental health: the younger the patient is, the more his mental health is negatively affected by AA. Furthermore, our study showed that unmarried patients had significantly altered scores in the dimension of mental health compared to married patients. Our results are in accordance with two recent studies [32, 38] which found that the impact of AA on the quality of life was more pronounced within younger age groups. Indeed, hair loss would entail more concern among those most vulnerable such as younger patients. These results denote that unestablished social life in younger and unmarried patients makes them worry about their future resulting in more psychological distress.

In our study, we found a relationship between the severity of AA and poorer quality of life (Figure 1).

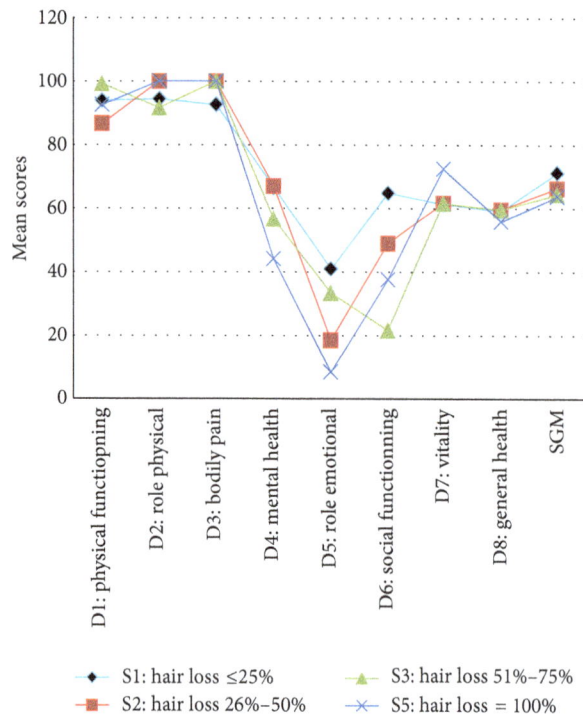

FIGURE 1: Mean scores SF-36 depending on the severity (SALT).

Legend:
- S1: hair loss ≤25%
- S2: hair loss 26%–50%
- S3: hair loss 51%–75%
- S5: hair loss = 100%

5. Conclusion

This study indicates that patients with AA experience a poor quality of life, which profoundly impacts their overall health and sense of well-being. Also, when examining a patient who is at high risk for poor quality of life, it would be reasonable to screen for psychiatric distress. Those with mild impairments should be encouraged to discuss their concerns at clinic visits or in a support-group setting. Moreover, the efficacy of any treatment must also consider the improvement in quality of life and not just see the percentage of hair regrowth. Studies of interventions such as counseling, psychoeducation, and psychotherapeutic interventions to reduce the impact of the disease may be warranted.

Conflict of Interests

The authors have no potential conflict of interests.

References

[1] E. Healy and S. Rogers, "PUVA treatment for alopecia areata—does it work? a retrospective review of 102 cases," *British Journal of Dermatology*, vol. 129, no. 1, pp. 42–44, 1993.

[2] S. A. Muller and R. K. Winkelmann, "Alopecia areata: an evaluation of 736 patients," *Archives of Dermatology*, vol. 88, pp. 290–297, 1963.

[3] V. H. Price and B. W. Colombe, "Heritable factors distinguish two types of alopecia areata," *Dermatologic Clinics*, vol. 14, no. 4, pp. 679–689, 1996.

[4] J. Shapiro, "Alopecia areata: update on therapy," *Dermatologic Clinics*, vol. 11, no. 1, pp. 35–46, 1993.

[5] R. B. Skinner Jr., W. H. Light, G. F. Bale, E. W. Rosenberg, and C. Leonardi, "Alopecia areata and presence of cytomegalovirus DNA," *Journal of the American Medical Association*, vol. 273, no. 18, pp. 1419–1420, 1995.

[6] E. Arca and Z. Kurumlu, "Etiopathogenesis, clinical features, and diagnosis in alopecia areata," *Dermatose*, vol. 2, pp. 83–89, 2003.

[7] D. A. De Berker, A. G. Messenger, and R. D. Sinclair, "Disorders of hair," in *Rook's Textbook of Dermatology*, T. Burns, S. Breathnach, N. Cox, and C. Griffiths, Eds., vol. 4, pp. 36–63, Blackwell Scientific Publications, Oxford, UK, 2004.

[8] L. A. Drake, R. I. Ceilley, R. L. Cornelison et al., "Guidelines of care for alopecia areata," *Journal of the American Academy of Dermatology*, vol. 26, no. 2, pp. 247–250, 1992.

[9] V. H. Price, "Alopecia areata: clinical aspects," *Journal of Investigative Dermatology*, vol. 96, no. 5, p. 68, 1991.

[10] A. Nanda, A. S. Al-Fouzan, and F. Al-Hasawi, "Alopecia areata in children: a clinical profile," *Pediatric Dermatology*, vol. 19, no. 6, pp. 482–485, 2002.

[11] N. Hunt and S. McHale, "The psychological impact of alopecia," *British Medical Journal*, vol. 331, no. 7522, pp. 951–953, 2005.

[12] F. Poot, "Psychological consequences of chronic hair diseases," *Revue Medicale de Bruxelles*, vol. 25, no. 4, pp. 286–288, 2004.

[13] G. Kiebert, S. V. Sorensen, D. Revicki et al., "Atopic dermatitis is associated with a decrement in health-related quality of life," *International Journal of Dermatology*, vol. 41, no. 3, pp. 151–158, 2002.

The domains referring to psychological and social components were particularly affected in patients with severe forms of AA. Indeed, given the psychological importance of hair, patients with severe forms of AA might find it more difficult to cope with their hair loss. According to Tan et al. [19], patients who presented limited AA appeared to be less affected than those who had an extensive AA. This shows that if AA is more severe, its impact on quality of life is more important. However, the relationship between disease severity and impaired quality of life has not been confirmed by all studies [39]. A study by Krueger et al. [40] revealed that AA areas in particularly visible locations had a more severe impact on quality of life than an area of the same size in a less visible location. Interestingly, a study by Reid et al. [41] showed that patients' quality of life was strongly correlated with the patient's perception of hair loss rather than with the clinical severity of hair loss. Generally, patients tend to perceive their hair loss as worse than clinical assessment, but patients and physicians seem to have synchronous scales of severity.

This lack of parallelism between clinical severity, patients' perception of hair loss, and psychological impact might be partly responsible for the frequent underestimation of psychological distress [42].

There are some limitations to our study that should be taken into consideration. First, the sample size was relatively small. Furthermore, it could have been interesting to assess the quality of life with a scale specially designed for dermatologic patients. However, to our knowledge, there is no such instrument translated in Arabic language so far.

[14] H. O. Beard, "Social and psychological implications of alopecia areata," *Journal of the American Academy of Dermatology*, vol. 14, no. 4, pp. 697–700, 1986.

[15] A. Firooz, M. R. Firoozabadi, B. Ghazisaidi, and Y. Dowlati, "Concepts of patients with alopecia areata about their disease," *BMC Dermatology*, vol. 5, 2005.

[16] M. A. Gupta and A. K. Gupta, "Depression and suicidal ideation in dermatology patients with acne, alopecia areata, atopic dermatitis and psoriasis," *British Journal of Dermatology*, vol. 139, no. 5, pp. 846–850, 1998.

[17] E. A. Olsen, M. K. Hordinsky, V. H. Price et al., "Alopecia areata investigational assessment guidelines—part II," *Journal of the American Academy of Dermatology*, vol. 51, no. 3, pp. 440–447, 2004.

[18] C. Allouche, L'indice SF36 de la qualité de vie: traduction en langue arabe et étude des qualités métrologiques. Doctoral dissertation in medicine. Sfax 2007. Number 2553.

[19] E. Tan, Y.-K. Tay, C.-L. Goh, and Y. C. Giam, "The pattern and profile of alopecia areata in Singapore—a study of 219 Asians," *International Journal of Dermatology*, vol. 41, no. 11, pp. 748–753, 2002.

[20] A. Kavak, N. Yeşildal, A. H. Parlak et al., "Alopecia areata in Turkey: demographic and clinical features," *Journal of the European Academy of Dermatology and Venereology*, vol. 22, no. 8, pp. 977–981, 2008.

[21] K. P. Kyriakis, K. Paltatzidou, E. Kosma, E. Sofouri, A. Tadros, and E. Rachioti, "Alopecia areata prevalence by gender and age," *Journal of the European Academy of Dermatology and Venereology*, vol. 23, no. 5, pp. 572–573, 2009.

[22] S. Madani and J. Shapiro, "Alopecia areata update," *Journal of the American Academy of Dermatology*, vol. 42, no. 4, pp. 549–570, 2000.

[23] D. Wasserman, D. A. Guzman-Sanchez, K. Scott, and A. Mcmichael, "Alopecia areata," *International Journal of Dermatology*, vol. 46, no. 2, pp. 121–131, 2007.

[24] N. Hunt and S. McHale, "Reported experiences of persons with alopecia areata," *Journal of Loss and Trauma*, vol. 10, no. 1, pp. 33–50, 2005.

[25] M. Dubois, K. Baumstarck-Barrau, C. Gaudy-Marqueste et al., "Quality of life in alopecia areata: a study of 60 cases," *Journal of Investigative Dermatology*, vol. 130, no. 12, pp. 2830–2833, 2010.

[26] A. T. Gulec, N. Tanriverdi, D. Dürü et al., "The role of psychological factors in alopecia areata and the impact of the disease on the quality of life," *International Journal of Dermatology*, vol. 43, no. 5, pp. 352–356, 2004.

[27] A. Firooz, M. R. Firoozabadi, B. Ghazisaidi, and Y. Dowlati, "Concepts of patients with alopecia areata about their disease," *BMC Dermatology*, vol. 5, 2005.

[28] T. F. Cash, "The psychosocial consequences of androgenetic alopecia: a review of the research literature," *British Journal of Dermatology*, vol. 141, no. 3, pp. 398–405, 1999.

[29] T. F. Cash, "The psychology of hair loss and its implications for patient care," *Clinics in Dermatology*, vol. 19, no. 2, pp. 161–166, 2001.

[30] Assouly P. Pelade. Encycl Med Chir, Dermatologie. 2006, 37-400-C-10.

[31] L. Papadopoulos and R. Bor, *Psychological Approaches to dermatology*, BPS Books/in lived experience of AA, Leicester, UK, 1999.

[32] N. Al-Mutairi and O. N. Eldin, "Clinical profile and impact on quality of life: seven years experience with patients of alopecia areata," *Indian Journal of Dermatology, Venereology and Leprology*, vol. 77, no. 4, pp. 489–493, 2011.

[33] D. Williamson, M. Gonzalez, and A. Y. Finlay, "The effect of hair loss in quality of life," *Journal of the European Academy of Dermatology and Venereology*, vol. 15, no. 2, pp. 137–139, 2001.

[34] N. Wolf, *The Beauty Myth*, William Morrow and Company, New York, NY, USA, 1991.

[35] G. L. Patzer, "Psychologic and sociologic dimensions of hair: an aspect of the physical attractiveness phenomenon," *Clinics in Dermatology*, vol. 6, no. 4, pp. 93–101, 1988.

[36] F. M. Camacho and M. Garcia-Hernandez, "Psychological features of androgenetic alopecia," *Journal of the European Academy of Dermatology and Venereology*, vol. 16, no. 5, pp. 476–480, 2002.

[37] J. Y. M. Koo, W. V. R. Shellow, C. P. Hallman, and J. E. Edwards, "Alopecia areata and increased prevalence of psychiatric disorders," *International Journal of Dermatology*, vol. 33, no. 12, pp. 849–850, 1994.

[38] T. Cartwright, N. Endean, and A. Porter, "Illness perceptions, coping and quality of life in patients with alopecia," *British Journal of Dermatology*, vol. 160, no. 5, pp. 1034–1039, 2009.

[39] M. A. Gupta and A. K. Gupta, "Psychiatric and psychological co-morbidity in patients with dermatologic disorders: epidemiology and management," *American Journal of Clinical Dermatology*, vol. 4, no. 12, pp. 833–842, 2003.

[40] G. G. Krueger, S. R. Feldman, C. Camisa et al., "Two considerations for patients with psoriasis and their clinicians: what defines mild, moderate, and severe psoriasis? what constitutes a clinically significant improvement when treating psoriasis?" *Journal of the American Academy of Dermatology*, vol. 43, no. 2 I, pp. 281–285, 2000.

[41] E. E. Reid, A. C. Haley, J. H. Borovicka et al., "Clinical severity does not reliably predict quality of life in women with alopecia areata, telogen effluvium, or androgenic alopecia," *Journal of the American Academy of Dermatology*, vol. 66, no. 3, pp. e97–e102, 2012.

[42] S. G. Consoli, M. Chastaing, and L. Misery, "Psychiatrie et dermatologie," Encycl Med Chir. 2010, 98-874-A-10.

16

Decreased Circulating T Regulatory Cells in Egyptian Patients with Nonsegmental Vitiligo: Correlation with Disease Activity

Doaa Salah Hegab[1] and Mohamed Attia Saad Attia[2]

[1]*Faculty of Medicine, Dermatology and Venereology Department, Tanta University Hospitals, El Geish Street, Tanta 31111, Egypt*
[2]*Faculty of Medicine, Clinical Pathology Department, Tanta University Hospitals, El Geish Street, Tanta 31111, Egypt*

Correspondence should be addressed to Doaa Salah Hegab; doaasalahhegab@yahoo.com

Academic Editor: Elizabeth Helen Kemp

Background. Vitiligo is an acquired depigmentary skin disorder resulting from autoimmune destruction of melanocytes. Regulatory T cells (Tregs), specifically $CD4^+CD25^+$ and Forkhead box P3$^+$ (FoxP3$^+$) Tregs, acquired notable attention because of their role in a variety of autoimmune pathologies. Dysregulation of Tregs may be one of the factors that can break tolerance to melanocyte self-antigens and contribute to vitiligo pathogenesis. *Methods.* In order to sustain the role of Tregs in pathogenesis and disease activity of vitiligo, surface markers for $CD4^+CD25^+$ and FoxP3$^+$ peripheral Tregs were evaluated by flow cytometry in 80 Egyptian patients with nonsegmental vitiligo in addition to 60 healthy control subjects and correlated with clinical findings. *Results.* Vitiligo patients had significantly decreased numbers of both peripheral $CD4^+CD25^+$ and FoxP3$^+$ T cells compared to control subjects (11.49% ± 8.58% of $CD4^+$ T cells versus 21.20% ± 3.08%, and 1.09% ± 0.96% versus 1.44% ± 0.24%, resp., $P < 0.05$ for both). Peripheral numbers of $CD4^+CD25^+$ and FoxP3$^+$ Tregs correlated negatively with VIDA score. *Conclusion.* Treg depletion with impaired immune downregulatory function might play a key role in the autoimmune conditions beyond nonsegmental vitiligo particularly in active cases. Effective Treg cell-based immunotherapies might be a future hope for patients with progressive vitiligo.

1. Introduction

Vitiligo is an acquired cutaneous disorder characterized by progressive, selective destruction of melanocytes and clinically characterized by the development of milky white macules and patches [1]. It is a multifactorial polygenic disorder and several theories have been proposed about the pathogenesis of vitiligo including autoimmune hypothesis, reactive oxygen species model, zinc-α2-glycoprotein deficiency hypothesis, viral theory, intrinsic theory, and biochemical, molecular, and cellular alterations accounting for loss of functioning melanocytes [2]. The integration of epidemiological, clinical, histoimmunological, and therapeutic data strongly supports immunological pathomechanism in vitiligo, which is commonly associated with autoimmune diseases like autoimmune thyroid diseases, insulin-dependent diabetes mellitus, alopecia areata, and pernicious anemia [3–5].

T regulatory cells (Tregs) are a component of the immune system that constitutes a key mechanism in maintaining peripheral self-tolerance through the control of autoreactive lymphocyte activation and the prevention of harmful effects of such activation. These cells are involved in shutting down immune responses after they have successfully eliminated invading organisms [6]. Natural Tregs express the transcriptional factor Forkhead box P3 (FoxP3), which serves as the dedicated mediator of the genetic program for Tregs development and function. FoxP3$^+$ is a reliable and specific marker of Tregs [7]. Natural and induced Tregs have many subsets with the most well-understood being those that express CD4, CD25, and FoxP3 ($CD4^+CD25^+$ FoxP3$^+$ Tregs), which had acquired notable attention because of their role in a variety of autoimmune pathologies, inflammatory disorders such as asthma and colitis, and immune responses to tissue transplants, tumors, and various infectious agents pathologies [8]. There are several other subpopulations of Tregs such as Treg17 cells [9]; interleukin 10- (IL-10-) producing "Tr1" cells; transforming growth factor-β- (TGF-β-) producing T

TABLE 1: Demographic and clinical characteristics of study participants.

	Vitiligo patients $n = 80$	Control group $n = 60$
Range of age in years, mean (SD)	9–60, 27.25 (14.32)	20–50, 33.9 (9.5)
Gender, n (%)		
Male	36 (45)	36 (60)
Female	44 (55)	24 (40)
Range of disease duration in years, mean (SD)	0.33–49, 5.34 (4.81)	NA
Type of vitiligo, n (%)		
Localised	36 (45)	
Generalised	32 (40)	NA
Acrofacial	12 (15)	
Range of VASI score, mean (SD)	10–90, 42.3 (26.7)	NA
VIDA score, n (%)		
0	16 (20)	
+1	12 (15)	
+2	32 (40)	NA
+3	16 (20)	
+4	4 (5)	

NA: not applicable. SD: standard deviation.

helper type 3 cells; CD8$^+$ T suppressor cells; natural killer T cells; CD4$^-$CD8$^-$ T cells; and $\gamma\delta$ T cells [10].

An altered generation of Tregs or a decrease in their suppressive functions may tip the balance towards autoimmunity, triggering the destruction of melanocytes and development of vitiligo [11].

This study aimed to evaluate the alterations in the numbers of peripheral CD4$^+$CD25$^+$ and FoxP3$^+$ Treg lymphocytes by flow cytometry in a sample of Egyptian patients with nonsegmental vitiligo versus health controls and to correlate these alterations with clinical findings of cases including vitiligo disease severity and activity.

2. Materials and Methods

2.1. Study Groups. The present case-control study enrolled 80 Egyptian patients with nonsegmental vitiligo, including 36 males (45%) and 44 females (55%), in addition to 60 age- and sex-matched healthy volunteers as control subjects, including 36 males (60%) and 24 females (40%). Table 1 shows the included subjects' demographic and clinical features. Vitiligo Area Scoring Index (VASI) [12] and Vitiligo Index of Disease Activity (VIDA) score [13] were determined for vitiligo patients. Patients who received systemic steroids or phototherapy for vitiligo in the preceding 6 weeks were excluded. Patients with comorbidities of other dermatologic or systemic diseases that may affect Tregs were also excluded. Two mL of peripheral venous blood was collected from all included subjects during their visits to the outpatient clinics of Dermatology and Venereology Department of Tanta University Hospitals after signing an informed written consent. Research approval was obtained from the Institutional Ethical Committee of Tanta University.

2.2. Antibodies Used and Flow Cytometric Analysis. The following monoclonal antibodies to human cell-surface molecules were used: anti-CD4-PerCP, anti-CD25-PE, and anti-FoxP3-APC, while the negative controls used were goat IgG-PerCP, IgG-PE, and IgG-APC (Becton-Dickinson Immunocytometry Systems, San Jose, CA, USA). Fluorocytometry was performed with a flow cytometer (FACSCalibur; Becton-Dickinson Immunocytometry Systems) equipped with a 488 nm blue laser (488-nm) and a red diode laser (635 nm) for multicolour fluorescence, plus forward-scatter and side-scatter measurements. Automated CellQuest Pro software (Becton-Dickinson Immunocytometry Systems) was used for fluorocytometric data analysis and graphic display, and the instrument was set by using calibrated beads provided. A minimum of 10.000 cells was measured in each analysis.

2.3. Statistical Analysis. Data were statistically analyzed by using Statistical Package for Social Sciences (SPSS Version 18). Data were expressed as the mean ± standard deviation, unless otherwise specified. Flow cytometric data were compared statistically among the groups by using the Mann-Whitney U test. The correlation coefficient (r) was generated by using Spearman's rank correlation. A P value of less than 0.05 was considered a statistically significant difference.

3. Results

3.1. Numbers of Peripheral CD4$^+$CD25$^+$ T Cells in Study Participants. Treg cells were identified within peripheral CD4$^+$ T-cell population according to their expression level of CD25 (Figures 1(a) and 1(b)). CD4$^+$CD25$^+$ T cells were CD4$^+$ T-cell subsets with bright CD25 surface expression and

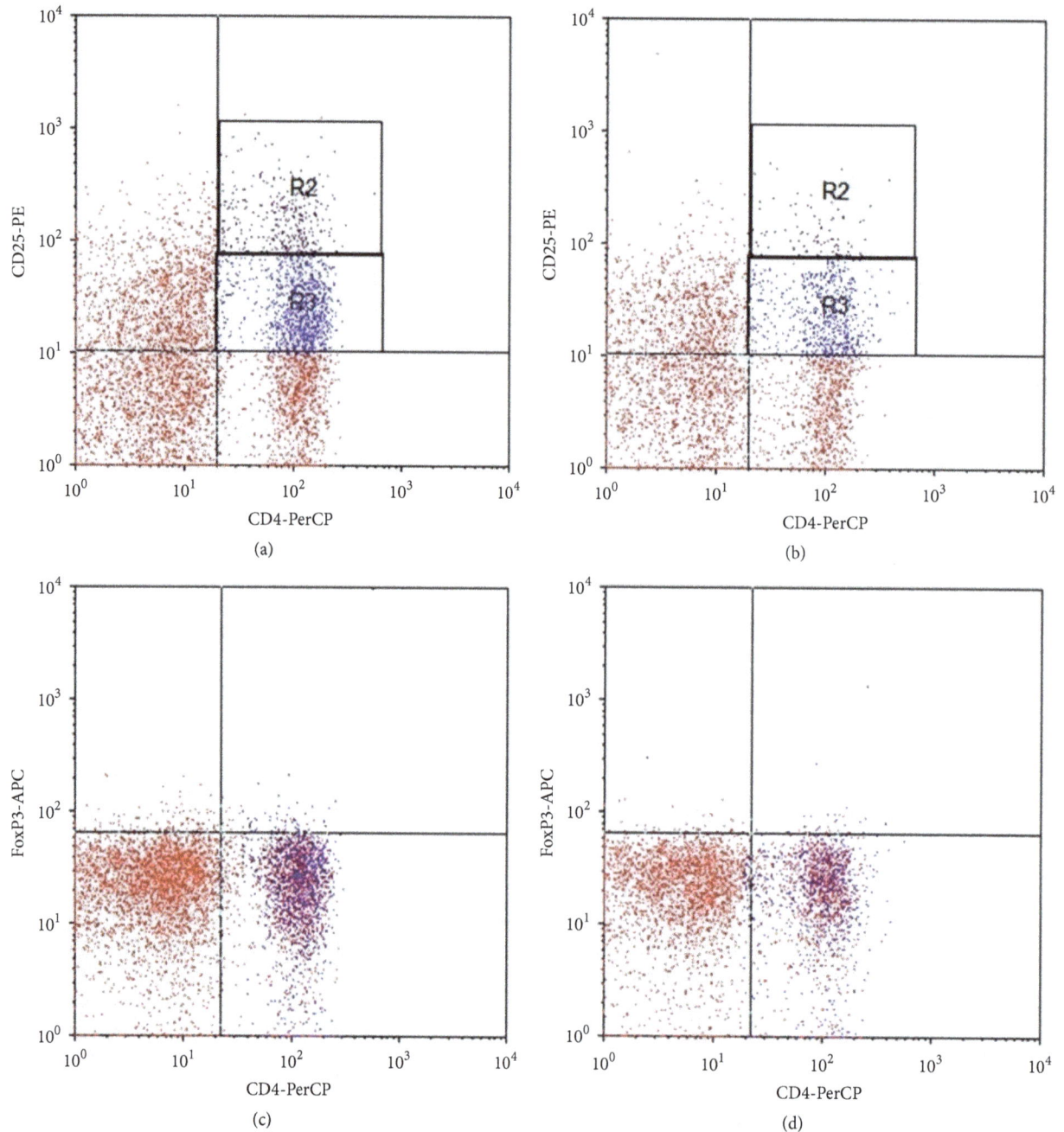

FIGURE 1: Frequency of circulating $CD4^+CD25^+$ Tregs and $CD4^+FoxP3^+$ T cells in healthy subjects and nonsegmental vitiligo patients by flow cytometry dot plot. (a) and (b) Representative profiles demonstrating Tregs as the $CD4^+CD25^{high}$ (R2) and $CD4^+CD25^{low}$ (R3) T-cell fraction by FACS analysis ((a) in a healthy subject, (b) in a vitiligo patient). (c) and (d) Representative profiles demonstrating Tregs as $FoxP3^+$ CD4 T cells ((c) in a healthy subject, (d) in a vitiligo patient).

were defined accordingly (including both $CD4^+CD25^{low}$ and, more importantly, $CD4^+CD25^{high}$).

Our results showed a statistically significant decrease in the percentage of peripheral $CD4^+CD25^+$ T cells in vitiligo patients (range from 2.9% to 34% of $CD4^+$ T cells with a mean of 11.49% ± 8.58%) compared to healthy controls (range from 17% to 27% with a mean of 21.20% ± 3.08%) with P value <0.05 (Figure 2(a)).

3.2. Numbers of Peripheral $FoxP3^+$ Tregs in Study Participants. FoxP3 expression was determined among the peripheral $CD4^+$ T cells (Figures 1(c) and 1(d)). The percentage of peripheral $FoxP3^+$ Tregs in vitiligo patients group ranged from 0.6% to 2.1% of $CD4^+$ T cells with a mean of 1.09% ± 0.96% which was significantly lower than that of control group which ranged from 0.04% to 2.0% with a mean of 1.44% ± 0.24% ($P < 0.05$) (Figure 2(b)).

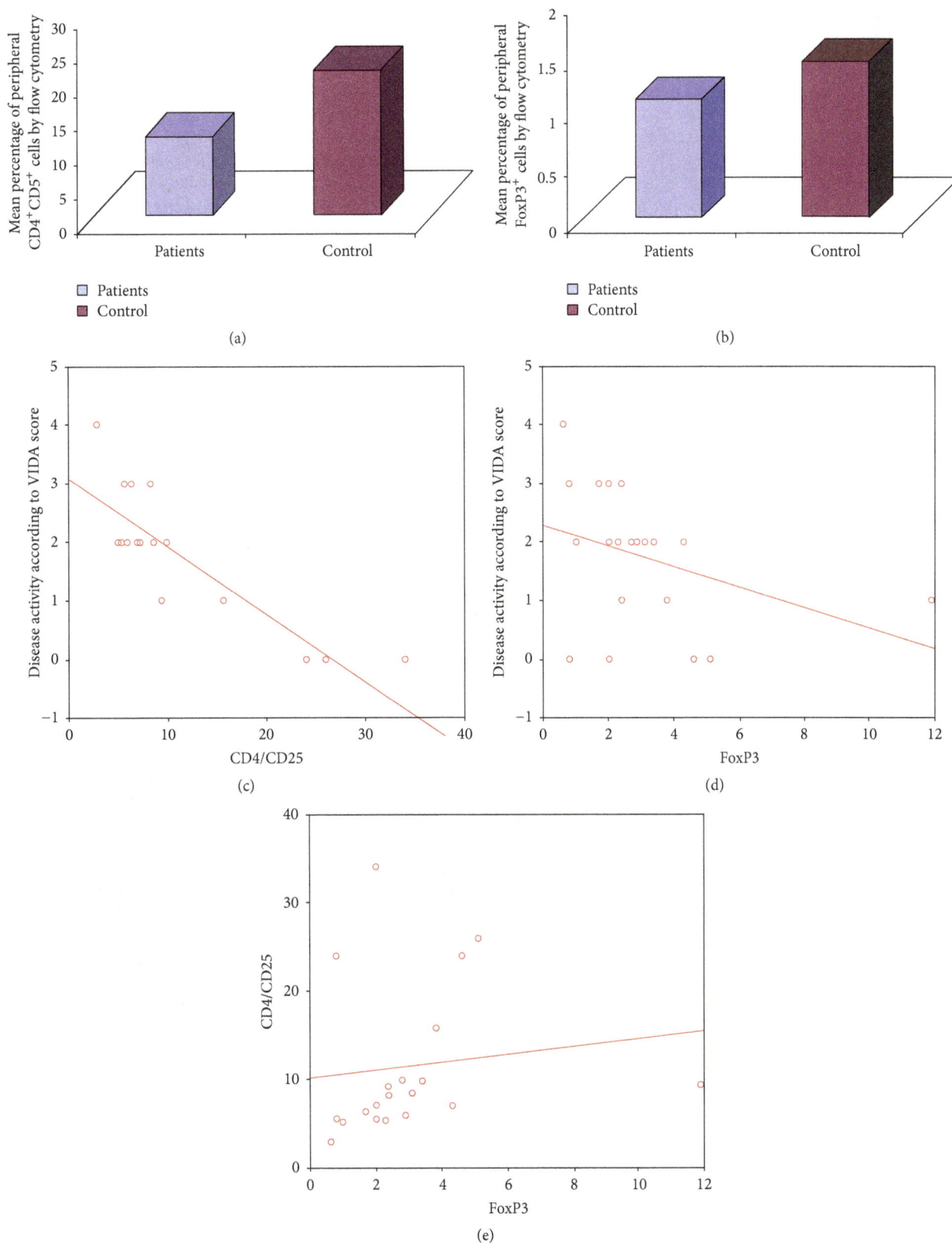

FIGURE 2: (a) The mean percentage of peripheral CD4$^+$CD25$^+$ Treg was significantly reduced in vitiligo compared to healthy controls. (b) The mean percentage of peripheral FoxP3$^+$ T cells from total peripheral CD4$^+$ cells was significantly reduced in vitiligo patients compared to controls. (c) Correlation between percentage of peripheral CD4$^+$CD25$^+$ lymphocytes and VIDA score. (d) Correlation between percentage of peripheral FoxP3$^+$ lymphocytes and VIDA score. (e) Correlation between percentage of peripheral FoxP3$^+$ lymphocytes in vitiligo patients group and the percentage of CD4$^+$CD25$^+$ lymphocytes in vitiligo patients.

3.3. Correlation of the Numbers of Peripheral CD4⁺CD25⁺ T Cells and FoxP3⁺ Tregs with the Patients' Clinical Findings and with Each Other. A statistically significant negative correlation was observed between the percentage of CD4⁺CD25⁺ T cells and FoxP3⁺ Tregs in the peripheral blood of vitiligo patients and vitiligo disease activity according to VIDA score ($r = -0.851$, $P < 0.001$ and $r = -0.512$, $P < 0.05$, resp.) (Figures 2(c) and 2(d)), while a statistically significant positive correlation was observed between peripheral percentage of FoxP3⁺ Tregs and the percentage of CD4⁺CD25⁺ cells in vitiligo patients ($r = 0.369$, $P < 0.05$) (Figure 2(e)).

Each of circulating CD4⁺CD25⁺ Tregs percentage and FoxP3⁺ Tregs percentage did not correlate with patients' age, vitiligo disease duration, or VASI score.

4. Discussion

Immunological self-tolerance is maintained not only by deletion of self-reactive lymphocytes in the central lymphoid organs but also by the control of their activation and expansion in the periphery [14]. As a key mechanism of such peripheral self-tolerance, naturally occurring Tregs suppress the expansion/activation of self-reactive T cells which have escaped thymic negative selection. The majority of these Tregs constitutively express CD25⁺ (IL-2R α-chain) and constitute about 5–10% of peripheral CD4⁺ T cells in mice and humans [15]. FoxP3⁺ can be specifically expressed in CD4⁺CD25⁺ Treg cells and it is associated with their development and function [16].

The role of Tregs in vitiligo pathogenesis has been a recent topic of research, and there is evidence that Tregs are jeopardized in vitiligo patients [2]. However, there is some contradicting data and this subject demands further investigation.

In our study, the percentage of CD4⁺CD25⁺ T cells in the peripheral blood of vitiligo patients was significantly lower than healthy controls. This matches the results of several previous reports [17–19].

On the other hand, some other studies had reported a nonsignificant increase in the peripheral percentage of CD4⁺CD25⁺ T cells in vitiligo patients compared to healthy controls [20, 21]. In another report, the percentage of CD4⁺CD25⁺ T cells was significantly elevated in the vitiligo patient cohort relative to normal control donors and this finding had been considered as a protective mechanism against the autoimmune process. Nevertheless, their observation that peripheral blood levels of these cells apparently did not correlate with severity of the disease or its rate of progression suggested that they may be induced simply by occurrence of the disease and do not correlate directly with autoimmune processes [22].

In the current study a negative correlation was observed between the percentage of peripheral CD4⁺CD25⁺ T cells in vitiligo patients and disease activity according to VIDA score. This result is in agreement with previous studies that detected reduced percentage of CD4⁺CD25⁺ T cells in peripheral blood of progressive vitiligo patients compared to the patients with stable vitiligo, and functional analysis of peripheral Tregs in vitiligo patients showed a correlation of

Tregs functions with the disease status [18, 20]. Moreover, Lili et al. observed that the percentage of circulating Treg cells increased significantly after treatment-induced disease stabilization [19].

In the present study the percentage of peripheral FoxP3⁺ cells in vitiligo patients was also significantly low compared to healthy controls and this matches previous reports [18, 23]. On the other hand, Ben Ahmed et al. suggested a recruitment of Tregs from the peripheral blood to the site of vitiligo which was further corroborated by the significant increase of FoxP3 expression in the vitiliginous skin of patients [20].

Among the clinical parameters of our vitiligo patients, a significant negative correlation was detected between the percentage of FoxP3⁺ cells in peripheral blood and VIDA score. This comes in agreement with a previous study in which VASI, VIDA, and stress scores correlated negatively with FoxP3⁺ cell levels both in peripheral blood (by real time PCR) and in skin samples (by immunohistochemistry) [23]. However, no evidence of a correlation between Tregs and either activity or duration of vitiligo was found by Moftah et al. in 2014 [24].

In the current study, a significant positive correlation was observed between the peripheral percentage of FoxP3⁺ cells and that of CD4⁺CD25⁺ T cells in vitiligo patients. This matches the results of previous studies [18, 25]. Yagi et al. showed in their study that FoxP3⁺ is preferentially and stably expressed in Tregs cells in humans and that ex vivo retroviral gene transfer of FoxP3⁺ can convert human naive CD4⁺ T cells into a regulatory T-cell phenotype similar to CD4⁺CD25⁺ Tregs cells, indicating that FoxP3⁺ may be a master regulatory gene for the function of CD4⁺CD25⁺ Treg cells in humans [26].

In vitiligo, the dysfunction of Tregs could result from the alteration of generation, peripheral survival, activation, suppressor mechanisms, or migratory behavior of these cells [27, 28]. Decreased percentage of peripheral CD4⁺CD25⁺ Tregs and decreased expression of FoxP3⁺ might impair the suppressive activity of Treg cells on cell proliferation with breakage of tolerance to melanocyte self-antigens which could contribute to the pathogenesis of vitiligo [17]. A previous study had indicated that an imbalance of CD8⁺ cytotoxic T lymphocytes and natural Tregs in frequency and function might be involved in the progression of generalized vitiligo. The deficiency and dysfunction of natural Treg cell subpopulations were thought to help in a global expansion and widespread activation of CD8⁺ T-cell population, which could result in the destruction of melanocytes and an elevated frequency of associated autoimmune diseases in generalized vitiligo patients [19].

Regulatory cytokines produced by Treg cells, such as IL-10 and TGF-β, are suggested to be related to the stability of vitiligo [29]. In 2013, Tembhre et al. detected increased serum levels of IL-10, IL-13, and IL-17A and decreased concentrations of TGF-β1 in patients with vitiligo and that might facilitate the melanocyte cytotoxicity; meanwhile treatment with NB-UVB was capable of elevating TGF-β levels, suggesting that Treg cytokines might play an important role in repigmentation [30]. Hegazy et al. proposed that restoration of the balance between Th17 and Tregs might represent a novel pathway for the improvement that NB-UVB exerts in vitiligo patients [31]. In the same regard, Eby et al. hypothesized that promoting Treg skin homing through enhanced expression of CCL22 might suppress depigmentation in vitiligo [32]. There is a future potential to utilize Treg and Treg-friendly therapies to replace current general immunosuppressives and induce tolerance as a path towards a drug-free strategy without associated toxicities in autoimmune diseases including vitiligo [33].

In conclusion, our results suggest that peripheral Treg depletion with impaired immune downregulatory function might participate in the autoimmune conditions beyond the pathophysiology and activity of nonsegmental vitiligo. Effective Treg cell-based immunotherapies might be a future hope for patients with progressive vitiligo. Larger scale studies might provide a better understanding of Tregs populations and functions, and that might help in successful treatment of autoimmune responses in active vitiligo based on induction or expansion of antigen-specific Tregs.

Conflict of Interests

The authors declare that there is no conflict of interests regarding the publication of this paper.

References

[1] A. Alikhan, L. M. Felsten, M. Daly, and V. Petronic-Rosic, "Vitiligo: a comprehensive overview Part I. Introduction, epidemiology, quality of life, diagnosis, differential diagnosis, associations, histopathology, etiology, and work-up," *Journal of the American Academy of Dermatology*, vol. 65, no. 3, pp. 473–491, 2011.

[2] G. F. Mohammed, A. H. Gomaa, and M. S. Al-Dhubaibi, "Highlights in pathogenesis of vitiligo," *World Journal of Clinical Cases*, vol. 3, no. 3, pp. 221–230, 2015.

[3] K. Ongenae, N. Van Geel, and J.-M. Naeyaert, "Evidence for an autoimmune pathogenesis of vitiligo," *Pigment Cell Research*, vol. 16, no. 2, pp. 90–100, 2003.

[4] J. Kasznicki and J. Drzewoski, "A case of autoimmune urticaria accompanying autoimmune polyglandular syndrome type III associated with Hashimoto's disease, type 1 diabetes mellitus, and vitiligo," *Endokrynologia Polska*, vol. 65, no. 4, pp. 320–323, 2014.

[5] N. Oiso, T. Suzuki, K. Fukai, I. Katayama, and A. Kawada, "Nonsegmental vitiligo and autoimmune mechanism," *Dermatology Research and Practice*, vol. 2011, Article ID 518090, 7 pages, 2011.

[6] Í. Caramalho, H. Nunes-Cabaço, R. B. Foxall, and A. E. Sousa, "Regulatory T-cell development in the human thymus," *Frontiers in Immunology*, vol. 6, article 395, 2015.

[7] K. E. Birch, M. Vukmanovic-Stejic, J. R. Reed, A. N. Akbar, and M. H. A. Rustin, "The immunomodulatory effects of regulatory T cells: implications for immune regulation in the skin," *British Journal of Dermatology*, vol. 152, no. 3, pp. 409–417, 2005.

[8] S. Sakaguchi, "Naturally arising CD4$^+$ regulatory T cells for immunologic self-tolerance and negative control of immune responses," *Annual Review of Immunology*, vol. 22, pp. 531–562, 2004.

[9] B. Singh, J. A. Schwartz, C. Sandrock, S. M. Bellemore, and E. Nikoopour, "Modulation of autoimmune diseases by interleukin (IL)-17 producing regulatory T helper (Th17) cells,"

[10] Q. Tang and J. A. Bluestone, "The Foxp3+ regulatory T cell: a jack of all trades, master of regulation," *Nature Immunology*, vol. 9, no. 3, pp. 239–244, 2008.

[11] R. D'Amelio, C. Frati, A. Fattorossi, and F. Aiuti, "Peripheral T-cell subset imbalance in patients with vitiligo and in their apparently healthy first-degree relatives," *Annals of Allergy*, vol. 65, no. 2, pp. 143–145, 1990.

[12] I. Hamzavi, H. Jain, D. McLean, J. Shapiro, H. Zeng, and H. Lui, "Parametric modeling of narrowband UV-B phototherapy for vitiligo using a novel quantitative tool: the Vitiligo Area Scoring Index," *Archives of Dermatology*, vol. 140, no. 6, pp. 677–683, 2004.

[13] T. Kawakami and T. Hashimoto, "Disease severity indexes and treatment evaluation criteria in vitiligo," *Dermatology Research and Practice*, vol. 2011, Article ID 750342, 3 pages, 2011.

[14] E. M. Shevach, "CD4$^+$CD25$^+$ suppressor T cells: more questions than answers," *Nature Reviews Immunology*, vol. 2, no. 6, pp. 389–400, 2002.

[15] F. Annunziato, L. Cosmi, F. Liotta et al., "Phenotype, localization, and mechanism of suppression of CD4$^+$CD25$^+$ human thymocytes," *The Journal of Experimental Medicine*, vol. 196, no. 3, pp. 379–387, 2002.

[16] S. Hori, T. Nomura, and S. Sakaguchi, "Control of regulatory T cell development by the transcription factor *Foxp3*," *Science*, vol. 299, no. 5609, pp. 1057–1061, 2003.

[17] A. Richetta, S. D'Epiro, M. Salvi et al., "Serum levels of functional T-regs in vitiligo: our experience and mini-review of the literature," *European Journal of Dermatology*, vol. 23, no. 2, pp. 154–159, 2013.

[18] M. Dwivedi, N. C. Laddha, P. Arora, Y. S. Marfatia, and R. Begum, "Decreased regulatory T-cells and CD4$^+$/CD8$^+$ ratio correlate with disease onset and progression in patients with generalized vitiligo," *Pigment Cell & Melanoma Research*, vol. 26, no. 4, pp. 586–591, 2013.

[19] Y. Lili, W. Yi, Y. Ji, S. Yue, S. Weimin, and L. Ming, "Global activation of CD8+ cytotoxic T lymphocytes correlates with an impairment in regulatory T cells in patients with generalized vitiligo," *PLoS ONE*, vol. 7, no. 5, Article ID e37513, 2012.

[20] M. Ben Ahmed, I. Zaraa, R. Rekik et al., "Functional defects of peripheral regulatory T lymphocytes in patients with progressive vitiligo," *Pigment Cell and Melanoma Research*, vol. 25, no. 1, pp. 99–109, 2012.

[21] J. Klarquist, C. J. Denman, C. Hernandez et al., "Reduced skin homing by functional Treg in vitiligo," *Pigment Cell and Melanoma Research*, vol. 23, no. 2, pp. 276–286, 2010.

[22] F. Mahmoud, H. Abul, D. Haines, C. Al-Saleh, M. Khajeji, and K. Whaley, "Decreased total numbers of peripheral blood lymphocytes with elevated percentages of CD4+CD45RO+ and CD4+CD25+ of T-helper cells in non-segmental vitiligo," *The Journal of Dermatology*, vol. 29, no. 2, pp. 68–73, 2002.

[23] M. A. Elela, R. A. Hegazy, M. M. Fawzy, L. A. Rashed, and H. Rasheed, "Interleukin 17, interleukin 22 and FoxP3 expression in tissue and serum of non-segmental vitiligo: a case-controlled study on eighty-four patients," *European Journal of Dermatology*, vol. 23, no. 3, pp. 350–355, 2013.

[24] N. H. Moftah, R. A. H. El-Barbary, M. A. Ismail, and N. A. M. Ali, "Effect of narrow band-ultraviolet B on CD4$^+$ CD25^{high} FoxP3$^+$T-lymphocytes in the peripheral blood of vitiligo patients," *Photodermatology Photoimmunology and Photomedicine*, vol. 30, no. 5, pp. 254–261, 2014.

Indian Journal of Medical Research, vol. 138, no. 5, pp. 591–594, 2013.

[25] G. Roncador, P. J. Brown, L. Maestre et al., "Analysis of FOXP3 protein expression in human CD4$^+$CD25$^+$ regulatory T cells at the single-cell level," *European Journal of Immunology*, vol. 35, no. 6, pp. 1681–1691, 2005.

[26] H. Yagi, T. Nomura, K. Nakamura et al., "Crucial role of *FOXP3* in the development and function of human CD25$^+$CD4$^+$ regulatory T cells," *International Immunology*, vol. 16, no. 11, pp. 1643–1656, 2004.

[27] L. J. Chi, H. B. Wang, and W. Z. Wang, "Impairment of circulating CD4$^+$CD25$^+$ regulatory T cells in patients with chronic inflammatory demyelinating polyradiculoneuropathy," *Journal of the Peripheral Nervous System*, vol. 13, no. 1, pp. 54–63, 2008.

[28] M. A. Kriegel, T. Lohmann, C. Gabler, N. Blank, J. R. Kalden, and H.-M. Lorenz, "Defective suppressor function of human CD4$^+$CD25$^+$ regulatory T cells in autoimmune polyglandular syndrome type II," *Journal of Experimental Medicine*, vol. 199, no. 9, pp. 1285–1291, 2004.

[29] A. C. Abreu, G. G. Duarte, J. Y. Miranda, D. G. Ramos, C. G. Ramos, and M. G. Ramos, "Immunological parameters associated with vitiligo treatments: a literature review based on clinical studies," *Autoimmune Diseases*, vol. 2015, Article ID 196537, 5 pages, 2015.

[30] M. K. Tembhre, V. K. Sharma, A. Sharma, P. Chattopadhyay, and S. Gupta, "T helper and regulatory T cell cytokine profile in active, stable and narrow band ultraviolet B treated generalized vitiligo," *Clinica Chimica Acta*, vol. 424, pp. 27–32, 2013.

[31] R. A. Hegazy, M. M. Fawzy, H. I. Gawdat, N. Samir, and L. A. Rashed, "T helper 17 and Tregs: a novel proposed mechanism for NB-UVB in vitiligo," *Experimental Dermatology*, vol. 23, no. 4, pp. 283–286, 2014.

[32] J. M. Eby, H. Kang, S. T. Tully et al., "CCL22 to activate treg migration and suppress depigmentation in vitiligo," *Journal of Investigative Dermatology*, vol. 135, no. 6, pp. 1574–1580, 2015.

[33] J. A. Bluestone, E. Trotta, and D. Xu, "The therapeutic potential of regulatory T cells for the treatment of autoimmune disease," *Expert Opinion on Therapeutic Targets*, vol. 19, no. 8, pp. 1091–1103, 2015.

17

Skin Disorders among Elder Patients in a Referral Center in Northern Iran (2011)

Abbas Darjani,[1] **Zahra Mohtasham-Amiri,**[2] **Kiarash Mohammad Amini,**[1] **Javad Golchai,**[1] **Shahryar Sadre-Eshkevari,**[1] **and Narges Alizade**[1]

[1] *Department of Dermatology, Medical Faculty of Guilan University, Rasht, Iran*
[2] *Department of Preventive and Community Medicine, Medical Faculty of Guilan University, 4163545851 Rasht, Iran*

Correspondence should be addressed to Zahra Mohtasham-Amiri; mohtashamaz@yahoo.com

Academic Editor: Giuseppe Argenziano

Background. Geriatric health care has become a worldwide concern, but a few statistical studies were carried out about skin diseases in this age group. In this study, we set out to determine the frequency as well as the age and gender distribution of dermatological diseases in geriatric patients. *Materials and Methods.* In a cross-sectional study, all patients over 60 years who were accepted to department of dermatology in north of Iran participated in this study. Baseline information and clinical examination were done by a group of dermatologists. Biopsy, Pathological and laboratory methods were used in order to confirm the diagnosis. *Results.* 440 patients were accepted to the department that 232 patients were male (52.7%). Benign neoplasm was as the common skin disease among patients (65%), followed by erythemo-squamous (35.3%) and precancerous lesions (26.1%). The most common precancerous lesion was actinic keratosis (24.3%). BCC by 8.8% was the most prevalent skin carcinoma. Pruritus was the common problem in other dermatological disease (22%). *Conclusion.* Skin disorders especially precancerous lesion are among those important health problems in elderly patients in this geographic area. Increasing general awareness about risk factors of these diseases and doing more researches in other regions are highly recommended.

1. Introduction

From 2000 until 2050, the world's population aged 60 and over will more than triple from 600 million to 2 billion. Most of this increase will occur in less developed countries, where the number of older people will rise from 400 million in 2000 to 1.7 billion by 2050 [1].

In the most countries of the world, the proportion of people of over 60 years old is growing faster than any other age group: this fact is happening as a result of both longer life expectancy and also of what we can determine as the declining fertility rates. This population ageing can be seen as a success story for public health policies and for socioeconomic development; on the other hand, it also challenges society to adapt, in order to maximize the health and functional capacity of older people [2].

The United Nations statistical projections demonstrate a rapid growth of elderly population in Iran. While the proportion of people with 60 years old age and above in Iran was 5.4 percent in 1975, it will increase to 10.5 percent in 2025 and 21.7 percent in 2050 [3]. According to the Census of Population and Housing 2006 of Iran, population of the Guilan province in north of Iran was 2404861 people with 242850 (10.09%) aged 60 years and above. Indeed, the province of Guilan has the highest elderly rate in Iran [4].

In aging, a decline in the regular functions of skin is observed, including cell replacement capacity, barrier function, chemical clearance capacity, sensory perception, mechanical protection, wound healing, immune responsiveness, thermoregulation, sweat production, sebum production, vitamin D production, and capacity to repair DNA. As a result, some inevitable changes, such as roughness, wrinkling, and laxity of the skin, and atypical presentations of dermatologic diseases are observed in elderly patients [5].

Geriatric health care has absorbed a worldwide attention, but few statistical studies were carried out about skin diseases in this age group. 30 years ago, the American HANES survey demonstrated that the frequency of skin disorders increases with age so that at the age of 70 some 70% had a significant skin condition and many others had multiple skin problems [6].

In this study, we attempted to determine the frequency as well as the age and gender distributions of dermatological diseases in geriatric patients who attended dermatologic center of an educational hospital in Rasht, Iran.

2. Methods and Materials

In a cross-sectional study, 440 patients over 60 years old have participated in this study between March 2010 and March 2011. Informed consent was received from all patients. Baseline information on sociodemographic variables, past medical history, and medication was all gathered by medical staff during a face-to-face interview before doing any examination. Each patient was examined carefully by two dermatologists. Biopsy, pathological, and laboratory methods were used to confirm the diagnosis of suspected lesions or disease. The diseases were categorized into seven different groups including erythematosquamous diseases (such as psoriasis, lichen planus, seborrheic dermatitis, contact dermatitis, paederus dermatitis, stasis dermatitis, lichen simplex chronics, and pilaris rubra pityriasis), infectious diseases (fungal, bacterial, and viral infections, infestations), benign neoplasm (pillar cyst, keloids, lipoma, seborrheic keratosis, pyogenic granuloma, epidermal cyst, keratoacantom, and skin tag), precancerous lesions (leukoplakia, actinic keratosis, and bowen), skin cancer (basal cell carcinoma BCC, Squamish cell carcinoma SCC, mycosis fungoides, and kaposis sarcoma), age-related skin changes (xerosis, senile lentigo, senile comedon, angioma, and nail ridging), and the others (leg ulcer, insect bite, sarcoidosis, ingrowing toe nail, corn, vasculitis, and vitiligo).

Data analysis was carried out with the SPSS Software, version 18. Descriptive statistics for the prevalence of skin disease were calculated, and gender differences in skin disease prevalence are investigated using a chi-square testing all the analyses; a P-value of <0.05 was considered statistically significant.

3. Results

During the study period, 4231 patients were accepted to the department. Among the patients who were enrolled in this study, 440 persons (10.4%) were older than 60 years; meanwhile 232 patients were males (52.7%) and the others were females (47.3%). Most of them were in the age group 60–69 years (57%), and 10% were above 80 years. Hypertension (27%), diabetes mellitus (18%), and heart disease (11%) were the most prevalent underlying diseases. Most of the participants were farmers (41%), retirees (13%), drivers (10%), and fishermen (4%), respectively.

Benign neoplasm was the common skin disease among patients (65%), followed by erythematosquamous (35.3%), and precancerous lesions (26.1%). Most of the patients (76%)

had more than one skin disease. Age-related skin changes were seen in all patients (Table 1).

The most frequent diseases of erythematosquamous diseases were defined as dermatitis (16.6%), psoriasis (12.3%), lichen planus (5.45%) and pilaris rubra pityriasis (1.1%). Fungal infections (tinea, candidiasis) were the most common infectious diseases (8.2%) followed by viral infections (herpes zoster) (4.5%) and infestations (scabies) (4.3%). The most common precancerous lesion was actinic keratosis (24.3%). BCC by 8.8% was the most prevalent skin carcinoma. Skin tag (48.8%) and seborrheic keratosis (8%) were the most common benign neoplasm. 69% of patients with skin tag were females. Pruritus was the common problem in other dermatological diseases (22%). The most frequent diseases according to age groups were shown in Table 2.

4. Discussion

Dermatologic clinic of Razi hospital is the referral clinic of dermatology in Guilan that covers in-hospital and outpatients dermatologic diseases in the most part of northern area of Iran. Since the majority of outpatient skin disorders are referred to private section and are not reported to the public official sector, the hospital-base data is the only accessible source. On the other hand, it is possible that differences between the distributions of the diseases were seen here with other community-based studies.

The majority of patients were exposed to sunlight due to their jobs. Also more than 62% of the patients had at least one underlying disease that was under medication to treat. Some of these medications can cause or aggravate skin diseases.

In our study, the above mentioned benign neoplasm group was the most common skin disease defined among the patients who have been taken into consideration; this disease affected almost two-thirds of them (65%). Seborrheic keratosis (8%) was the most common benign neoplasm. This rate is different from other studies of elderly populations, where its prevalence of 1.7% to 85% has been recorded [5, 7–11]. Seborrheic keratosis is the most common benign epithelial tumor of adulthood. These differences may be related to different settings of the participants (population-base, clinic-base or nursing home), different climate, and different jobs of participants. It seems that sunlight exposure may play a role because seborrheic keratoses are common on sun exposed areas such as the back, arms, face, and neck [12, 13]. Two-thirds of patients with skin tag were females. Obesity and overweight (even temporary increases in weight) dramatically increase the chances of having skin tags [14]. Unfortunately, we did not record weights and heights of patients to reveal the relation between skin tag and obesity in our patients.

In our study, actinic keratosis was the most common skin disease after age-related skin changes with 24.3% prevalence rate. Actinic keratosis is a precursor lesion to squamous cell carcinoma, and lifetime sun exposure is an important risk factor for it, and various studies cite a <1–20% risk of transformation to squamous cell carcinoma (SCC) for an individual lesion over the course of a year [15]. This rate is

TABLE 1: The distributions of all skin diseases according to gender.

Disease	Total n (440)		Male n (232)		Female n (208)		P value
	n	%	n	%	n	%	
Age-related skin changes	440	100	232	100	208	100	NS
Erythematosquamous diseases	156	35.3	84	36.2	72	34.6	NS
Infectious diseases	89	20.2	40	17.2	49	23.6	NS
Benign neoplasm	286	65	149	64.2	137	65.7	NS
Precancerous lesions	115	26.1	62	26.7	53	25.5	NS
Skin carcinomas	68	15.4	47	20.3	21	10.1	0.001
Others	223	50.7	114	49.1	109	52.4	NS

TABLE 2: The most prevalent skin diseases according to age groups.

Disease	Age group					
	60–69 years no. (250)		70–79 years no. (144)		≥80 years no. (46)	
	No.	%	No.	%	No.	%
Age-related nails changes	209	83.6	125	86.8	40	86.9
Senile angioma	133	53.2	76	52.7	22	47.8
Lentigo	113	45.2	68	47.2	26	56.5
Skin tag	118	47.2	70	48.6	27	58.7
Actinic keratosis	61	24.4	36	25	10	21.7
Pruritus	52	20.8	33	22.9	12	26
Dermatitis	40	16	20	13.8	13	28.3
Psoriasis	36	14.4	13	9	5	10.9
Xerosis	30	12	14	9.7	7	15.2
BCC	20	8	13	9	6	13
Fungal infection	20	8	10	6.9	6	13
Pemphigus vulgaris	25	10	10	6.9	2	4.3
Seborrheic keratosis	19	7.6	12	8.3	5	10.9
Lichen planus	15	6	6	4.2	3	6.5
Herpes zoster	11	4.4	6	4.2	3	6.5
Scabies	10	4	5	3.5	4	8.7
Callosity	10	4	5	3.5	3	6.5
SCC	10	4	5	3.5	2	4.4
Leg ulcer	8	3.2	6	4.2	3	6.5
Mycosis fungoides	5	2	3	2.1	1	2.2
Keratoacantom	5	2	1	0.7	1	2.2

higher than the reported rates of this disease in Tehran [16] and Italy [17] but consistent with other studies in old aging in Taiwan, Croatia, and Australia with, respectively, 22.4% (8), 22.3% (10) and 25% [11]. This similar rate may be due to similar climate in these area, and exposure to sunlight.

Pruritus with high rate as 22% was a common problem in our study. Pruritus in the elderly can be caused by a variety of dermatological and systemic conditions, but the most common cause is dry skin [18]. Low humidity combined with hot showers and overuse of soaps results in dryness and cracking of the skin. This rate is different from other studies of elderly populations, where its prevalence of 6.4% in Tunisia [9], 8.8%–11.5% in Turkey [5, 7], 14.2% in Taiwan [8], 18.9% in Italy [17], and 49.6% in India [19] has been recorded [5, 7–11].

Xerosis also was reported from 11.6% of patients. This disease was shown as 1.5% in Japan [20], 5.4% in Turkey [7], 18.2% in Hong Kong [19], 28% in Tehran [16], 29.5% in Australia [21], 58.3% in Taiwan [22], and 77% in a systematic review [11]. Differences in humidity and lifestyle can describe the wide difference of these complaints in the elderly.

Dermatitis was another common problem in this study that was affected 16.6%. Other studies have shown different rates from 1.5% to 58.7% [5, 7, 10, 19–24]. Contact dermatitis (most common form of dermatitis) is a delayed-type hypersensitivity reaction to an antigen (allergen) that contacts the skin; indeed, the higher incidence of dermatitis in this age group may happen due to more contact with the environmental and physical factors.

Cutaneous malignant tumors were found in 15.4% of prominently, in male patients in comparison with female (*P* value <0.001). BCC was diagnosed in 8.8% that was the most prevalent skin carcinoma. Basal cell carcinoma is the most common skin cancer (~75%) and is related to chronic ultraviolet light exposure.

The proportion of skin tumor cases in this study was much higher than other studies which have been done in western and eastern parts of the country [8, 9, 19, 21–23]. Type of the clinic as referral clinic and jobs of patients may be the most causes of this high rate of malignancy.

Fungal infections were the most common infectious diseases in our study that were found out in 8.2%. Other studies showed different rates from 4.4% to 61.6% [8, 9, 19–23]. Fungal infection depends on underlying diseases such as diabetes, bedridden status, and also hygiene level of patients. It seems that infection diseases are more prevalent among nursing home care patients in comparison with community-dowelling patients.

Overall, our research supports the opinion that skin diseases are a common and inevitable consequence of aging. A lifetime of solar radiation exposure, combined with intrinsic changes in the dermal structures, predisposes geriatric individual to a wide variety of skin diseases; we witnessed many of them during this research.

References

[1] World Health Organization, "What are the public health implications of global ageing?" 2012, http://www.who.int/features/qa/42/en/index.html.

[2] World Health Organization, "Aging," 2012, http://www.who.int/topics/ageing/en/.

[3] "United Nations World Population Ageing: 1950–2050, Countries of area: Iran (Islamic Republic of Iran)," http://www.un.org/esa/population/publications/worldageing19502050/pdf/113iran%28.pdf.

[4] M. Abbasi kakroodi, F. Farzad, and F. Pakdaman, *Picture of Old Ages in Guilan*, Rasht, Guilan, Iran, 1st edition, 2011.

[5] B. Yalçin, E. Tamer, G. G. Toy, P. Öztaş, M. Hayran, and N. Alli, "The prevalence of skin diseases in the elderly: analysis of 4099 geriatric patients," *International Journal of Dermatology*, vol. 45, no. 6, pp. 672–676, 2006.

[6] R. Marks, "Skin disease in the elderly," *European Journal of Dermatology*, vol. 16, no. 4, pp. 460–461, 2006.

[7] S. G. Bilgili, A. S. Karadag, H. U. Ozkol, O. Calka, and N. Akdeniz, "The prevalence of skin diseases among the geriatric patients in Eastern Turkey," *Journal of the Pakistan Medical Association*, vol. 62, no. 6, pp. 535–539, 2012.

[8] Y. H. Liao, K. H. Chen, M. P. Tseng, and C.-C. Sun, "Pattern of skin diseases in a geriatric patient group in Taiwan: a 7-year survey from the Outpatient Clinic of a University Medical Center," *Dermatology*, vol. 203, no. 4, pp. 308–313, 2001.

[9] A. Souissi, F. Zeglaoui, N. El Fekih, B. Fazaa, B. Zouari, and M. R. Kamoun, "Skin diseases in the elderly: a multicentre Tunisian study," *Annales de Dermatologie et de Venereologie*, vol. 133, no. 3, pp. 231–234, 2006.

[10] H. Cvitanović, E. Kneževic, I. Kuljanac, and E. Jančić, "Skin disease in a geriatric patients group in outpatient dermatologic clinic Karlovac, Croatia," *Collegium Antropologicum*, vol. 34, no. 2, pp. 247–251, 2010.

[11] D. R. Smith and P. A. Leggat, "Prevalence of skin disease among the elderly in different clinical environments," *Australasian Journal on Ageing*, vol. 24, no. 2, pp. 71–76, 2005.

[12] C. S. Landefeld, R. M. Palmer, M. A. G. Johnson, C. B. Johnston, and W. L. Lyons, *Current Geriatric Diagnosis & Treatment*, McGraw-Hill, New York, NY, USA, 1st edition, 2004.

[13] T. P. Habif, Ed., *Clinical Dermatology*, Mosby Elsevier, Philadelphia, Pa, USA, 5th edition, 2009.

[14] C. S. William Jr., "What is a skin tag?" 2012, http://www.medicinenet.com/skin_tag/article.htm.

[15] C. S. Landefeld, R. M. Palmer, M. A. G. Johnson et al., *Current Geriatric Diagnosis & Treatment*, McGraw-Hill, 1st edition, 2004.

[16] M. R. Roodsari and F. Malekzad, "The prevalence of skin diseases among nursing-home patients in north tehran," *Clinical Dermatology: Retinoids and other Treatments*, vol. 24, no. 3, pp. 43–45, 2008.

[17] P. Rubegni, S. Poggiali, N. Nami, M. Rubegni, and M. Fimiani, "Skin diseases in geriatric patients: our experience from a public skin outpatient clinic in Siena," *Giornale Italiano di Dermatologia e Venereologia*, vol. 147, no. 6, pp. 631–636, 2012.

[18] T. G. Berger and M. Steinhoff, "Pruritus in elderly patients-eruptions of senescence," *Seminars in Cutaneous Medicine and Surgery*, vol. 30, no. 2, pp. 113–117, 2011.

[19] P. C. Durai, D. M. Thappa, R. Kumari, and M. Malathi, "Aging in elderly: chronological versus photoaging," *Indian Journal of Dermatology*, vol. 57, pp. 343–352, 2012.

[20] D. R. Smith, H. Kubo, S. Tang, and Z. Yamagata, "Skin disease among staff in a Japanese nursing home," *Journal of Occupational Health*, vol. 45, no. 1, pp. 60–62, 2003.

[21] D. R. Smith, R. Atkinson, S. Tang, and Z. Yamagata, "A survey of skin disease among patients in an Australian nursing home," *Journal of Epidemiology*, vol. 12, no. 4, pp. 336–340, 2002.

[22] D. R. Smith, H.-M. Sheu, F.-S. Hsieh, Y.-L. Lee, S.-J. Chang, and Y. L. Guo, "Prevalence of skin disease among nursing home patients in southern Taiwan," *International Journal of Dermatology*, vol. 41, no. 11, pp. 754–759, 2002.

[23] S. W. Chan, "Prevalence of skin problems in elderly homes residents in Hong Kong," *Hong Kong Journal of Dermatology and Venereology*, vol. 14, no. 2, pp. 66–70, 2006.

[24] K. Weismann, R. Krakauer, and B. Wanscher, "Prevalence of skin diseases in old age," *Acta Dermato-Venereologica*, vol. 60, no. 4, pp. 352–353, 1980.

18

Clinical Features and Drug Characteristics of Patients with Generalized Fixed Drug Eruption in the West of Iran (2005–2014)

Hossein Kavoussi,[1] **Mansour Rezaei,**[2] **Katayoun Derakhshandeh,**[3] **Alireza Moradi,**[3] **Ali Ebrahimi,**[1] **Harif Rashidian,**[4] **and Reza Kavoussi**[4]

[1]*Dermatology Department, Imam Reza Hospital, Kermanshah University of Medical Sciences (KUMS), Kermanshah 6714415333, Iran*
[2]*Health School, Family Health Research Center of Kermanshah University of Medical Sciences (KUMS), Kermanshah 6714415333, Iran*
[3]*Department of Pharmaceutics, School of Pharmacy, Hamadan University of Medical Sciences, Hamadan, Iran*
[4]*Kermanshah University of Medical Sciences (KUMS), Kermanshah 6714415333, Iran*

Correspondence should be addressed to Hossein Kavoussi; hkawosi@kums.ac.ir

Academic Editor: Craig G. Burkhart

Background. Generalized fixed drug eruption is a specific variant of fixed drug eruption with multifocal lesions. Diagnosis of this drug reaction is straightforward, but occasionally recognition of the causative drug is not possible. This study was aimed at evaluating the clinical features and culprit drugs in generalized fixed drug eruptions in the west of Iran. *Method.* This cross-sectional study was carried out on 30 patients with criteria of generalized fixed drug eruption over 9 years. Demographic, clinical, and drug intake information were collected. *Results.* Out of 30 patients (17 females and 13 males) with the mean age of 26.67 ± 10.21 years, 28 (93.3%) and 2 (6.7%) cases had plaque and bullous clinical presentation, respectively. Upper limbs were the most common (90%) site of involvement. The antibiotic group, especially cotrimoxazole (26.1%), was reported to be the most common offending drug, but the causative drug was not determined in 7 (23.3%) patients. *Conclusion.* Many cases of generalized fixed drug eruption firstly presented as limited lesions and led to generalized lesion due to repeated intake of the causative drug. No causative drug was found in some patients, which might be associated with concurrent intake of several drugs, multiple FDE, and peculiarity of the patch test.

1. Introduction

Fixed drug eruption (FDE) is a specific drug reaction which characteristically recurs in the same location after reexposure to the same or related medications [1–4].

FDE is a common type of drug eruption whose incidence has tended to increase in the recent years [4].

Although diagnosis of FDE is easy for dermatologists, recognition of the offending drugs may be problematic [3, 4].

Generalized fixed drug eruption (GFDE) is a clinical variant of FDE that is presented with numerous multifocal lesions. Skin lesion is usually manifested with well-defined erythematous to violaceous round or oval plaque as generalized nonbullous fixed drug eruption and is occasionally vesicular or bullous as generalized bullous fixed drug eruption [5–7].

GFDE is not often fatal but sometimes results in cosmetic problems [1, 4, 7].

In this study, the patients with GFDE were evaluated to identify the caustic drugs, clinical type, number of episodes, location of lesions, and some demographic data of patients.

2. Method and Material

This cross-sectional (descriptive-analytic) study was done at Imam Reza referral hospital of Kermanshah University of Medical Sciences over 9 years, from 2005 to 2014.

TABLE 1: Demographic data and clinical features of patients with generalized fixed drug eruption.

Variables	
Mean of age (years)	26.67 ± 10.21
Gender (F/M)	17/13
Mean of episode	3.77 ± 2.11
Location	
Face and head (n%)	10 (33.3%)
Upper limbs (n%)	27 (90.0%)
Trunk (n%)	20 (66.7%)
Lower limbs (n%)	21 (70.0%)
Genital area (n%)	9 (30.0%)
Mucous membrane (n%)	8 (26.7%)
Clinical feature	
Nonbullous (n%)	28 (93.3%)
Bullous (n%)	2 (6.7%)

TABLE 2: Drug behavior and offending drugs.

Behavior of drug intake	
Monodrug intake (n%)	5 (16.7%)
Multiple drug intake (n%)	25 (83.3%)
Recognized caustic drug (n%)	23 (73.3%)
Antibiotic (n%)	14 (60. 9%)
Cotrimoxazole (n%)	6 (26.1%)
Metronidazole (n%)	4 (17.4%)
Doxicyclin (n%)	2 (8.7%)
Azithromycin (n%)	1 (4.3%)
Nitrofurantoin (n%)	1 (4.3%)
Analgesic (n%)	7 (30.4%)
Ibuprofen (n%)	3 (13.0%)
Mefenamic acid (n%)	1 (3.4%)
Meloxicam (n%)	1 (3.4%)
Novafen (n%)	1 (3.4%)
Miscellaneous (n%)	2 (8.7%)
Unrecognized caustic drug (n%)	7 (26.7%)

The patients with typical clinical manifestation or histopathological documentation for FDE were enrolled in this study. Also, the patients had to suffer from at least three involved locations and a minimum of 10 lesions.

The offending drugs were identified by taking a meticulous history or performing the patch test at the site of previous FDE lesions with the medications consumed over the last 30 days.

Demographic data such as age, gender, history of medications, number of episodes, clinical features, and causative drug were recorded.

Analysis of data was carried out by SPSS (version 22) software. Analysis of qualitative data was done by Chisquare and Fisher's exact test. For quantitative variables, firstly, one sample KS test was used to measure the normality and later was applied based on the results of Leven's and independent t-test or Mann-Whitney U test. Significance level was considered 0.05 for analysis of the tests.

3. Results

A total of 30 patients, 17 (56.7%) females and 13 (43.3%) males (Table 1), were recruited in this study.

The age range of the patients was 13–57 years with the mean age of 26.67 ± 10.21 years. Fourteen (46.7%) patients stood in the third decade. The mean age in bullous variant (44.5±17.8) was more than that of nonbullous variant (25.39± 9.78) of GFDE, but there was no statistically significant difference between them.

Most of the patients (73.3%) were diagnosed by their typical clinical manifestation, but 27.8% of patients were diagnosed through histopathologic documentation.

The range of FDE episode was 1–10 times with the mean of 3.77 ± 2.11. Most of the subjects (39%) had 3 episodes (Table 1). The number of episodes was more in females and nonbullous GFDE. There was a significant difference between episode and gender (PV = 0.043) but not clinical features (PV = 0.225).

Involvement of the upper limbs, as the most common location of distribution, was seen in 27 (90%) cases. GFDE lesions were located on lower limbs in 21 (70%) cases, on trunk in 20 (66.7%) cases, and on face and scalp in 10 (33.3%) cases (Table 1).

FDE lesions were seen in 9 (30%) and 8 (26.7%) cases in genital and oral mucosa areas, respectively (Table 1).

As for the clinical presentation, 28 (93.3%) patients had plaque skin lesions, while bullous lesions were found in 2 (6.7%) cases (Table 1).

There was no significant difference between clinical features and gender (PV = 0.492), multiple drug intake (PV = 0.1), and mucous membrane involvement (PV = 0.492).

When the patients were referred to the clinic, multidrug consumption was reported in 25 (83.3%) patients, but only 5 (16.7%) of them had monodrug intake (Table 2).

Although recognition of the offending drugs was distinguished in 23 (76.6%) cases, it was not distinguished in 7 (23.3%) patients (Table 2). Patch test was not positive in any patients with medication intake in the last 30 days.

The category of causative drugs included 14 (60.9%) antibiotics, 7 (30.4%) analgesics, and 2 (8.7%) miscellaneous cases. The most common offending drugs were cotrimoxazole in 6 (26.1%) cases, metronidazole in 4 (17.4%) cases, and ibuprofen in 3 (13%) cases (Table 2). GBFDE was seen in two females, one due to metronidazole and the other due to cotrimoxazole.

4. Discussion

Our findings indicated that the majority of patients with GFDE were females with concurrent multidrug intake, involvement of upper limbs, experience of several episodes, and antibiotic intake, especially cotrimoxazole.

Our results showed most of the patients were females in the third decade of their life. Jung et al. [3] and Ognongo-Ibiaho and Atanda [8] reported a higher frequency of FDE for males in their fourth decade of life, but Mahboob and Haroon [9] found equal rates in both sexes.

In a study from Taiwan [10], most patients had previous events of FDE. Also, Jung et al. [3] found a mean episode of 2.6 in their patients. In our patients, the high frequency of episode may be related to the existence of atypical cases of FDE and unfamiliarity of doctors of medicine, especially general practitioners, with FDE.

We performed biopsy and histopathologic evaluation in some patients for definite diagnosis because of atypical forms of FDE such as GBFDE [5–7] and nonpigmented variant [11] that required histopathologic documentation.

FDE sometimes presents with a solitary lesion. However, with reuse of causative drugs and induction of new attack, in addition to previous lesions, new lesions appear [1, 3, 4, 9–11]. In some studies, extremities have been reported as the most common site of involvement [1, 3, 11]. Also, Lee et al. [10] reported upper extremities as the most common involved location. In our patients, consistent with previous studies, the lesions were mostly located on upper extremities.

In FDE, genital area involvement is most frequently caused by cotrimoxazole [12]. However, involvement of penis is uncommon [13] and a retrospective study showed, from 321 cases, 16.5% of them had genital area involvement [14]. High frequency of genital area involvement (30%) in our study was related to the presence of bullous variant (6.7%), cotrimoxazole as the most common causative medication (26.1%), and multiple attacks in our patients.

Mucous membrane FDE lesions may be alone or in association with skin involvement [15], but mucous membrane involvement is more common in the bullous variant than in nonbullous variant of GFDE (66.7% versus 30%) [10]. Twenty-six percent of our patients showed erosion in oral mucous membrane, which is consistent with other results of studies.

The patients with GFDE usually take multiple drugs at a time [10, 16], which is consistent with the results of our study. We tend to think that, in drug reactions, taking multiple drugs concurrently is one of the problems that impede the accurate recognition of the causative drug.

We could not determine the offending drug in approximately one-fourth of the patients. Offending drug was not recognized by Lee [4] and Lee et al. [10] in 71.6% and 23% of patients, respectively. Concurrent intake of multiple drugs [10, 16], multiple FDE [17], controversial usefulness of patch test [18], self-medication, and inaccurate past medical history reported by the patients [19] are the most important impediments for determination of culprit drugs.

In most studies, multifocal or generalized FDE is not common [4, 10, 16], and bullous type of GFDE is its rare form, which must be differentiated from Stevens-Johnson syndrome and toxic epidermal necrolysis [7, 10]. Repeated intake of causative drug or related drugs, in addition to old lesions, induces new lesions which occasionally become generalized [1, 19]. We think dissemination in most of our cases may be associated with atypical presentation, unawareness of FDE on the part of general practitioners, self-medication, and confusing history reported by the patients, which resulted in delay in diagnosis and avoidance of culprit drug.

Consistent with several studies [9, 14, 20, 21], our findings showed antibiotic drugs, especially cotrimoxazole, were the most common culprit drugs in FDE. But in other studies, analgesics medications [2, 3, 22] have been frequently reported as offending drugs in this type of drug reaction. In a case series by Patro et al. [16] and another study by Lee et al. [10], recognition of incremental drug was not possible in most of the patients with multifocal FDE or GFDE because of multiple drug intake. The difference of causative drugs in various areas may be dependent on self-medication in the community [20], genetic predisposition [23], concurrent intake of multiple drugs [16], and popular drugs in each region [19].

In conclusion, it seems that many cases of GFDE other than bullous GFDE are first presented as FDE with limited lesions, which result in disseminated FDE by repeated exposure to the causative drug. The most common offending drug belonged to antibiotic group, especially cotrimoxazole, and the most involved site was reported as the upper limb. Sometimes the causative drug is not recognized, which may be due to concurrent intake of several drugs, multiple FDE, and absence of distinctive paraclinic assessment for recognition of causative drugs. We suggest detailed education of medical students about drug reactions, especially FDE, multiple FDE as a unique drug reaction during concurrent intake of several drugs, and obtaining a detailed history of patients to determine the offending drug.

Conflict of Interests

The authors declare that there is no conflict of interests regarding the publication of this paper.

Acknowledgment

This paper results from student's thesis.

References

[1] S. M. Breathnach, "Drug reactions," in *Rook's Textbook of Dermatology*, T. Burns, S. Breathnach, N. Cox, and C. Griffiths, Eds., pp. 28–177, Blackwell Science, Oxford, UK, 8th edition, 2010.

[2] Y. K. Heng, Y. W. Yew, D. S. Y. Lim, and Y. L. Lim, "An update of fixed drug eruptions in Singapore," *Journal of the European Academy of Dermatology and Venereology*, vol. 29, no. 8, pp. 1539–1544, 2015.

[3] J.-W. Jung, S.-H. Cho, K.-H. Kim, K.-U. Min, and H.-R. Kang, "Clinical features of fixed drug eruption at a tertiary hospital in Korea," *Allergy, Asthma and Immunology Research*, vol. 6, no. 5, pp. 415–420, 2014.

[4] A.-Y. Lee, "Fixed drug eruptions. Incidence, recognition, and avoidance," *American Journal of Clinical Dermatology*, vol. 1, no. 5, pp. 277–285, 2000.

[5] Y. Sawada, M. Nakamura, and Y. Tokura, "Generalized fixed drug eruption caused by pazufloxacin," *Acta Dermato-Venereologica*, vol. 91, no. 5, pp. 600–601, 2011.

[6] C. Can, E. Akkelle, B. Bay, Ö. Arıcan, Ö. Yalçın, and M. Yazicioglu, "Generalized fixed drug eruption in a child due to trimethoprim/sulfamethoxazole," *Pediatric Allergy and Immunology*, vol. 25, no. 4, pp. 413–415, 2014.

[7] S. Lipowicz, P. Sekula, S. Ingen-Housz-Oro et al., "Prognosis of generalized bullous fixed drug eruption: comparison with Stevens-Johnson syndrome and toxic epidermal necrolysis," *British Journal of Dermatology*, vol. 168, no. 4, pp. 726–732, 2013.

[8] A. N. Ognongo-Ibiaho and H. L. Atanda, "Epidemiological study of fixed drug eruption in Pointe-Noire," *International Journal of Dermatology*, vol. 51, supplement 1, pp. 30–31, 2012.

[9] A. Mahboob and T. S. Haroon, "Drugs causing fixed eruptions: a study of 450 cases," *International Journal of Dermatology*, vol. 37, no. 11, pp. 833–838, 1998.

[10] C.-H. Lee, Y.-C. Chen, Y.-T. Cho, C.-Y. Chang, and C.-Y. Chu, "Fixed-drug eruption: a retrospective study in a single referral center in northern Taiwan," *Dermatologica Sinica*, vol. 30, no. 1, pp. 11–15, 2012.

[11] W. B. Shelley and E. D. Shelley, "Nonpigmenting fixed drug eruption as a distinctive reaction pattern: examples caused by sensitivity to pseudoephedrine hydrochloride and tetrahydrozoline," *Journal of the American Academy of Dermatology*, vol. 17, no. 3, pp. 403–407, 1987.

[12] E. Özkaya-Bayazit, "Specific site involvement in fixed drug eruption," *Journal of the American Academy of Dermatology*, vol. 49, no. 6, pp. 1003–1007, 2003.

[13] N. Lawrentschuk, D. Pan, and A. Troy, "Fixed drug eruption of the penis secondary to sulfamethoxazole-trimethoprim," *TheScientificWorldJournal*, vol. 6, pp. 2319–2322, 2006.

[14] B. Saka, K. Kombaté, B.-H. Médougou et al., "Fixed drug eruption in dermatology setting in Lomé (Togo): a retrospective study of 321 cases," *Bulletin de la Societe de Pathologie Exotique*, vol. 105, no. 5, pp. 384–387, 2012.

[15] V. K. Jain, V. B. Dixit, and Archana, "Fixed drug eruption of the oral mucous membrane," *Annals of Dentistry*, vol. 50, no. 1, pp. 9–11, 1991.

[16] N. Patro, M. Panda, M. Jena, and S. Mishra, "Multifocal fixed drug eruptions: a case series," *International Journal of Pharmaceutical Sciences Review and Research*, vol. 23, no. 1, pp. 63–66, 2013.

[17] J. Verbov, "Fixed drug eruption due to a drug combination but not to its constituents," *Dermatologica*, vol. 171, no. 1, pp. 60–61, 1985.

[18] S. Ohtoshi, Y. Kitami, H. Sueki, and T. Nakada, "Utility of patch testing for patients with drug eruption," *Clinical and Experimental Dermatology*, vol. 39, no. 3, pp. 279–283, 2014.

[19] S. Padmavathi, K. Manimekalai, and S. Ambujam, "Causality, severity and preventability assessment of adverse cutaneous drug reaction: a prospective observational study in a tertiary care hospital," *Journal of Clinical and Diagnostic Research*, vol. 7, no. 12, pp. 2765–2767, 2013.

[20] V. N. Sehgal and G. Srivastava, "Fixed drug eruption (FDE): changing scenario of incriminating drugs," *International Journal of Dermatology*, vol. 45, no. 8, pp. 897–908, 2006.

[21] R. Sharma, D. Dogra, and N. Dogra, "A study of cutaneous adverse drug reactions at a tertiary center in Jammu, India," *Indian Dermatology Online Journal*, vol. 6, no. 3, pp. 168–171, 2015.

[22] S. R. Shukla, "Drugs causing fixed drug eruptions," *Dermatologica*, vol. 163, no. 2, pp. 160–163, 1981.

[23] M. Tohkin, A. Ishiguro, N. Kaniwa, Y. Saito, K. Kurose, and R. Hasegawa, "Prediction of severe adverse drug reactions using pharmacogenetic biomarkers," *Drug Metabolism and Pharmacokinetics*, vol. 25, no. 2, pp. 122–133, 2010.

19

Exploring the Physiological Link between Psoriasis and Mood Disorders

Cody J. Connor,[1,2] Vincent Liu,[3,4] and Jess G. Fiedorowicz[5,6,7]

[1]Department of Family Medicine, Broadlawns Medical Center, Des Moines, IA 50314, USA
[2]Carver College of Medicine, University of Iowa, Iowa City, IA 52242, USA
[3]Department of Dermatology, University of Iowa, Iowa City, IA 52242, USA
[4]Department of Pathology, University of Iowa, Iowa City, IA 52242, USA
[5]Department of Psychiatry, University of Iowa, Iowa City, IA 52242, USA
[6]Department of Internal Medicine, University of Iowa, Iowa City, IA 52242, USA
[7]Department of Epidemiology, College of Public Health, University of Iowa, Iowa City, IA 52242, USA

Correspondence should be addressed to Cody J. Connor; cody_jc_14@hotmail.com

Academic Editor: Desmond Tobin

Psoriasis is a chronic, immune-mediated skin condition with a high rate of psychiatric comorbidity, which often goes unrecognized. Beyond the negative consequences of mood disorders like depression and anxiety on patient quality of life, evidence suggests that these conditions can worsen the severity of psoriatic disease. The mechanisms behind this relationship are not entirely understood, but inflammation seems to be a key feature linking psoriasis with mood disorders, and physiologic modulators of this inflammation, including the hypothalamic-pituitary-adrenal axis and sympathetic nervous system, demonstrate changes with psychopathology that may be contributory. Cyclical disruptions in the secretion of the sleep hormone, melatonin, are also observed in both depression and psoriasis, and with well-recognized anti-inflammatory and antioxidant activity, this aberration may represent a shared contributor to both conditions as well as common comorbidities like diabetes and cardiovascular disease. While understanding the complexities of the biological mechanisms at play will be key in optimizing the management of patients with comorbid psoriasis and depression/anxiety, one thing is certain: recognition of psychiatric comorbidity is an imperative first step in effectively treating these patients as a whole. Evidence that improvement in mood decreases psoriasis severity underscores how psychological awareness can be critical to clinicians in their practice.

1. Introduction

Psoriasis vulgaris is a chronic, autoimmune, inflammatory skin disorder phenotypically characterized by clearly demarcated, salmon-colored plaques surfaced by micaceous, silvery scale. It is considered to be immune-mediated, arising with increase and activation of cutaneous T cells and dendritic cells [1]. Following migration to the skin, these immune cells release proinflammatory cytokines, such as interleukin-1 (IL-1), IL-6, and tumor necrosis factor α (TNF-α), which promote inflammation and keratinocyte proliferation. These keratinocytes accumulate without shedding, resulting in the distinctive patches of thickened, scaly skin. Although often underappreciated, psoriasis can result in considerable

disability to afflicted patients, and some estimate that the burden imparted is comparable to other major diseases like chronic heart failure, chronic obstructive pulmonary disease, and cancer [2].

Psychiatric comorbidity is estimated to affect over 30% of patients with dermatologic disease [3]. The prevalence of depression and anxiety in those with psoriasis, specifically, is significantly higher than that observed in the general population [4], and in comparison to many other dermatologic conditions, psychiatric morbidity is higher and quality of life scores are lower [5–9]. One might attribute the association between psoriasis and mood disorders as simply resulting from the related embarrassment, shame, and social anxiety incurred from the physical manifestations of disease;

however, the fact that the prevalence of mood symptoms in psoriasis is higher than that observed with many other disfiguring skin disorders [5–9] begs for investigation of common or overlapping mechanisms linking both conditions.

2. The Role of Inflammation

There is a growing body of literature supporting some link between major depressive disorder and inflammation [10]. Elevations in proinflammatory cytokines like prostaglandin E2 (PGE2), C-reactive protein (CRP), TNF-α, IL-1β, IL-2, and IL-6 have been reported in major depressive disorder and, at times, have shown a dose-response with severity of depression [10, 11]. These findings, however, cannot distinguish whether the depression is causing the inflammation or vice versa. In exploring this question of temporality, there is evidence and biological plausibility for both directions.

2.1. Depression Causing Inflammation. Could depressive states induce elevations in the inflammatory cytokines previously mentioned? A randomized controlled trial revealed that antidepressant treatment with the selective serotonin reuptake inhibitor (SSRI), sertraline, significantly decreased not only depression scores, but also baseline measurements of CRP and IL-6 in depressed subjects [12]. A large meta-analysis also demonstrated that psychological stress elevates inflammatory markers like CRP, TNF-α, IL-1β, and IL-6 [13]. The net effect is an acute increase in the proinflammatory potential of the circulating immune system, and in the setting of psoriasis, this could mean exacerbation of disease. In fact, 40–80% of cases of psoriasis onset or exacerbation have been attributed to psychosocial factors, revealing a significant role for mood in modulating disease [14]. While there has been limited empirical study of those with cooccurring depression and psoriasis, a case report describes a young adult woman with schizoaffective disorder who experienced consistent worsening of psoriasis during periods of increased depression and suicidality with improvement during periods of normal mood [15]. Exacerbation of psoriasis with worsening depression and anxiety is common, and a variety of physiological pathways may be involved in mediating this relationship.

One particularly plausible pathway involves abnormal activation of the hypothalamic-pituitary-adrenal (HPA) axis. Various studies have identified chronically elevated baseline levels of corticotropin releasing hormone (CRH), adrenocorticotropic hormone (ACTH), and cortisol in depressed individuals [16]. This HPA-axis hyperactivity may result from changes in the number and function of cortisol receptors functioning in negative feedback. The effects of cortisol are mediated by two different types of intracellular receptors, the mineralocorticoid receptor (MR, type I) and the glucocorticoid receptor (GR, type II) [17]. MRs have a much higher affinity (10x) for endogenous glucocorticoids like cortisol. GRs, on the other hand, bind strongly to synthetic steroids like dexamethasone. Given these profiles, MRs are believed to primarily moderate cortisol's effects and its feedback on the HPA axis when cortisol levels are low. During periods of acute stress, cortisol levels may increase 100-fold, effectively

saturating the MRs and leaving the GRs as the main regulators of glucocorticoid action and HPA activity [18].

Decreases in the number or function of GRs may thus result in decreased negative feedback by cortisol, leading to the HPA hyperactivity demonstrated in depressed individuals. This mechanism is supported by reports of cortisol nonsuppression following administration of dexamethasone—which, recall, normally has strong GR affinity—in subjects with major depression: an effect that disappears with clinical recovery from depression [16]. Hypercortisolemia appears to produce negative effects on mood and cognition. These effects may be mediated mainly through MRs, or possibly through GRs that have not lost their functional capacity as the ones in the hypothalamus, which participate in HPA autoregulation.

2.2. HPA Axis and Sympathetic Nervous System Effects on Skin and Inflammation. HPA hyperactivity appears not only to influence mood, but also to effect changes in the skin. CRH has been shown to stimulate local cutaneous production of cytokines like IL-6 and IL-11 [19], and it also amplifies cytokine-stimulated keratinocyte expression of the immune trafficking adhesion molecules, hCAM and ICAM-1, and the major histocompatibility complex II receptor, HLA-DR [20]. In addition, CRH activates the proinflammatory protein complex NF-κB (nuclear factor kappa-light-chain-enhancer of activated B cells), which is present in almost all cell types and modulates DNA transcription and immune reaction in response to stimuli like stress, UV light, free radicals, and bacterial/viral infection [21]. Through all of these changes, CRH effectively shifts keratinocytes into an immunoactive state [20] and thus may contribute to inflammatory skin conditions, such as psoriasis. In fact, biopsies of psoriatic lesions show significantly increased expression of CRH compared to normal skin, suggesting a possible role of CRH in the underlying pathophysiologic mechanism of the disease [22].

Evidence suggests that peripheral CRH is part of an HPA-like system that functions locally within the skin and hair follicles [23, 24]. Whether produced locally or delivered by peripheral nerves, CRH may be a key component of the "brain-skin axis," mediating interactions between the central and peripheral stress response pathways [24]. Downstream HPA products, like cortisol, are also known to act peripherally within this cutaneous system. Administration of systemic glucocorticoids in rodents has been shown to cause adverse changes in the skin, including disruption of epidermal cell proliferation [25] and barrier homeostasis [26]. These cutaneous effects are blocked by simultaneous administration of the steroid hormone receptor antagonist, RU-486, effectively identifying glucocorticoids as the mediators through which stress may disturb cutaneous quiescence [26].

The way in which the HPA axis is affected appears to differ amongst psoriasis patients depending on whether they suffer from depression or anxiety. Those with depression have chronically elevated levels of CRH, ACTH, and cortisol, while those with stress-responsive psoriasis (psoriasis that worsens during periods of high stress) have been shown to have a blunted HPA-stress response, with less cortisol released into circulation following acute stress [27]. Even so, it may be that depression and anxiety both worsen the severity of psoriasis, only through separate mechanisms. In those with stress-responsive psoriasis, acute anxiety may cause the production of inflammatory cytokines without the appropriate release of anti-inflammatory cortisol to mitigate the cutaneous response [27].

One study found that chronic psychological stress prolongs epidermal permeability barrier recovery following intentional disruption by repeated stripping with cellophane tape, and the extent of this prolongation was directly correlated with the patients' measured stress levels [28]. This demonstrates the influence that stress can have on the skin and is of particular importance in psoriasis, which has been associated with abnormalities in epidermal barrier function that are directly related to severity of the psoriatic lesions [29]. It is interesting to consider that this observed prolongation of barrier recovery may be due to an overall effect of anxiety on healing in general. It is true that chronic psychological stress has been observed to delay wound healing both in rats [30] and in humans [31, 32]. The consequence of this effect may be particularly meaningful in psoriasis, where the Koebner phenomenon (lesions forming at sites of trauma) is a commonly observed source of worsening disease. By disrupting normal barrier homeostasis and slowing wound healing, anxiety may sensitize the psoriatic patient to the formation of trauma-induced plaques and/or cause delay in resolution of such lesions [28].

Beyond HPA axis contributions, there may also be a role for autonomic modulation via the sympathetic nervous system (SNS). Anxiety, in particular, has been extensively correlated with sympathetic activation and vagal inhibition [33]. Likewise, those with depression demonstrate increased sympathetic tone, with elevated muscle sympathetic nervous system activity (MSNA) both at rest and during mental stress: an effect that is more pronounced as depression scores worsen and is reduced by treatment with sertraline [34]. Plasma norepinephrine—another measure of SNS activity—is also higher in those with major depression, and this normalizes after treatment with antidepressants like SSRIs [35] and desipramine [36].

The SNS innervates both primary and secondary lymphoid organs and is known to promote inflammation [37]. Studies have revealed sympathetic-mediated upregulation of proinflammatory cytokines like IL-6 and IL-1β [38], as well as increased mobilization and release of bone-marrow-derived hematopoietic stem and progenitor cells into circulation [39]. In particular, norepinephrine appears to be the main effector in this sympathetic enhancement of immune activity [40]. Saint-Mezard et al. demonstrated that psychological stress experienced prior to immunization afforded an "adjuvant" effect upon the resulting inflammatory reaction by augmenting dendritic cell response and consequently increasing primary and memory T-cell activation [40]. Through selective depletion of NE, they were able to further determine that this effect was mediated by NE and not stress-induced glucocorticoid release, as NE depletion effectively normalized dendritic cell migratory activity and the ensuing hypersensitivity reaction. Psoriatic patients have been found to secrete excess NE in response to stress as compared to

control patients [41, 42]: a finding that might help explain the apparent stress responsiveness of the condition and the characteristic cytokine milieu of elevated TNF-α and IFN with increased trafficking of lymphocytes and dendritic cells to the skin.

Of the receptor subtypes involved in the sympathetic stress response, the alpha adrenergic receptors (α-ARs) have been repeatedly revealed as the mediators bringing about increased cytokine production and proinflammatory changes [43]. Norepinephrine released in response to stress activates α-ARs present in macrophages and dendritic cells, subsequently leading to increased release of TNF-α and suppression of anti-inflammatory IL-10 [43]. Of course, such an effect would reasonably lead to exacerbation of an inflammatory condition already brewing in a patient, such as psoriasis. In contrast, activation of β_2-ARs in these same immune cells elicits a suppression of TNF-α release and promotes IL-10 production, and in T cells, β_2 activation inhibits production of IL-2, which is needed for lymphocyte proliferation required to mount an ample immune response [43].

Given the opposing actions of these two AR subclasses, the particular immunologic stress reaction imparted in an individual is dependent upon the differential expression of α- and β-ARs within that subject and the ultimate balance of their effects as a whole. Lubahn et al. discovered that, in the chronic inflammatory disease, rheumatoid arthritis, treatment with β_2-agonists did not significantly elicit a change in cytokine profiles or immune function while administration of an α-antagonist did produce such an effect [43]. They concluded that chronic inflammatory disease alters the ability of the SNS to regulate immunoreactivity through ordinary β_2-AR signal transduction, effectively shifting toward α-ARs as the primary receptor class regulating immune function in such conditions. As psoriasis, like rheumatoid arthritis, is a disease of chronic inflammation, it is not unreasonable to imagine that a similar mechanism may explain the stress-responsiveness of the disease. In fact, use of β-blocker medication has been well-reported in the literature to cause onset of psoriasis and exacerbation of already present disease [44, 45], providing evidence that this may indeed be the case.

Presumably by further diminishing the anti-inflammatory effects of β-AR stimulation, β-blockers appear to augment the inflammatory actions of α-ARs, causing worsening of disease. While the downstream effects on TNF-α and IL-10 have already been indicated as key components of this pathway, there also appears to be a role for fibroblast growth factor 10 (FGF10) in determining the influence of the SNS on psoriasis. Studies have found that FGF10 causes keratinocyte proliferation as seen in psoriatic disease [46, 47], and immunostaining has discovered increased expression of FGF10 in psoriatic lesions, positively correlating with the amount of T-cell infiltrate detected [46]. In further exploring the influence of FGF10 in psoriasis, Yao et al. found that neutralization of FGF10 with a monoclonal antibody significantly improved β-blocker-induced psoriasis in guinea pigs, in terms of both epidermal thickness and monocyte infiltrate [47]. This reaffirmed that FGF10 exerts an effect on psoriasis severity and that disruption of normal β-AR activity—as observed in chronic diseases like rheumatoid arthritis or psoriasis—can allow for this effect to rise above the normal anti-inflammatory actions, otherwise keeping it in check. The overarching conclusion conveyed by these studies is that SNS activity, triggered by acute stress, generates NE that disproportionately activates proinflammatory α-ARs in the setting of chronic disease, and in psoriasis, this can lead to worsening of disease by means of various chemical messengers including TNF-α and FGF10.

Some have theorized that the adjuvant-like effect of acute stress on immunoreactivity is an evolutionary adaptation, the purpose of which is to prepare the body to fight off infection following injury [48, 49]. The interesting thing about mankind is that each individual interprets their environment through their own eyes, affected by their personal set of experiences, wisdom, coping mechanisms, fears, and expectations. It is the subjective interpretation of a stressor that dictates one's reaction and subsequent immune response, suggesting that inflammatory responses should be less likely in those that "go with the flow" or do not become as anxious in the face of stressors as others [48]. Research has shown that this is indeed the case. Carroll et al. found that task related increases in anxiety and anger are directly correlated with serum levels of inflammatory IL-6, demonstrating that affective responses are instrumental in determining the degree of subsequent immune reactivity in an individual [50]. Others have reproduced this same result and, in addition, discovered that perceived social support diminishes the relationship between subjective stress experience and IL-6 increase [51].

This discussion is highly pertinent when considering the way that depression might influence psoriasis, as those with depression suffer from cognitive distortions that alter the ways in which they interpret their environment [52, 53]. This includes decreases in perceived degree of social support among depressed subjects: an effect that improves with effective treatment and resolution of depressive symptoms [53]. While the increased stress immune responsiveness of patients with low social support might be an evolutionarily advantageous adaptation, it becomes detrimental when the immune system is already active and directed in a pathological process, such as psoriasis. Under such circumstances, acute stress only amplifies the present disease process and worsens disease severity rather than enhancing infection defenses as evolutionary pressures intended.

Beyond the effects of acute stress, chronic stress is likely to be a predominant issue for patients with depression/anxiety. How do the consequences of chronic stress differ, and how might they alternatively impact the course of inflammatory disease? There is ample evidence that chronic stress can result in immunosuppression or immune dysregulation [49], with the exact effect determined by a number of individual factors. As similarly discussed in regard to depression, chronic stress results in lasting HPA axis hyperactivity with elevated baseline levels of ACTH, CRH, and cortisol. Physiologic levels of glucocorticoids, unlike pharmacologic levels, have been found to actually enhance immune responses by increasing T-cell responsiveness to IL-2, promoting production of cytokines like IL-1 and IL-6, and supporting biological

sensitivity to cytokines like granulocyte colony-stimulating factor, granulocyte macrophage colony-stimulating factor, and IFN-γ [49]. In addition, HPA axis response to acute stress is blunted, meaning anti-inflammatory cortisol does not appropriately elevate, and the normal diurnal cycle of cortisol secretion in the body is also disrupted [54]. These changes appear to correlate with the harmful effects of chronic stress [49]—including decreased wound healing, as previously reviewed, and promotion of inflammation through increased production of inflammatory cytokines and a shift toward type 2 cytokine-mediated immune responses [49, 55]—and are thought to be the primary means by which stress induces or exacerbates autoimmune and allergic diseases.

With all considered, depression and anxiety likely contribute to the worsening of inflammatory disorders, like psoriasis, via both HPA axis and SNS hyperactivity. Those with mood disorders demonstrate baseline disruptions in these physiologic systems that contribute to ongoing immunopathology. Additionally, these populations show increased responsiveness to acute stressors, which further alters immune function and can acutely worsen chronic disorders of inflammation and autoimmunity.

2.3. Inflammation Causing Depression. While the discussion thus far has centered on the ways in which depressive or anxious states appear to increase inflammation, induction of an inflammatory state, as in psoriasis, can also precipitate changes in mood, including depressive symptoms. One study found that healthy volunteers vaccinated for *Salmonella typhi* subsequently displayed increases in inflammatory markers, like IL-6, TNF-α, and IL-1Ra, as well as depressive symptoms without signs of physical sickness [56]. Other researchers have witnessed the induction of "sickness behavior" in rats following injection of IL-1 and lipopolysaccharide (LPS). This "sickness behavior" included decreases in energy, sleep, appetite, interest exploring, and sexual activity: a presentation reminiscent of major depression [57]. Furthermore, baseline CRP and IL-6 measurements have been observed to effectively predict future depression at 12-year follow-up, while baseline symptoms of depression were not predictive of future inflammatory markers [58]. A randomized control trial using the TNF-α inhibitor, etanercept, revealed that treatment of inflammation in the setting of psoriasis results in measured improvements in fatigue and depressive symptoms [59]. While decreases in fatigue were correlated with decreased joint pain, improvements in depressive symptoms were less correlated with psoriasis and arthritis severity, suggesting the presence of an alternative mechanism to explain this particular effect: potentially the physiologic changes associated with decreased systemic inflammation as opposed to the psychological effects of decreased psoriasis severity. All of these studies demonstrate the potential for inflammation, and thus psoriasis, to induce depression, and one possible mechanism to explain this effect involves alterations in the metabolism of serotonin.

Cytokines, more specifically IL-2 and IFN-α, have been shown to directly increase the enzymatic activity of indoleamine 2,3-dioxygenase (IDO), which increases the conversion of tryptophan to kynurenine [60]. Shunting of tryptophan toward kynurenine consequently decreases the production of serotonin from tryptophan, resulting in a functional serotonin deficit that might produce depressive symptoms. Compounding this effect, tryptophan metabolites, including kynurenine, have been found to independently induce depressive symptoms [61]. Besides activation via inflammatory cytokines, this pathway is also activated following induction of tryptophan 2,3-dioxygenase (TDO) by glucocorticoids: another potential explanation for how the hypercortisolemia seen in depression may contribute to symptomatology [61]. Inflammatory cytokines like IL-6 have also been found to increase the breakdown of serotonin [62]. Thus, inflammation may affect mood by simultaneously decreasing production and increasing degradation of serotonin.

3. The Role of Melatonin

Inflammatory cytokines are not the only biomarkers linking depression and psoriasis. Depression is associated with disruptions in the secretion of melatonin [63], which physiologically follows a circadian rhythm with elevated levels at night, usually peaking in the early morning between 2 and 4 a.m. [64]. Melatonin is well known for regulating the daily sleep cycle, but it also modulates immune function. By reducing levels of TNF-α, IL-6, and IL-8, melatonin can theoretically attenuate the severity of inflammatory disorders [65, 66]. Melatonin dysregulation has been observed in other inflammatory conditions, as well, including sarcoidosis and, indeed, psoriasis vulgaris [67, 68]. Such disruptions in cyclic melatonin secretion could contribute to the inflammation observed in these disease states. Nighttime melatonin levels have been recorded to be significantly lower in patients with psoriasis than in healthy controls [64]. Decreased melatonin levels could contribute to the previously mentioned Koebner phenomenon responsible for exacerbating psoriasis, as absence of melatonin through pinealectomy has been shown to delay wound healing in rats, while melatonin replacement in these rats effectively eradicated this effect [69].

In those with depression, decreased melatonin levels and a dysfunctional circadian rhythm may disinhibit the release of melanocyte stimulating hormone (MSH), which has been linked to seborrhea in rats and may play a role in psoriasis [15, 70]. In addition, hypersecretion of CRH results in the production of ACTH from its precursor molecule, proopiomelanocortin (POMC). As a byproduct of ACTH synthesis from POMC, MSH levels would be expected to increase under such circumstances: an effect seen in Cushing's disease where the overproduction of ACTH can, through associated elevations in MSH, physically manifest itself as generalized hyperpigmentation [71].

Thus, MSH may be elevated in depression due to both low melatonin levels and hypersecretion of CRH, and this could contribute to the presentation of patients with psoriasis. Interestingly, studies have implicated MSH as a contributor to depressive symptoms [72, 73], and administration of an MSH inhibitor has been observed to significantly improve depressive symptoms [74]. Further research is certainly needed to

better characterize the role that cyclic changes in melatonin play in depression and psoriasis, and the mechanism by which this role is achieved.

Low melatonin may also play a role in the morbidity of psoriasis. A prospective cohort study with 14,128 subjects demonstrated a significantly increased risk for developing diabetes mellitus type II (DMII) in psoriasis patients versus the comparison group, and this risk was directly related to the severity of the psoriasis [75]. Interestingly, melatonin has been shown to participate in the regulation of blood glucose levels via melatonin receptors within the pancreatic beta cells and insulin receptors in the pituitary gland [76]. The interrelationship has been demonstrated in DMII, where increased levels of insulin are accompanied by decreased levels of melatonin, decreased expression of pineal insulin receptors, and increased pancreatic expression of melatonin receptors [76]. In fact, there is evidence for a circadian rhythm of insulin secretion, which demonstrates an inverse relationship between insulin and melatonin levels [77]. The link between melatonin and diabetes has not yet been fully elucidated, but DMII is associated with decreased levels of melatonin, and recent genome-wide association studies have demonstrated that single nucleotide polymorphisms of the MT2 melatonin receptor locus significantly increase the risk for developing DMII [78–80]. Others have demonstrated that pinealectomy in rats results in insulin resistance and decreased expression of GLUT 4 receptors, with return to control values following melatonin replacement [81].

The mechanism behind the apparent protective effects of melatonin is not established, but available evidence offers some clues. Some studies have found that melatonin might sensitize pancreatic beta cells [82] or even induce regeneration and proliferation of beta cells that have been destroyed in streptozotocin-induced type I diabetes [83–85]. Its activity as a free radical scavenger [86, 87] provides protection to pancreatic beta cells which, themselves, have low antioxidative capacity and are thus susceptible to oxidative damage [88]. Several publications support the notion that diabetes creates a state of increased free radical production [89–91], so decreased melatonin may represent a possible contributing factor as well as a target for intervention via melatonin supplementation. In fact, melatonin has been shown to decrease insulin resistance in rats with DMII, reportedly by improving lipid metabolism [92].

Insulin resistance has also been associated with major depression, a condition which, as discussed, also demonstrates abnormalities in melatonin secretion and is a common comorbidity of psoriasis. Might abnormalities in melatonin be the link between psoriasis, depression, and diabetes? This conclusion cannot be drawn by the simple associations observed, but melatonin levels naturally decline with age, and this may contribute to the incidence of diabetes as well as the other inflammatory conditions mentioned, including psoriasis. Both later-onset (type II) psoriasis [93] and DMII develop with age in those predisposed, and this may partially result from a drop in melatonin levels beyond a threshold necessary for counteracting the disease process. This is similar to the suggestion by some researchers that the age-related decline of melatonin may be contributory to the

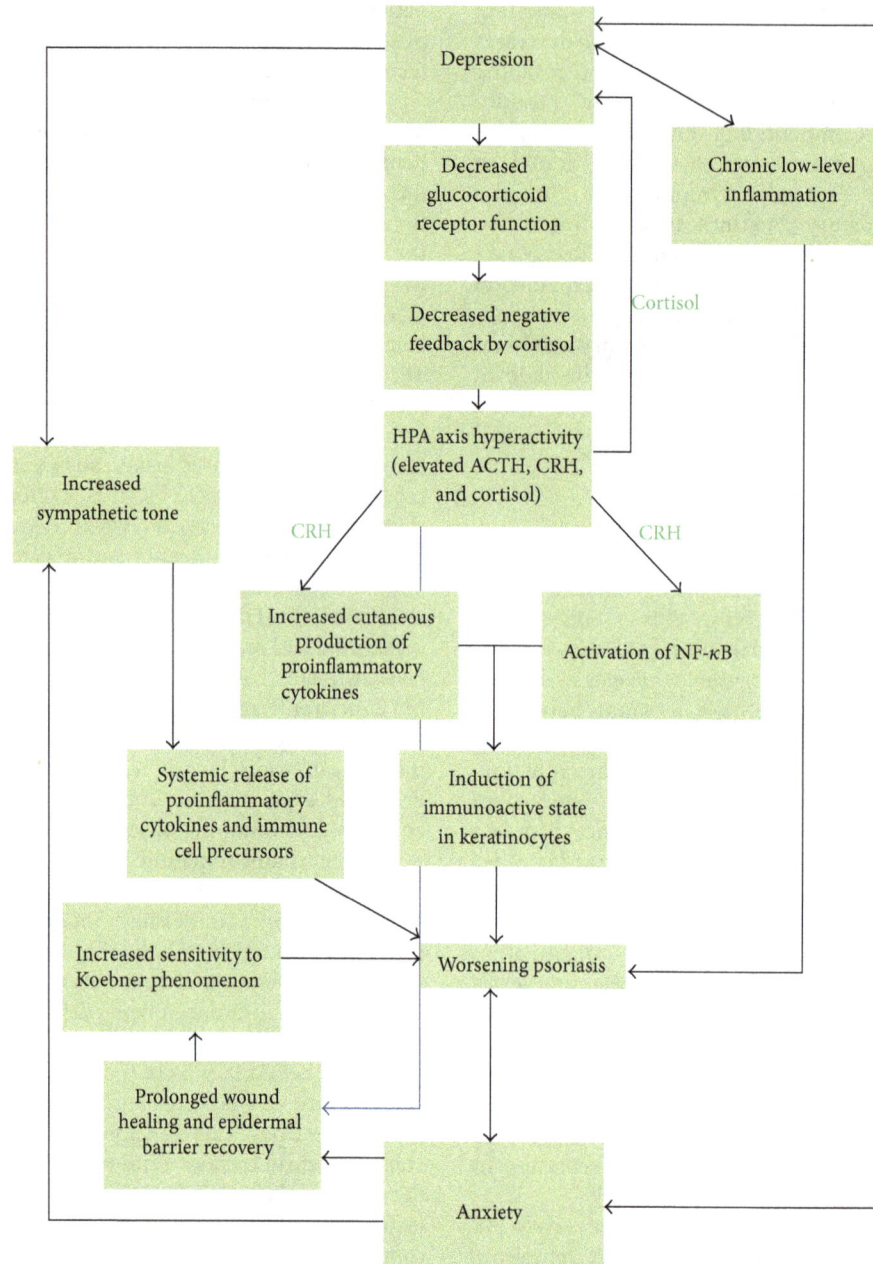

FIGURE 1: Overview: psoriasis and mood disorders. Depression and anxiety interact with psoriasis through associations with HPA axis hyperactivity, sympathetic hyperactivity, chronic inflammation, and delayed wound healing.

increased incidence of breast cancer in older women [94]. Of course, melatonin is not the only neuroendocrine factor that fluctuates with age, and it is likely that other such factors are also at play in modulating the relationship between psoriasis, diabetes, and inflammation.

In addition to depression and diabetes, psoriasis is associated with a variety of conditions in which chronic inflammation plays a pathophysiological role, including myocardial infarction, hypertension, stroke, metabolic syndrome, and cardiovascular mortality [75]. Melatonin may more directly affect these morbidities, and psoriasis itself, via its well-supported anti-inflammatory properties. For example, melatonin administration has been shown in multiple reports to decrease blood pressure in untreated, hypertensive men and

even in adolescents with type I diabetes [95–97]. In addition, it has also been observed to protect against endothelial dysfunction [98] and ischemic heart failure [99], further illustrating the potentially widespread clinical applications of melatonin, particularly in the at-risk psoriatic population.

Clinical practice may already hint at the significance of melatonin in both depression and psoriasis. Phototherapy is a common, and effective, treatment for depression, and it is also a current treatment for psoriatic lesions. The mechanism underlying its usefulness in psoriasis is not entirely known, but the current conceptual model implicates inhibition of keratinocyte proliferation, and more importantly, immunomodulation via altered cytokine composition and cytokine receptor expression decreased adhesion molecules necessary for immune cell trafficking, altered types and functions of antigen presenting cells, and induction of lymphocyte apoptosis [100–103]. Considering that sunlight serves as the main zeitgeber in setting the circadian rhythm of melatonin secretion, it is possible that normalization of melatonin derangement may be another benefit of phototherapy, as long as light exposure includes the retina. Melatonin may be a candidate for study as a treatment option for comorbid depression and psoriasis, given its potential to address the aberrations in cyclical melatonin secretion observed in both conditions. In fact, the melatonin receptor agonist, agomelatine, has already shown effectiveness in treating depressive symptoms, further demonstrating the influence this hormone has in mood disorders.

4. Integrated Treatment

Not only is managing depression important for enhancing the patient's quality of life, but it may also be helpful in improving his/her psoriasis. According to one study, three negative schemas—vulnerability to harm, defectiveness, and social isolation—predict anxiety and depression in psoriasis patients [104]. The apparent role of such cognitive distortions may support the use of cognitive behavioral therapy (CBT) in this population. A case-controlled study [105] involving 40 patients with psoriasis receiving adjunctive group CBT revealed greater reduction in depression and anxiety scores and nearly double the reductions in self-reported disability and life stress scores compared with the control group. Perhaps more interestingly, the treatment group also experienced a significant reduction in Psoriasis Area Severity Index (PASI) scores at 6 weeks and 6 months' follow-up, with 64% of patients achieving 75% psoriasis clearance at 6-month follow-up compared with 23% of the control group.

While SSRIs are often the first-line treatment for depression, fluoxetine has been observed to exacerbate psoriasis in some patients [106, 107]. Lithium, a common treatment for bipolar disorder, has also been reported to worsen psoriasis and even induce psoriasiform lesions in those without psoriasis [108, 109]. In both cases, standard psoriasis treatments are ineffective, with resolution ensuing only after lithium discontinuation [109]. To avoid aggravation of comorbid psoriasis in these sensitive populations, CBT might be an attractive alternative treatment to psychoactive medication, with a possible additional role for adjunctive melatonin supplementation.

5. Conclusion

Overall, psoriasis vulgaris and mood disorders are highly associated, and despite frequent underdiagnosis, this combination of comorbidities causes patients much disability. Interestingly, fluctuations in mood appear to affect the severity of psoriasis (Figure 1) and, thus, may serve as a potential target for intervention [15, 110]. By ensuring that patients are properly screened and referred when depression is suspected, treatment can begin, morbidity can be prevented, and the psoriasis itself may improve in kind. The overlapping inflammatory cascades in both conditions could also represent a potentially important point of intervention, as addressing this could theoretically have a synergistic effect on improving psoriasis by mitigating both the basal inflammatory state and the depression and anxiety that cause exacerbations. In addition, it is intriguing to note the potential that melatonin offers in modulating various associations with psoriasis and mood disorders, including HPA axis abnormalities, epidermal barrier function deficits, diabetes, and the cardiovascular comorbidities associated with the chronic inflammation characteristic of these conditions.

Conflict of Interests

The authors have no affiliations with or financial involvement in any organization or entity with a direct financial interest in the subject matter or materials discussed in the paper. The authors declare that there is no conflict of interests regarding the publication of this paper.

Acknowledgments

Jess G. Fiedorowicz is supported by the National Institute of Mental Health (K23MH083695) and the National Heart, Lung, and Blood Institute (P01HL014388).

References

[1] F. O. Nestle, D. H. Kaplan, and J. Barker, "Psoriasis," *The New England Journal of Medicine*, vol. 361, no. 5, pp. 496–509, 2009.

[2] S. R. Rapp, S. R. Feldman, M. L. Exum, A. B. Fleischer, and D. M. Reboussin, "Psoriasis causes as much disability as other major medical diseases," *Journal of the American Academy of Dermatology*, vol. 41, no. 3, part 1, pp. 401–407, 1999.

[3] M. A. Gupta and A. K. Gupta, "Psychiatric and psychological co-morbidity in patients with dermatologic disorders: epidemiology and management," *American Journal of Clinical Dermatology*, vol. 4, no. 12, pp. 833–842, 2003.

[4] S. K. Kurd, A. B. Troxel, P. Crits-Christoph, and J. M. Gelfand, "The risk of depression, anxiety, and suicidality in patients with psoriasis: a population-based cohort study," *Archives of Dermatology*, vol. 146, no. 8, pp. 891–895, 2010.

[5] M. Ghajarzadeh, M. Ghiasi, and S. Kheirkhah, "Associations between skin diseases and quality of life: a comparison of psoriasis, vitiligo, and alopecia areata," *Acta Medica Iranica*, vol. 50, no. 7, pp. 511–515, 2012.

[6] M. Karelson, H. Silm, and K. Kingo, "Quality of life and emotional state in vitiligo in an Estonian sample: comparison with psoriasis and healthy controls," *Acta Dermato Venereologica*, vol. 93, no. 4, pp. 446–450, 2013.

[7] V. Kumar, S. K. Mattoo, and S. Handa, "Psychiatric morbidity in pemphigus and psoriasis: a comparative study from India," *Asian Journal of Psychiatry*, vol. 6, no. 2, pp. 151–156, 2013.

[8] N. Sharma, R. V. Koranne, and R. K. Singh, "Psychiatric morbidity in psoriasis and vitiligo: a comparative study," *Journal of Dermatology*, vol. 28, no. 8, pp. 419–423, 2001.

[9] A. Mufaddel and A. E. Abdelgani, "Psychiatric comorbidity in patients with psoriasis, vitiligo, acne, eczema and group of patients with miscellaneous dermatological diagnoses," *Open Journal of Psychiatry*, vol. 4, no. 3, pp. 168–175, 2014.

[10] J. D. Rosenblat, D. S. Cha, R. B. Mansur, and R. S. McIntyre, "Inflamed moods: a review of the interactions between inflammation and mood disorders," *Progress in Neuro-Psychopharmacology and Biological Psychiatry*, vol. 53, pp. 23–34, 2014.

[11] Y. Dowlati, N. Herrmann, W. Swardfager et al., "A meta-analysis of cytokines in major depression," *Biological Psychiatry*, vol. 67, no. 5, pp. 446–457, 2010.

[12] C. Pizzi, S. Mancini, L. Angeloni, F. Fontana, L. Manzoli, and G. M. Costa, "Effects of selective serotonin reuptake inhibitor therapy on endothelial function and inflammatory markers in patients with coronary heart disease," *Clinical Pharmacology and Therapeutics*, vol. 86, no. 5, pp. 527–532, 2009.

[13] A. Steptoe, M. Hamer, and Y. Chida, "The effects of acute psychological stress on circulating inflammatory factors in humans: a review and meta-analysis," *Brain, Behavior, and Immunity*, vol. 21, no. 7, pp. 901–912, 2007.

[14] M. A. Gupta, A. K. Gupta, and H. F. Haberman, "Psoriasis and psychiatry: an update," *General Hospital Psychiatry*, vol. 9, no. 3, pp. 157–166, 1987.

[15] R. Sandyk and R. Pardeshi, "Mood-dependent fluctuations in the severity of tardive dyskinesia and psoriasis vulgaris in a patient with schizoaffective disorder: possible role of melatonin," *International Journal of Neuroscience*, vol. 50, no. 3-4, pp. 215–221, 1990.

[16] L. Arborelius, M. J. Owens, P. M. Plotsky, and C. B. Nemeroff, "The role of corticotropin-releasing factor in depression and anxiety disorders," *Journal of Endocrinology*, vol. 160, no. 1, pp. 1–12, 1999.

[17] M. Joëls and E. R. de Kloet, "Mineralocorticoid and glucocorticoid receptors in the brain. Implications for ion permeability and transmitter systems," *Progress in Neurobiology*, vol. 43, no. 1, pp. 1–36, 1994.

[18] L. Jacobson and R. Sapolsky, "The role of the hippocampus in feedback regulation of the hypothalamic-pituitary-adrenocortical axis," *Endocrine Reviews*, vol. 12, no. 2, pp. 118–134, 1991.

[19] B. Zbytek, A. Mysliwski, A. Slominski, J. Wortsman, E. T. Wei, and J. Mysliwska, "Corticotropin-releasing hormone affects cytokine production in human HaCaT keratinocytes," *Life Sciences*, vol. 70, no. 9, pp. 1013–1021, 2002.

[20] M.-E. Quevedo, A. Slominski, W. Pinto, E. Wel, and J. Wortsman, "Pleiotropic effects of corticotropin releasing hormone on normal human skin keratinocytes," *In Vitro Cellular and Developmental Biology: Animal*, vol. 37, no. 1, pp. 50–54, 2001.

[21] B. Zbytek, L. M. Pfeffer, and A. T. Slominski, "Corticotropin-releasing hormone stimulates NF-κB in human epidermal keratinocytes," *Journal of Endocrinology*, vol. 181, no. 3, pp. R1–R7, 2004.

[22] J. E. Kim, D. H. Cho, H. S. Kim et al., "Expression of the corticotropin-releasing hormone-proopiomelanocortin axis in the various clinical types of psoriasis," *Experimental Dermatology*, vol. 16, no. 2, pp. 104–109, 2007.

[23] N. Ito, T. Ito, A. Kromminga et al., "Human hair follicles display a functional equivalent of the hypothalamic-pituitary-adrenal axis and synthesize cortisol," *The FASEB Journal*, vol. 19, no. 10, pp. 1332–1334, 2005.

[24] M. O'Kane, E. P. Murphy, and B. Kirby, "The role of corticotropin-releasing hormone in immune-mediated cutaneous inflammatory disease," *Experimental Dermatology*, vol. 15, no. 3, pp. 143–153, 2006.

[25] T. Tsuchiya and I. Horii, "Epidermal cell proliferative activity assessed by proliferating cell nuclear antigen (PCNA) decreases

[26] M. Denda, T. Tsuchiya, P. M. Elias, and K. R. Feingold, "Stress alters cutaneous permeability barrier homeostasis," *The American Journal of Physiology—Regulatory Integrative and Comparative Physiology*, vol. 278, no. 2, pp. R367–R372, 2000.

[27] H. L. Richards, D. W. Ray, B. Kirby et al., "Response of the hypothalamic-pituitary-adrenal axis to psychological stress in patients with psoriasis," *British Journal of Dermatology*, vol. 153, no. 6, pp. 1114–1120, 2005.

[28] A. Garg, M.-M. Chren, L. P. Sands et al., "Psychological stress perturbs epidermal permeability barrier homeostasis: implications for the pathogenesis of stress-associated skin disorders," *Archives of Dermatology*, vol. 137, no. 1, pp. 53–59, 2001.

[29] R. Ghadially, J. T. Reed, and P. M. Elias, "Stratum corneum structure and function correlates with phenotype in psoriasis," *Journal of Investigative Dermatology*, vol. 107, no. 4, pp. 558–564, 1996.

[30] D. A. Padgett, P. T. Marucha, and J. F. Sheridan, "Restraint stress slows cutaneous wound healing in mice," *Brain, Behavior, and Immunity*, vol. 12, no. 1, pp. 64–73, 1998.

[31] M. Ebrecht, J. Hextall, L.-G. Kirtley, A. Taylor, M. Dyson, and J. Weinman, "Perceived stress and cortisol levels predict speed of wound healing in healthy male adults," *Psychoneuroendocrinology*, vol. 29, no. 6, pp. 798–809, 2004.

[32] J. K. Kiecolt-Glaser, P. T. Marucha, A. M. Mercado, W. B. Malarkey, and R. Glaser, "Slowing of wound healing by psychological stress," *The Lancet*, vol. 346, no. 8984, pp. 1194–1196, 1995.

[33] S. D. Kreibig, "Autonomic nervous system activity in emotion: a review," *Biological Psychology*, vol. 84, no. 3, pp. 394–421, 2010.

[34] A. Z. Scalco, M. U. P. B. Rondon, I. C. Trombetta et al., "Muscle sympathetic nervous activity in depressed patients before and after treatment with sertraline," *Journal of Hypertension*, vol. 27, no. 12, pp. 2429–2436, 2009.

[35] D. A. Barton, T. Dawood, E. A. Lambert et al., "Sympathetic activity in major depressive disorder: identifying those at increased cardiac risk?" *Journal of Hypertension*, vol. 25, no. 10, pp. 2117–2124, 2007.

[36] R. C. Veith, N. Lewis, O. A. Linares et al., "Sympathetic nervous system activity in major depression: basal and desipramine-induced alterations in plasma norepinephrine kinetics," *Archives of General Psychiatry*, vol. 51, no. 5, pp. 411–422, 1994.

[37] M. V. Singh, M. W. Chapleau, S. C. Harwani, and F. M. Abboud, "The immune system and hypertension," *Immunologic Research*, vol. 59, no. 1–3, pp. 243–253, 2014.

[38] K. M. Grebe, K. Takeda, H. D. Hickman et al., "Cutting edge: sympathetic nervous system increases proinflammatory cytokines and exacerbates influenza A virus pathogenesis," *Journal of Immunology*, vol. 184, no. 2, pp. 540–544, 2010.

[39] Y. Katayama, M. Battista, W.-M. Kao et al., "Signals from the sympathetic nervous system regulate hematopoietic stem cell egress from bone marrow," *Cell*, vol. 124, no. 2, pp. 407–421, 2006.

[40] P. Saint-Mezard, C. Chavagnac, S. Bosset et al., "Psychological stress exerts an adjuvant effect on skin dendritic cell functions in vivo," *The Journal of Immunology*, vol. 171, no. 8, pp. 4073–4080, 2003.

[41] A. Buske-Kirschbaum, M. Ebrecht, S. Kern, and D. H. Hellhammer, "Endocrine stress responses in TH1-mediated chronic inflammatory skin disease (psoriasis vulgaris)—do they parallel

following immobilization-induced stress in male Syrian hamsters," *Psychoneuroendocrinology*, vol. 21, no. 1, pp. 111–117, 1996.

stress-induced endocrine changes in TH2-mediated inflammatory dermatoses (atopic dermatitis)?" *Psychoneuroendocrinology*, vol. 31, no. 4, pp. 439–446, 2006.

[42] G. Schmid-Ott, R. Jacobs, B. Jäger et al., "Stress-induced endocrine and immunological changes in psoriasis patients and healthy controls. A preliminary study," *Psychotherapy and Psychosomatics*, vol. 67, no. 1, pp. 37–42, 1998.

[43] C. L. Lubahn, D. Lorton, J. A. Schaller, S. J. Sweeney, and D. L. Bellinger, "Targeting α- and β-adrenergic receptors differentially shifts Th1, Th2, and inflammatory cytokine profiles in immune organs to attenuate adjuvant arthritis," *Frontiers in Immunology*, vol. 5, article 346, 2014.

[44] K. H. Basavaraj, N. M. Ashok, R. Rashmi, and T. K. Praveen, "The role of drugs in the induction and/or exacerbation of psoriasis," *International Journal of Dermatology*, vol. 49, no. 12, pp. 1351–1361, 2010.

[45] S. Wu, J. Han, W.-Q. Li, and A. A. Qureshi, "Hypertension, antihypertensive medication use, and risk of psoriasis," *JAMA Dermatology*, vol. 150, no. 9, pp. 957–963, 2014.

[46] D. Kovacs, M. Falchi, G. Cardinali et al., "Immunohistochemical analysis of keratinocyte growth factor and fibroblast growth factor 10 expression in psoriasis," *Experimental Dermatology*, vol. 14, no. 2, pp. 130–137, 2005.

[47] N. Yao, J.-X. Xia, X.-M. Liu et al., "Topical application of a new monoclonal antibody against fibroblast growth factor 10 (FGF10) mitigates propranolol-induced psoriasis-like lesions in guinea pigs," *European Review for Medical and Pharmacological Sciences*, vol. 18, no. 7, pp. 1085–1091, 2014.

[48] F. S. Dhabhar, "Effects of stress on immune function: the good, the bad, and the beautiful," *Immunologic Research*, vol. 58, no. 2-3, pp. 193–210, 2014.

[49] F. S. Dhabhar, "Enhancing versus suppressive effects of stress on immune function: implications for immunoprotection and immunopathology," *NeuroImmunoModulation*, vol. 16, no. 5, pp. 300–317, 2009.

[50] J. E. Carroll, C. A. Low, A. A. Prather et al., "Negative affective responses to a speech task predict changes in interleukin (IL)-6," *Brain, Behavior, and Immunity*, vol. 25, no. 2, pp. 232–238, 2011.

[51] E. Puterman, E. S. Epel, A. O'Donovan, A. A. Prather, K. Aschbacher, and F. S. Dhabhar, "Anger is associated with increased IL-6 stress reactivity in women, but only among those low in social support," *International Journal of Behavioral Medicine*, vol. 21, no. 6, pp. 936–945, 2013.

[52] M. J. Maher, P. A. Mora, and H. Leventhal, "Depression as a predictor of perceived social support and demand: a componential approach using a prospective sample of older adults," *Emotion*, vol. 6, no. 3, pp. 450–458, 2006.

[53] E. Stice, P. Rohde, J. Gau, and C. Ochner, "Relation of depression to perceived social support: results from a randomized adolescent depression prevention trial," *Behaviour Research and Therapy*, vol. 49, no. 5, pp. 361–366, 2011.

[54] S. Sephton and D. Spiegel, "Circadian disruption in cancer: a neuroendocrine-immune pathway from stress to disease?" *Brain, Behavior, and Immunity*, vol. 17, no. 5, pp. 321–328, 2003.

[55] E. M. J. Peters, C. Liezmann, B. F. Klapp, and J. Kruse, "The neuroimmune connection interferes with tissue regeneration and chronic inflammatory disease in the skin," *Annals of the New York Academy of Sciences*, vol. 1262, no. 1, pp. 118–126, 2012.

[56] C. E. Wright, P. C. Strike, L. Brydon, and A. Steptoe, "Acute inflammation and negative mood: mediation by cytokine activation," *Brain, Behavior, and Immunity*, vol. 19, no. 4, pp. 345–350, 2005.

[57] A. J. Dunn, A. H. Swiergiel, and R. de Beaurepaire, "Cytokines as mediators of depression: what can we learn from animal studies?" *Neuroscience and Biobehavioral Reviews*, vol. 29, no. 4-5, pp. 891–909, 2005.

[58] D. Gimeno, M. Kivimäki, E. J. Brunner et al., "Associations of C-reactive protein and interleukin-6 with cognitive symptoms of depression: 12-year follow-up of the Whitehall II study," *Psychological Medicine*, vol. 39, no. 3, pp. 413–423, 2009.

[59] S. Tyring, A. Gottlieb, K. Papp et al., "Etanercept and clinical outcomes, fatigue, and depression in psoriasis: double-blind placebo-controlled randomised phase III trial," *The Lancet*, vol. 367, no. 9504, pp. 29–35, 2006.

[60] L. Capuron, G. Neurauter, D. L. Musselman et al., "Interferon-alpha-induced changes in tryptophan metabolism. Relationship to depression and paroxetine treatment," *Biological Psychiatry*, vol. 54, no. 9, pp. 906–914, 2003.

[61] M. Maes, B. E. Leonard, A. M. Myint, M. Kubera, and R. Verkerk, "The new '5-HT' hypothesis of depression: cell-mediated immune activation induces indoleamine 2,3-dioxygenase, which leads to lower plasma tryptophan and an increased synthesis of detrimental tryptophan catabolites (TRYCATs), both of which contribute to the onset of depression," *Progress in Neuro-Psychopharmacology and Biological Psychiatry*, vol. 35, no. 3, pp. 702–721, 2011.

[62] J. Wang and A. J. Dunn, "Mouse interleukin-6 stimulates the HPA axis and increases brain tryptophan and serotonin metabolism," *Neurochemistry International*, vol. 33, no. 2, pp. 143–154, 1998.

[63] R. P. Brown, J. H. Kocsis, S. Caroff et al., "Depressed mood and reality disturbance correlate with decreased nocturnal melatonin in depressed patients," *Acta Psychiatrica Scandinavica*, vol. 76, no. 3, pp. 272–275, 1987.

[64] L. B. Kartha, L. Chandrashekar, M. Rajappa et al., "Serum melatonin levels in psoriasis and associated depressive symptoms," *Clinical Chemistry and Laboratory Medicine*, vol. 52, no. 6, pp. e123–e125, 2014.

[65] A. Carrillo-Vico, P. J. Lardone, N. Álvarez-Śnchez, A. Rodriguez-Rodriguez, and J. M. Guerrero, "Melatonin: buffering the immune system," *International Journal of Molecular Sciences*, vol. 14, no. 4, pp. 8638–8683, 2013.

[66] E. Esposito and S. Cuzzocrea, "Antiinflammatory activity of melatonin in central nervous system," *Current Neuropharmacology*, vol. 8, no. 3, pp. 228–242, 2010.

[67] A. Miles and D. Philbrick, "Melatonin: perspectives in laboratory medicine and clinical research," *Critical Reviews in Clinical Laboratory Sciences*, vol. 25, no. 3, pp. 231–253, 1987.

[68] N. Mozzanica, G. Tadini, A. Radaelli et al., "Plasma melatonin levels in psoriasis," *Acta Dermato-Venereologica*, vol. 68, no. 4, pp. 312–316, 1988.

[69] M. Ozler, K. Simsek, C. Ozkan et al., "Comparison of the effect of topical and systemic melatonin administration on delayed wound healing in rats that underwent pinealectomy," *Scandinavian Journal of Clinical and Laboratory Investigation*, vol. 70, no. 6, pp. 447–452, 2010.

[70] A. J. Thody and S. Shuster, "Control of sebaceous gland function in the rat by α melanocyte stimulating hormone," *Journal of Endocrinology*, vol. 64, no. 3, pp. 503–510, 1975.

[71] K. R. Feingold and P. M. Elias, "Endocrine-skin interactions. Cutaneous manifestations of adrenal disease, pheochromocytomas, carcinoid syndrome, sex hormone excess and deficiency, polyglandular autoimmune syndromes, multiple endocrine neoplasia syndromes, and other miscellaneous disorders," *Journal of the American Academy of Dermatology*, vol. 19, no. 1, part 1, pp. 1–20, 1988.

[72] S. N. Goyal, D. M. Kokare, C. T. Chopde, and N. K. Subhedar, "Alpha-melanocyte stimulating hormone antagonizes antidepressant-like effect of neuropeptide Y in Porsolt's test in rats," *Pharmacology Biochemistry and Behavior*, vol. 85, no. 2, pp. 369–377, 2006.

[73] D. M. Kokare, M. P. Dandekar, P. S. Singru, G. L. Gupta, and N. K. Subhedar, "Involvement of alpha-MSH in the social isolation induced anxiety- and depression-like behaviors in rat," *Neuropharmacology*, vol. 58, no. 7, pp. 1009–1018, 2010.

[74] R. H. Ehrensing and A. J. Kastin, "Melanocyte-stimulating hormone-release inhibiting hormone as a antidepressant. A pilot study," *Archives of General Psychiatry*, vol. 30, no. 1, pp. 63–65, 1974.

[75] M.-S. Lee, R.-Y. Lin, and M.-S. Lai, "Increased risk of diabetes mellitus in relation to the severity of psoriasis, concomitant medication, and comorbidity: a nationwide population-based cohort study," *Journal of the American Academy of Dermatology*, vol. 70, no. 4, pp. 691–698, 2014.

[76] E. Peschke and E. Mühlbauer, "New evidence for a role of melatonin in glucose regulation," *Best Practice & Research Clinical Endocrinology & Metabolism*, vol. 24, no. 5, pp. 829–841, 2010.

[77] G. Boden, J. Ruiz, J.-L. Urbain, and X. Chen, "Evidence for a circadian rhythm of insulin secretion," *American Journal of Physiology—Endocrinology and Metabolism*, vol. 271, part 1, no. 2, pp. E246–E252, 1996.

[78] V. Lyssenko, C. L. F. Nagorny, M. R. Erdos et al., "Common variant in MTNR1B associated with increased risk of type 2 diabetes and impaired early insulin secretion," *Nature Genetics*, vol. 41, no. 1, pp. 82–88, 2009.

[79] I. Prokopenko, C. Langenberg, J. C. Florez et al., "Variants in *MTNR1B* influence fasting glucose levels," *Nature Genetics*, vol. 41, no. 1, pp. 77–81, 2009.

[80] T. Sparsø, A. Bonnefond, E. Andersson et al., "G-allele of intronic rs10830963 in MTNR1B confers increased risk of impaired fasting glycemia and type 2 diabetes through an impaired glucose-stimulated insulin release: studies involving 19,605 Europeans," *Diabetes*, vol. 58, no. 6, pp. 1450–1456, 2009.

[81] M. M. Zanquetta, P. M. Seraphim, D. H. Sumida, J. Cipolla-Neto, and U. F. Machado, "Calorie restriction reduces pinealectomy-induced insulin resistance by improving GLUT4 gene expression and its translocation to the plasma membrane," *Journal of Pineal Research*, vol. 35, no. 3, pp. 141–148, 2003.

[82] D. M. Kemp, M. Ubeda, and J. F. Habener, "Identification and functional characterization of melatonin Mel 1a receptors in pancreatic β cells: potential role in incretin-mediated cell function by sensitization of cAMP signaling," *Molecular and Cellular Endocrinology*, vol. 191, no. 2, pp. 157–166, 2002.

[83] P. L. Montilla, J. F. Vargas, I. F. Túnez et al., "Oxidative stress in diabetic rats induced by streptozotocin: protective effects of melatonin," *Journal of Pineal Research*, vol. 25, no. 2, pp. 94–100, 1998.

[84] H. Vural, T. Sabuncu, S. Oktay Arslan, and N. Aksoy, "Melatonin inhibits lipid peroxidation and stimulates the antioxidant status of diabetic rats," *Journal of Pineal Research*, vol. 31, no. 3, pp. 193–198, 2001.

[85] M. Kanter, H. Uysal, T. Karaca, and H. O. Sagmanligil, "Depression of glucose levels and partial restoration of pancreatic beta-cell damage by melatonin in streptozotocin-induced diabetic rats," *Archives of Toxicology*, vol. 80, no. 6, pp. 362–369, 2006.

[86] R. J. Reiter, D.-X. Tan, S. J. Kim et al., "Augmentation of indices of oxidative damage in life-long melatonin—deficient rats," *Mechanisms of Ageing and Development*, vol. 110, no. 3, pp. 157–173, 1999.

[87] R. J. Reiter, D.-X. Tan, and S. Burkhardt, "Reactive oxygen and nitrogen species and cellular and organismal decline: amelioration with melatonin," *Mechanisms of Ageing and Development*, vol. 123, no. 8, pp. 1007–1019, 2002.

[88] M. Tiedge, S. Lortz, J. Drinkgern, and S. Lenzen, "Relation between antioxidant enzyme gene expression and antioxidative defense status of insulin-producing cells," *Diabetes*, vol. 46, no. 11, pp. 1733–1742, 1997.

[89] D. Giugliano, A. Ceriello, and G. Paolisso, "Oxidative stress and diabetic vascular complications," *Diabetes Care*, vol. 19, no. 3, pp. 257–267, 1996.

[90] C. J. Mullarkey, D. Edelstein, and M. Brownlee, "Free radical generation by early glycation products: a mechanism for accelerated atherogenesis in diabetes," *Biochemical and Biophysical Research Communications*, vol. 173, no. 3, pp. 932–939, 1990.

[91] S. P. Wolff, "Diabetes mellitus and free radicals. Free radicals, transition metals and oxidative stress in the aetiology of diabetes mellitus and complications," *British Medical Bulletin*, vol. 49, no. 3, pp. 642–652, 1993.

[92] S. Nishida, T. Segawa, I. Murai, and S. Nakagawa, "Long-term melatonin administration reduces hyperinsulinemia and improves the altered fatty-acid compositions in type 2 diabetic rats via the restoration of Delta-5 desaturase activity," *Journal of Pineal Research*, vol. 32, no. 1, pp. 26–33, 2002.

[93] R. G. B. Langley, G. G. Krueger, and C. E. M. Griffiths, "Psoriasis: epidemiology, clinical features, and quality of life," *Annals of the Rheumatic Diseases*, vol. 64, no. 2, pp. ii18–ii25, 2005.

[94] S. M. Hill, C. Cheng, L. Yuan et al., "Age-related decline in melatonin and Its MT1 receptor are associated with decreased sensitivity to melatonin and enhanced mammary tumor growth," *Current Aging Science*, vol. 6, no. 1, pp. 125–133, 2013.

[95] A. Cavallo, S. R. Daniels, L. M. Dolan, J. A. Bean, and J. C. Khoury, "Blood pressure-lowering effect of melatonin in type 1 diabetes," *Journal of Pineal Research*, vol. 36, no. 4, pp. 262–266, 2004.

[96] F. A. J. L. Scheer, G. A. Van Montfrans, E. J. W. Van Someren, G. Mairuhu, and R. M. Buijs, "Daily nighttime melatonin reduces blood pressure in male patients with essential hypertension," *Hypertension*, vol. 43, no. 2, pp. 192–197, 2004.

[97] E. Grossman, M. Laudon, R. Yalcin et al., "Melatonin reduces night blood pressure in patients with nocturnal hypertension," *The American Journal of Medicine*, vol. 119, no. 10, pp. 898–902, 2006.

[98] M.-W. Hung, G. M. Kravtsov, C.-F. Lau, A. M.-S. Poon, G. L. Tipoe, and M.-L. Fung, "Melatonin ameliorates endothelial dysfunction, vascular inflammation, and systemic hypertension in rats with chronic intermittent hypoxia," *Journal of Pineal Research*, vol. 55, no. 3, pp. 247–256, 2013.

[99] A. Ö. Sehirli, D. Koyun, Ş. Tetik et al., "Melatonin protects against ischemic heart failure in rats," *Journal of Pineal Research*, vol. 55, no. 2, pp. 138–148, 2013.

[100] R. Johnson, L. Staiano-Coico, L. Austin, I. Cardinale, R. Nabeya-Tsukifuji, and J. G. Krueger, "PUVA treatment selectively induces a cell cycle block and subsequent apoptosis in human T-lymphocytes," *Photochemistry and Photobiology*, vol. 63, no. 5, pp. 566–571, 1996.

[101] T. J. Laing, B. C. Richardson, M. B. Toth, E. M. Smith, and R. M. Marks, "Ultraviolet light and 8-methoxypsoralen inhibit expression of endothelial adhesion molecules," *The Journal of Rheumatology*, vol. 22, no. 11, pp. 2126–2131, 1995.

[102] G. Sethi and A. Sodhi, "Role of p38 mitogen-activated protein kinase and caspases in UV-B-induced apoptosis of murine peritoneal macrophages," *Photochemistry and Photobiology*, vol. 79, no. 1, pp. 48–54, 2004.

[103] T. P. Singh, M. P. Schön, K. Wallbrecht et al., "8-Methoxypsoralen plus ultraviolet a therapy acts via inhibition of the IL-23/Th17 axis and induction of Foxp3$^+$ regulatory T cells involving CTLA4 signaling in a psoriasis-like skin disorder," *Journal of Immunology*, vol. 184, no. 12, pp. 7257–7267, 2010.

[104] A. Mizara, L. Papadopoulos, and S. R. McBride, "Core beliefs and psychological distress in patients with psoriasis and atopic eczema attending secondary care: the role of schemas in chronic skin disease," *British Journal of Dermatology*, vol. 166, no. 5, pp. 986–993, 2012.

[105] D. G. Fortune, H. L. Richards, B. Kirby, S. Bowcock, C. J. Main, and C. E. M. Griffiths, "A cognitive-behavioural symptom management programme as an adjunct in psoriasis therapy," *British Journal of Dermatology*, vol. 146, no. 3, pp. 458–465, 2002.

[106] C. Hemlock, J. S. Rosenthal, and A. Winston, "Fluoxetine-induced psoriasis," *Annals of Pharmacotherapy*, vol. 26, no. 2, pp. 211–212, 1992.

[107] L. T. P. Lin and S. K. Kwek, "Onset of psoriasis during therapy with fluoxetine," *General Hospital Psychiatry*, vol. 32, no. 4, pp. 446.e9–446.e10, 2010.

[108] D. Deandrea, N. Walker, M. Mehlmauer, and K. White, "Dermatological reactions to lithium: a critical review of the literature," *Journal of Clinical Psychopharmacology*, vol. 2, no. 3, pp. 199–204, 1982.

[109] V. J. Selmanowitz, "Lithium, leukocytes, and lesions," *Clinics in Dermatology*, vol. 4, no. 1, pp. 170–175, 1986.

[110] H.-S. Moon, A. Mizara, and S. R. McBride, "Psoriasis and psycho-dermatology," *Dermatology and Therapy*, vol. 3, no. 2, pp. 117–130, 2013.

20

In Vivo Noninvasive Imaging of Healthy Lower Lip Mucosa: A Correlation Study between High-Definition Optical Coherence Tomography, Reflectance Confocal Microscopy, and Histology

Alejandra García-Hernández, Rodrigo Roldán-Marín, Pablo Iglesias-Garcia, and Josep Malvehy

Melanoma Unit, Dermatology Department, Hospital Clínic, C/Villaroel 170, 08036 Barcelona, Spain

Correspondence should be addressed to Rodrigo Roldán-Marín; roroderm@yahoo.com

Academic Editor: Iris Zalaudek

In recent years, technology has allowed the development of new diagnostic techniques which allow real-time, *in vivo*, noninvasive evaluation of morphological changes in tissue. This study compares and correlates the images and findings obtained by high-definition optical coherence tomography (HD-OCT) and reflectance confocal microscopy (RCM) with histology in normal healthy oral mucosa. The healthy lip mucosa of ten adult volunteers was imaged with HD-OCT and RCM. Each volunteer was systematically evaluated by RCM starting in the uppermost part of the epithelium down to the lamina propia. Afterwards, volunteers were examined with a commercially available full-field HD-OCT system using both the "slice" and the "en-face" mode. A "punch" biopsy of the lower lip mucosa was obtained and prepared for conventional histology. The architectural overview offered by "slice" mode HD-OCT correlates with histologic findings at low magnification. In the superficial uppermost layers of the epithelium, RCM imaging provided greater cellular detail than histology. As we deepened into the suprabasal layers, the findings are in accordance with physiological cellular differentiation and correlate with the images obtained from conventional histology. The combined use of these two novel non-invasive imaging techniques provides morphological imaging with sufficient resolution and penetration depth, resulting in quasihistological images.

1. Introduction

In recent years, technology has allowed the development of new diagnostic techniques which allow real-time, *in vivo*, noninvasive acquisition of images to evaluate morphological changes in tissue. These techniques include high-frequency ultrasound, reflectance confocal microscopy (RCM), and optical coherence tomography (OCT). The use of these technologies has proven to have application in ophthalmology [1], cardiology [2], gastroenterology [3], dermatology [4–6], and vascular surgery [7].

Oral malignancy is particularly high among men and the 8th most common cancer worldwide [8]. It represents about 2% of cancers in the UK [9] and 3% of all cancers in men and 2% of all cancers in women within the United States [10]. Squamous cell carcinoma accounts for about 90%

of cases of oral cancer [11]. The majority of them develop from premalignant lesions, which generally appear as white patches (leukoplakia) or red patches (erythroplakia). Their malignant transformation rates are reported to be 0.9% to 17% and 14% to 50%, respectively [12]. The difficulty of determining whether such lesions are merely dysplasias or have already progressed to invasive carcinomas represents a constant therapeutic dilemma. Additionally, tumor detection is further complicated by the tendency toward field cancerization leading to multicentric lesions [13]. In the last 2 decades, diagnostic progress has been limited and overall patient survival has remained more or less unchanged. Unfortunately, advances in surgery, radiotherapy, medical oncology, and chemotherapy have offered limited progress in terms of overall survival. Until today, the single greatest determinant of long-term patient survival and quality of life remains early lesion detection and prompt and effective treatment [10].

Apart from excisional biopsy, there does not exist other validated methods for detecting malignant transformation *in vivo*. In such a manner, a sensitive diagnostic tool for non-invasive detection of oral malignancy and reliable screening of high-risk populations would be very helpful to identify patients at early, more treatable stages of the disease [14]. One of the main aims of these different, *in vivo*, noninvasive technologies is the identification of premalignant disorders and cancer at its earliest stage.

Optical coherence tomography (OCT) is a relatively new biomedical imaging modality that can generate high-resolution cross-sectional images of microstructures in biological systems, resembling vertical sections in histology [1]. Only recently has OCT been used more systematically for the investigation of oral cavity lesions [10, 15–17]. High-definition optical coherence tomography (HD-OCT) is a technique based on the principle of conventional OCT, specifically the ability to carry out optical imaging deeply within highly scattering media, with micrometre resolution in both transversal and axial directions. It uses a two-dimensional, infrared-sensitive (1000–1700 nm) imagining array for light detection. This enables focus tracking: the focal plane is continuously moved through the sample. The movements of the focal plane and the reference mirror are synchronized, and the refractive index of the sample is taken into account. This results in a high lateral resolution of 3 μm at all depths of the sample. A high axial resolution (3 μm in skin) is achieved using a broadband thermal light source combined with a special filter. Moreover, the system is capable of capturing a slice image and an en-face image in real time as well as fast (35 s) 3D acquisition. The spectral sensitivity makes it possible to work in the near infrared range above 1000 nm. The field of view is 1.8 × 1.5 mm. The tissue penetration depth goes up to 570 μm, and the total light power at the tissue is <3.5 mW. The system works in direct contact with the tissue using an optical matching gel comparable to ultrasound gel. The result is transferred to a computer and displayed using a greyscale or color palette, thereby generating an HD-OCT image.

Reflectance confocal microscopy (RCM) is an noninvasive imaging technique that enables an en-face (horizontal plane) visualization of the tissue with a resolution at the cellular level (0.5–1.0 μm in the lateral dimension and 4-5 μm in the axial ones) and therefore may provide an alternative to histopathology. The device uses a diode laser as a source of monochromatic and coherent light, which penetrates into the tissue and illuminates a small point inside. The light is reflected, goes through a small pinhole and forms an image in the detector. This small pinhole does not allow the reflected light (reflectance) to reach the detector from another point. Therefore, only reflected light from the focal region (confocal) is detected. Light from out-of-focus planes is rejected at the pinhole. The contrast in RCM images relies on the differences in the reflectivity of the tissue, which is depending on chemical and molecular structures. Due to these variations of the refractive index, only a certain portion of the light is reflected. Structures with a higher refractive index appear bright in RCM. Melanin and melanosomes are the strongest natural sources of contrast resulting white in RCM. The commercially used RCM Vivascope 1500 uses a laser diode with a near-infrared wavelength of 830 nm. Laser power of 830 nm causes no damage to tissue, but limits the imaging depth to 200–300 μm. The correlation between images of RCM and histopathology in oral mucosa has been previously reported [18, 19].

This study compares and correlates the images obtained by HD-OCT and RCM with histology findings in normal healthy oral lower lip mucosa. Thus, it serves as a foundation for the use of these noninvasive imaging techniques as screening tools for the early detection of oral cancer and precancer.

2. Materials and Methods

2.1. Subjects. The healthy oral lower lip mucosa of ten adult volunteers was imaged with HD-OCT and RCM. All gave their informed consent. The study population consisted of 7 women and 3 men ranging in age between 22 and 56 years old. Four subjects were skin phototype III, four were phototype IV, and two were phototype II. Demographic data of study population is summarized in Table 1.

2.2. Evaluation Protocol. A commercially available Reflectance Confocal Microscope (Vivascope 1500 Caliber I.D., New York, USA) was used for imaging. A detailed description of this technique and the device used has been previously published. Reflectance confocal microscopy evaluation was performed on the oral mucosa of the lower lip. Each volunteer was systematically evaluated by RCM: 6 individual images were obtained at previously set standardized depths with the reference mark (Z0) set in the uppermost part of the epithelium down to the lamina propia (Figure 1), and vertical mapping using a Vivastack was performed in 1.5 μm steps to a maximum depth of 150 μm beginning at the uppermost part of the epithelium into the lamina propia.

After the evaluation with RCM, all volunteers were examined with a commercially available full-field HD-OCT system (Skintell, Agfa Healthcare Morstel, Belgium and München, Germany). A detailed description of the technique and the device has been previously published. All volunteers were systematically evaluated. As a result of the large diameter of the HD-OCT probe, there was no possible identification mark within the mucosa. The probe was placed in the centre of the lower lip oral mucosa to allow a rough colocalization with the RCM and histological section. To make an image, the subject was positioned in front of the system. The probe was lifted from the holder, and optical gel (approximately 10 μL) was applied to the probe sensor lens. The probe sensor lens was then positioned on the patient's oral mucosa using mild pressure. Scanning automatically began in the slice mode. A live "slice" view of the mucosal tissue was displayed, the image was captured and saved. During scanning, the foot pedal was used to switch between slice mode and en-face mode. A 3D scan was was also performed. Characteristic features were documented.

TABLE 1: Demographic parameters of studied population.

Patients	Gender	Age	Phototype
1	F	29	III
2	M	37	IV
3	F	34	III
4	F	22	III
5	F	43	III
6	F	35	IV
7	F	56	II
8	M	31	IV
9	F	27	II
10	M	31	IV

F: Female; M: Male.

2.3. Histological Evaluation. Two volunteers underwent a 3 mm "punch" biopsy of the lower lip mucosa following local anesthesia with 2% lidocaine with epinephrine, and tissue sections were prepared as usual for conventional histology with H&E. The histological evaluation was performed by a board-certified pathologist and a dentist specialized in oral medicine and oral pathology (AGH).

3. Results

3.1. Epithelial Uppermost Layers. With RCM in the superficial uppermost layers of the epithelium (Z0), we visualized a highly scattering image where we observed mild scaling, and cells appeared flattened and ill-demarcated. Nuclei appeared bright and were surrounded by a dark halo (Figure 2).

The en-face mode of HD-OCT starting in the uppermost part of the epithelium demonstrated a highly scattering image where architectural epithelial structure could be appreciated, but horizontal imaging with HD-OCT did not achieve cellular detail resolution as RCM (Figure 3).

When imaging the oral mucosa with HD-OCT in real time "slice" view, the reflectivity of the tissue led to a signal-intense, bright band on the surface, which corresponds with the entrance signal. The thinly, partially parakeratinized layer appeared as a scattering homogenous layer, with a sharp demarcation line between it and the higher scattering epithelium. The architectural overview offered by "slice" mode HD-OCT correlates with histologic findings at low magnification (Figure 4).

Under the light microscope on conventional histology, the epithelium seemed as nonhomogenously parakeratinized. The cells in the uppermost layers of the epithelium appeared very eosinophilic, thin, and flat. Nuclei persisted and also became notoriously flattened. The large filament content of the cytoplasm may give the appearance of microfolds. The intercellular space between the epithelial cells is narrow (Figure 5).

3.2. Stratum Granulosum/Prickle Cell Layers. With RCM at the stratum granulosum cells appeared to have a granular aspect possibly related to the presence of cytoplasmic granules (Z1). Nuclei are easily distinguished as bright mostly

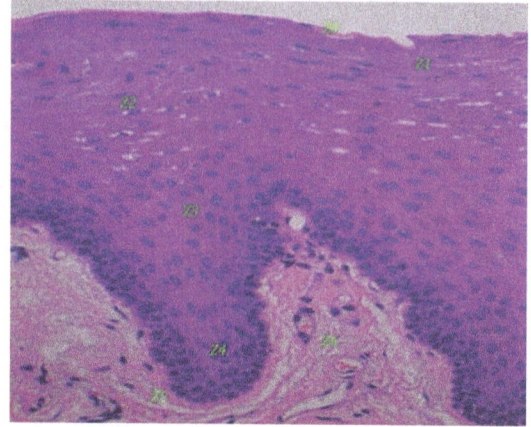

FIGURE 1: Histology image of healthy oral lower lip mucosa with reference marks (Z) showing where standardized depth reflectance confocal microscopy evaluation was peformed.

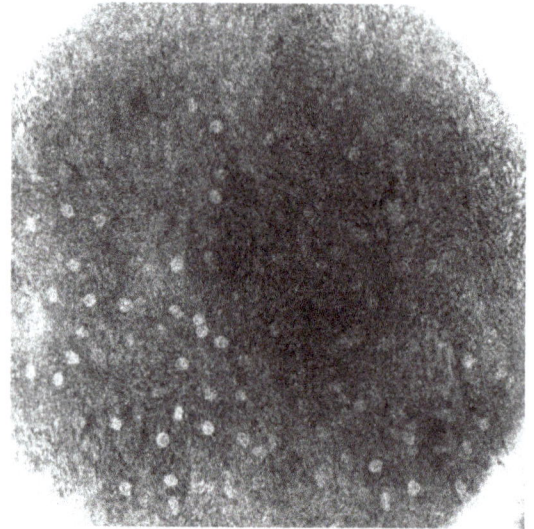

FIGURE 2: Reflectance confocal microscopy image at Z0 showing ill-demarcated cells with bright nuclei surrounded by a dark halo.

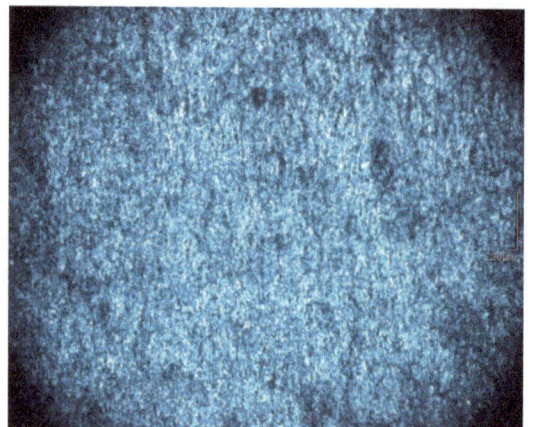

FIGURE 3: High-definition optical coherence tomography "en-face" image at supreficial epithelial layers.

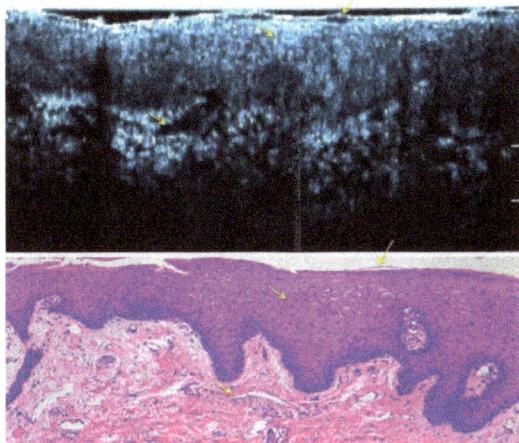

FIGURE 4: High-definition optical coherence tomography "slice" image with histologic correlation. Yellow arrows pinpoint the anatomical correlation between the "slice" image obtained with HD-OCT and the histology image.

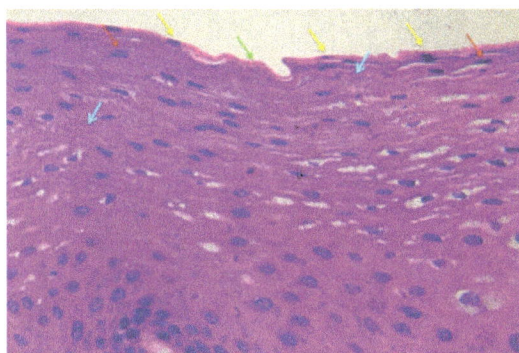

FIGURE 5: Conventional histology image under light microscopy showing the uppermost epithelial layers. Green arrow: non-keratinized area pinpointing abscence of nuclei. Yellow arrows: parakeratinized areas with presence of nuclei in the uppermost epithelial layer. Red arrows: flat nuclei in upper epithelial layers. Blue arrows: large filament content of cytoplasm giving appearance of microfolds.

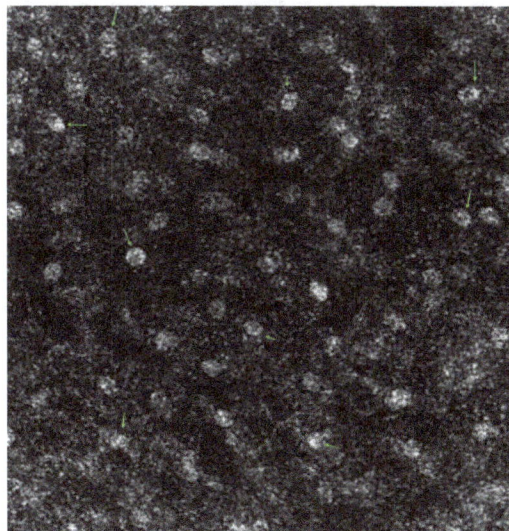

FIGURE 6: Reflectance confocal microscopy image at the stratum granulosum layer (Z1). Green arrows: nuclei display mostly as bright rounded structures and a fine granular apperance of the cytoplasm is observed.

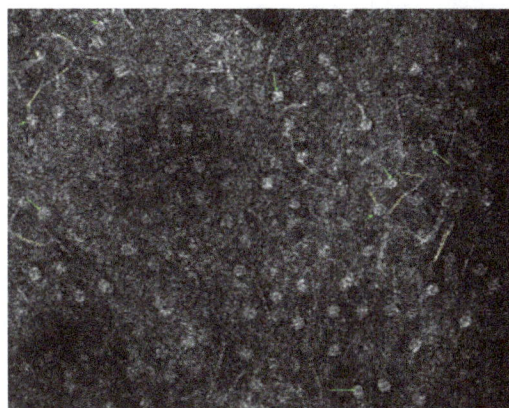

FIGURE 7: Reflectance confocal microscopy image at the prickle cell layer (Z2). Green arrows: signal bright rounded nuclei. Yellow lines: cytoplasmic border and intercellular junction.

round structures (Figure 6). As we deepened into the epithelium to the suprabasal layers (Z2 and Z3), cells appeared larger, more spherical, and hyporefractive. Nuclei occupied a greater proportion of the total area of the cell and were clearly visible as bright structures. Cell membranes start becoming visible, and intercellular borders and junctions (desmosomes) become apparent (Figure 7). At Z3 level, the epithelium acquires a more reticular or widened honeycomb pattern. Dermal papillae may start becoming visible (Figure 8). These findings are in accordance with physiological cellular differentiation and correlate with the image obtained from conventional histology.

When visualizing these layers with the "en-face" mode of HD-OCT, cells appeared small and also revealed a granular appearance at the stratum granulosum layer correlating properly with the RCM and histology findings. In the stratum spinosum cells were clustered giving the appearance of a honeycomb pattern.

The "slice" mode of HD-OCT showed that the epithelium reveals a less intense signal than the lamina propia.

On conventional histology, the granular layer is wanting. However, the transitional status of the cells is clearly recognized. Cells and nuclei become flat and irregularly shaped. Some nuclei acquire a dotted or pyknotic appearance. In the prickle cell layer, cells appear larger, round, or polygonal. Nuclei seem large and intensely basophilic and remain centrally located.

3.3. Basal Cell Layer and Epithelial Junction. With RCM, the basal cell layer (Z4 and Z5) at the interpapillary pegs cells appeared much smaller, condensed, and surrounding the papillae. In this plane, nuclei were visible as dark structures

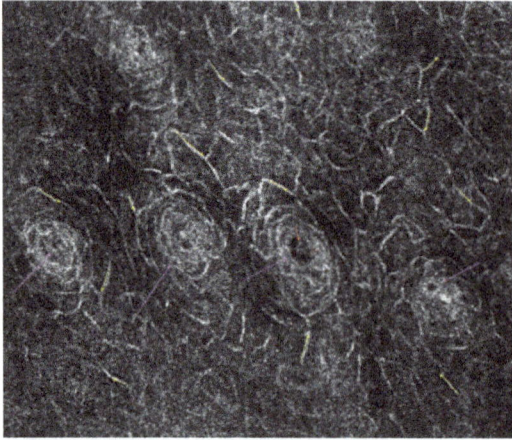

FIGURE 8: Reflectance confocal microscopy image at prickle cell layer (Z3). Yellow lines: reticular or wider honeycomb pattern, Purple arrows: dermal papillae, Red arrows: blood vessels.

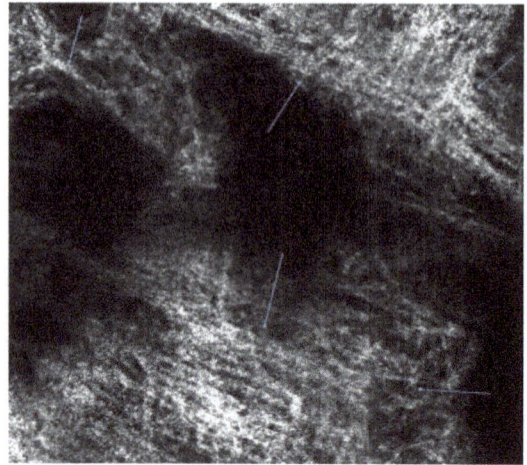

FIGURE 10: Reflectance confocal microscopy image at the lamina propia showing apperance of collagen fibers and bundles. Blue arrows: collagen fibers.

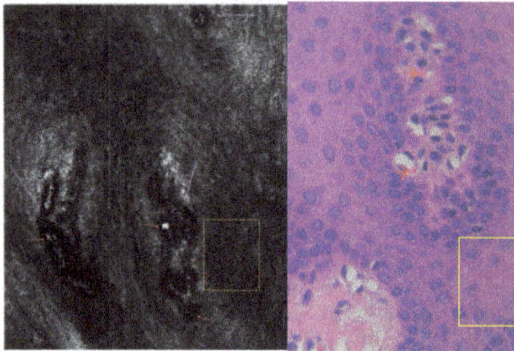

FIGURE 9: Reflectance confocal microscopy findings at the basal cell layer and epithelial junction with histologic correlation. Purple arrows: blood vessels, Red arrows: erythrocytes and blood vessel traffic, Yellow square: loss of honeycomb pattern.

within cells. Within the papillae, small bright cells corresponding to erythrocytes traveling inside the blood vessels were easily distinguished (Figure 9).

HD-OCT "en-face" mode at the epithelial junction provided the architectural appearance of rings of bright cells surrounding the dark dermal papillae. With the "slice" mode, the epithelial junction could be distinguished if the border was relatively flat and not overly serrated.

On conventional histology, at the basal cell layer, cells have a cuboidal shape containing large rounded nuclei. Mitotic activity can be easily distinguished.

3.4. Lamina Propia. With RCM at the lamina propia (Z6) collagen fibers and blood vessels with active blood flow were visible, showing proper correlation with histological sections (Figure 10).

In the lamina propia, "en-face" HD-OCT showed the refractive nature of collagen which makes it appear as white reticulated fibers with scattered blood vessels. It is worthwhile mentioning that the depth of penetration with which

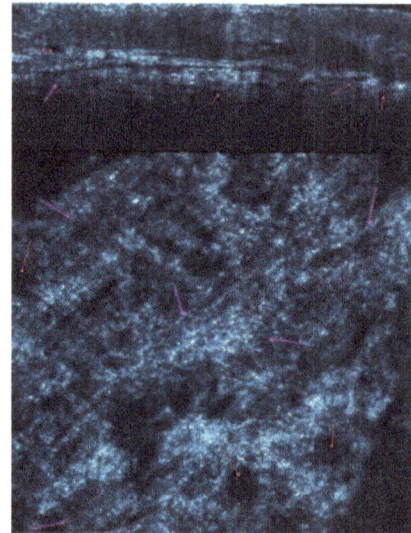

FIGURE 11: High-Definition Optical Coherence Tomography "slice" view and "en-face" image correlating findings at the level of the lamina propia. Purple arrows: collagen fibers, Red arrows: blood vessels.

an image with fair-enough resolution could be observed with HD-OCT was approximately 450 μm. While imaging with HD-OCT in "slice" mode the lamina propia appeared more signal-intense, with some signal poor cavities corresponding to blood vessels (Figure 11).

On conventional histology, the lamina propia is composed of loose connective tissue with a rich vascular supply. The deeper layers contain heavy bundles of collagen fibers.

4. Discussion

The diagnosis of oral cancer and precancer still requires taking a surgical biopsy to study the sampled tissue histologically. Oral biopsies can be painful and associated with bleeding

TABLE 2: Technical data on swept source-optical coherence tomography, high definition-optical coherence tomography, and reflectance confocal microscopy.

Technical data	SS-OCT Vivo Sight	HD-OCT Skintell	RCM VivaScope 1500
Light source	Santec HSL-2000-12-MDL	Halogen lamp with Gaussian filter	Diode laser
Wavelength	1310 nm	1300 nm	830 nm
Lateral resolution	<7.5 μm	3 μm	0.5 to 1.0 μm
Axial resolution	<5 μm	3 μm	4 to 5 μm
Penetration depth	1200 to 2000 μm	570 μm	200–300 μm
Field of view (en-face)	6 × 6 mm	1.8 × 1.5 mm	0.5 × 0.5 mm 8 mm × 8 mm VivaStack
3D Imaging	Yes	Yes	No

nm: nanometre; μm: micrometre; mm: millimetre.

TABLE 3: Reflectance confocal microscopy, high-definition optical coherence tomography, and conventional histology morphological characteristics in lip mucosa according to tissue depth.

Reference mark	Depth	RCM characteristics	HD-OCT "en-face" characteristics	Histology
Z0	0 μm	Highly scattering homogenous	Highly scattering homogenous layer	Nonhomogenously parakeratinized
Z1	4.96 μm	Cytoplasmic granular appearance	Granular appearance and high scattering	Wanting granular layer. Cells appear very eosinophilic, thin and flat. Narrow intercellular spaces
Z2	29.79 μm	Cytoplasmic border becomes apparent	Cytoplasmic granular appearance and areas with honeycomb pattern	Cells and nuclei become flat and irregularly shaped. Nuclei acquire pyknotic appearance
Z3	84.36 μm	Wider honeycomb pattern. May be difficult to clearly distinguish nuclei. Dermal papillae may start becoming visible	Dermal papillae may start becoming visible	In the prickle layer, cells appear round or polygonal. Nuclei seem intensely basophilic and centrally located
Z4	124.00 μm	Loss of honeycomb pattern. Nuclei become dark and are not clearly distinguished	Dermal papillae	Basal cell layer cells have a cuboidal shape containing large rounded nuclei. Mitotic activity can be easily distinguished
Z5	173.00 μm	Epithelial junction, ill-defined papillae and collagen fibers	Transitional epithelium	
Z6	193.69 μm	Collagen fibers	Collagen fibers	Loose connective tissue with a rich vascular supply. The deeper layers contain heavy bundles of collagen fibers

and difficulties in eating and speaking. Alternatively, different noninvasive optical diagnostic techniques have emerged.

Reflectance confocal microscopy has revolutionized the noninvasive technique for morphological investigation of living tissue on a microscopic level. Unlike routine histology, the images obtained with RCM are parallel to the surface (horizontal or en-face), rather than cross-sectional (vertical or slice). They are greyscale images, similar to radiographic images. The field of view with reflectance confocal microscopy is 500-500 μm across. The level being imaged can be identified by the morphological appearance of the tissue at a given depth. On the other hand, the depth of the section can be measured using a micrometre attached to the Z stage of the objective lens. With this system it is possible to image normal tissue to a depth of 200 μm. The boundaries of individual cells are easily visualized because of the high lateral resolution of approximately 1 μm and the axial resolution (section thickness) of 3–5 μm. Reflectance confocal microscopy findings of healthy oral mucosa had been previously documented. However, these findings until now had not been validated. Our results confirm the validity of RCM imaging as an appropriate noninvasive tool to assess tissue architecture and cellular morphology of the oral cavity. According to our results in the vast majority of cases we were unable to achieve imaging with appropriate resolution beyond 195 μm, and at this penetration depth our findings

TABLE 4: Cellular features in lower lip mucosa evaluated *in vivo* by reflectance confocal microscopy and high-definition optical coherence tomography.

Reference mark (μm)	Cellular structure	RCM image from Vivastack sets (μm)	HD-OCT image from "slice" mode (μm)
Z0	Nuclei (where visible)	10–13.2	NA
Z1	Nuclei	12–14.3	9.7–13.5
Z2	Nuclei	11–16.8	12–17.6
Z3	Nuclei	10–14	10.9–16.9
Z4	Nuclei	NA	NA
Z5	Nuclei	NA	NA
Z6	Nuclei	NA	NA
Z0	Cytoplasmic border	21–34.2	24.6–29.4
Z1	Cytoplasmic border	22–27	21–22.9
Z2	Cytoplasmic border	23–35.4	22.4–35
Z3	Cytoplasmic border	25–34	21.9–33.8
Z4	Cytoplasm	21–32	18.8–20.2
Z5	Cytoplasm	16–22	NA
Z6	Cytoplasm	NA	NA
Z5-Z6	Junctional epithelium	16–32	20.5–29

NA: not applicable.

TABLE 5: Mean measurements of cellular and morphologic features in lower lip mucosa *in vivo* by reflectance confocal microscopy and high-definition optical coherence tomography.

Structure	Histology image (μm)	RCM image (μm)	HD-OCT image (μm)
Epithelium thickness (μm)	100–245	153–194	151–232
Interpapillary space	33–203.7	NA	57.4–498
Papillae diameter (shortest/longest) (μm)	99/265	NA	150/287.1
Capillary diameter (longest/shortest) (μm)	200/34	208/33	261.9/36.7
Collagen fiber bundles	Regularly dispossessed reticular pattern	Regularly dispossessed reticular pattern	Regularly dispossessed reticular pattern

were consistent with structures found in the lamina propia. In contrast, White et al. [18] report lamina propia findings at a penetration depth of 350–450 μm. It is possible that these disagreements in depth are related to the variability of epithelial thickness among subjects but also possibly related to differences in the illumination source. They used an Nd:YAG laser confocal microscope at 1064 nm, while we used a diode laser at 830 nm, thus penetration discordance may be expected.

Just very recently, Contaldo et al. have published RCM features in different healthy oral mucosal sites (lips, cheek, gingivae, and tongue) and provided further evidence on the usefulness and applicability of the handheld version of RCM (Vivascope 3000, Lucid, Rochester, NY) as an adjunct tool in the clinical evaluation and management of patients with oral diseases [19].

Despite the significant progress in the *in vivo* analysis, RCM does have limitations. Firstly, images are only parallel to the tissue surface, and the penetration depth is limited. Moreover, RCM image interpretation requires a fair amount of specialized training; results remain strongly user dependent and reproducibility of results may vary between investigators. Furthermore, unfortunately RCM equipment is expensive and currently only available in few selected centres. Yet, interest in the field of confocal microscopy is growing and its usefulness is becoming increasingly evident.

OCT has been recently used to assess oral cavity lesions and to distinguish benign from malignant lesions. However, these studies have been performed with SS-OCT and *ex vivo* tissue samples. To the best of our knowledge, this is the first study using HD-OCT in the *in vivo* examination of healthy oral mucosa. Table 2 summarizes technical data differences between RCM, SS-OCT, and HD-OCT.

In contrast to RCM, images obtained with HD-OCT are both horizontal (en-face) and vertical (slice). The images generated are displayed using either greyscale or a color palette. The field of view of the en-face mode (parallel to the surface) is 1.8–1.5 mm across. A lateral resolution of 3 μm allows the identification of individual cells. The high bandwidth of the lightsource leads to a high axial (depth) resolution of 3 μm, which is comparable to that of RCM. With this system it is possible to visualize tissue to a depth of up to 570 μm, which is almost three times deeper than with RCM. The main limitation for the use of HD-OCT to examine oral mucosal tissue is the size and weight of the probe which makes it impossible to access certain areas of the oral cavity.

Another relevant and interesting finding from our results is that the lining mucosa of the lower lip revealed a thinly, nonhomogenously, parakeratinized epithelium. The majority of histology textbooks mention that the epithelium in this anatomical area is nonkeratinized. This may be due to a certain anatomical variability of this basic pattern in adults, as exemplified by the thinly keratinized linea alba ("white line") at the level of the occlusal plane.

The combined use of these two novel noninvasive imaging techniques provides morphological imaging with sufficient resolution and penetration depth (Tables 3, 4, and 5), resulting in quasihistological images. One can only imagine that in a near future the advances in noninvasive imaging techniques will allow *in vivo*, easy, fast, painless examination of inflammatory and proliferative diseases of the oral cavity.

In conclusion, our findings suggest that high-definition optical coherence tomography and reflectance confocal microscopy allow examination of healthy oral lower lip mucosa with adequate histological correlation. Further studies are needed to assess the validity of these avant-garde diagnostic techniques in diseased oral tissue.

Conflicts of Interests

The authors declare that they have no conflict of interests.

References

[1] D. Huang, E. A. Swanson, C. P. Lin et al., "Optical coherence tomography," *Science*, vol. 254, no. 5035, pp. 1178–1181, 1991.

[2] S. K. Nadkarni, M. C. Pierce, B. H. Park et al., "Measurement of collagen and smooth muscle cell content in atherosclerotic plaques using polarization-sensitive optical coherence tomography," *Journal of the American College of Cardiology*, vol. 49, no. 13, pp. 1474–1481, 2007.

[3] B. J. Vakoc, M. Shishko, S. H. Yun et al., "Comprehensive esophageal microscopy by using optical frequency-domain imaging (with video)," *Gastrointestinal Endoscopy*, vol. 65, no. 6, pp. 898–905, 2007.

[4] C. Carrera, S. Puig, and J. Malvehy, "In vivo confocal reflectance microscopy in melanoma," *Dermatology and Therapy*, vol. 25, pp. 410–422, 2012.

[5] M. Boone, G. B. Jemec, and V. Del Marmol, "High-definition optical coherence tomography enables visualization of individual cells in healthy skin: comparison to reflectance confocal microscopy," *Experimental Dermatology*, vol. 21, pp. 740–744, 2012.

[6] T. Maier, M. Braun-Falco, T. Hinz, M. H. Schmid-Wendtner, T. Ruzicka, and C. Berking, "Morphology of basal cell carcinoma in high definition optical coherence tomography: En-face and slice imaging mode, and comparison with histology," *Journal of the European Academy of Dermatology and Venereology*, vol. 27, no. 1, pp. 97–104, 2012.

[7] N. A. Patel, X. Li, D. L. Stamper, J. G. Fujimoto, and M. E. Brezinski, "Guidance of aortic ablation using optical coherence tomography," *International Journal of Cardiovascular Imaging*, vol. 19, no. 2, pp. 171–178, 2003.

[8] P. E. Petersen, "Strengthening the prevention of oral cancer: the WHO perspective," *Community Dentistry and Oral Epidemiology*, vol. 33, no. 6, pp. 397–399, 2005.

[9] Z. Hamdoon, W. Jerjes, R. Al-Delayme, G. McKenzie, A. Jay, and C. Hooper, "Structural validation of oral mucosal tissue using optical coherence tomography," *Head & Neck Oncology*, vol. 4, p. 29, 2012.

[10] J. M. Ridgway, W. B. Armstrong, S. Guo et al., "In vivo optical coherence tomography of the human oral cavity and oropharynx," *Archives of Otolaryngology—Head and Neck Surgery*, vol. 132, no. 10, pp. 1074–1081, 2006.

[11] J. S. Cooper, K. Porter, K. Mallin et al., "National cancer database report on cancer of the head and neck: 10-year update," *Head and Neck*, vol. 31, no. 6, pp. 748–758, 2009.

[12] S. Grajewski, D. Quarcoo, S. Uibel, C. Scutaru, D. Groneberg, and M. Spallek, "A scientometric analysis of leukoplakia and erythroplakia," *Laryngo-Rhino-Otologie*, vol. 89, no. 4, pp. 210–215, 2010.

[13] D. P. Slaughter, H. W. Southwick, and W. Smejkal, "Field cancerization in oral stratified squamous epithelium; clinical," *Cancer*, vol. 6, no. 5, pp. 963–968, 1953.

[14] M. DeCoro and P. Wilder-Smith, "Potential of optical coherence tomography for early diagnosis of oral malignancies," *Expert Review of Anticancer Therapy*, vol. 10, no. 3, pp. 321–329, 2010.

[15] P. Wilder-Smith, W.-G. Jung, M. Brenner et al., "In vivo optical coherence tomography for the diagnosis of oral malignancy," *Lasers in Surgery and Medicine*, vol. 35, no. 4, pp. 269–275, 2004.

[16] H. Kawakami-Wong, S. Gu, M. J. Hammer-Wilson, J. B. Epstein, Z. Chen, and P. Wilder-Smith, "In vivo optical coherence tomography-based scoring of oral mucositis in human subjects: a pilot study," *Journal of Biomedical Optics*, vol. 12, no. 5, Article ID 051702, 2007.

[17] M. T. Tasi, C. K. Lee, H. C. Lee et al., "Differentiating oral lesions in different carcinogenesis stages with optical coherence tomography," *Journal of Biomedical Optics*, vol. 14, Article ID 044028, 2009.

[18] M. W. White, M. Rajadhyaksha, S. González, R. L. Fabian, and R. R. Anderson, "Noninvasive imaging of human oral mucosa in vivo by confocal reflectance microscopy," *Laryngoscope*, vol. 109, no. 10, pp. 1709–1717, 1999.

[19] M. Contaldo, M. Agozzino, E. Moscarella, S. Esposito, R. Serpico, and M. Ardigo, "In vivo characterization of healthy oral mucosa by reflectance confocal microscopy: a translational research for optical biopsy," *Ultrastructural Pathology*, vol. 37, pp. 151–158, 2013.

21

A 3-Month, Randomized, Double-Blind, Placebo-Controlled Study Evaluating the Ability of an Extra-Strength Marine Protein Supplement to Promote Hair Growth and Decrease Shedding in Women with Self-Perceived Thinning Hair

Glynis Ablon

Ablon Skin Institute Research Center, Manhattan Beach, CA 90266, USA

Correspondence should be addressed to Glynis Ablon; grablonmd@gmail.com

Academic Editor: Bruno A. Bernard

An oral marine protein supplement (MPS) is designed to promote hair growth in women with temporary thinning hair (Viviscal Extra Strength; Lifes2good, Inc., Chicago, IL). This double-blind, placebo-controlled study assessed the ability of MPS to promote terminal hair growth in adult women with self-perceived thinning hair associated with poor diet, stress, hormonal influences, or abnormal menstrual cycles. Adult women with thinning hair were randomized to receive MPS (N = 30) or placebo (N = 30) twice daily for 90 days. Digital images were obtained from a $4\,cm^2$ area scalp target area. Each subject's hair was washed and shed hairs were collected and counted. After 90 days, these measures were repeated and subjects completed Quality of Life and Self-Assessment Questionnaires. MPS-treated subjects achieved a significant increase in the number of terminal hairs within the target area ($P < 0.0001$) which was significantly greater than placebo ($P < 0.0001$). MPS use also resulted in significantly less hair shedding ($P = 0.002$) and higher total Self-Assessment ($P = 0.006$) and Quality of Life Questionnaires scores ($P = 0.035$). There were no reported adverse events. MPS promotes hair growth and decreases hair loss in women suffering from temporary thinning hair. This trial is registered with ClinicalTrials.gov Identifier: NCT02297360.

1. Introduction

Hair loss in women is often an overlooked and underappreciated condition that affects women almost as frequently as it affects men. In the United States, 40% of people with hair loss are women and 40% of women have visible hair loss by age of 40. Hair loss may begin in women as early as their teens [1] or 20s [2] and increases significantly with age. In one study, 6% of women aged under 50 years were diagnosed as having female pattern hair loss, increasing to 38% in subjects aged 70 years and over [3].

Reasons for female pattern hair loss include medical conditions, medications, and physiologic or emotional stress [4–6]. A recent study of twins showed that significant factors associated with hair loss in women included divorce or separation, multiple marriages, more children, longer sleep duration, higher stress severity, smoking, higher income, and various medical conditions [7]. Regardless of the cause, the psychological impact of hair loss in women is well-known [8–11]. The psychological impact of hair loss is also more severe for women than men.

Nutritional deficiencies are also a known cause of hair loss [4] and may include inadequate intake of proteins, minerals, essential fatty acids, and vitamins [12]. Dietary zinc deficiency may be a cause of alopecia [13, 14]. Compared to normal controls, serum zinc concentrations were shown to be significantly lower among women with female pattern hair loss [15], which can be halted or improved with zinc supplements [14, 16]. Zinc supplements can increase hair growth in patients with alopecia areata [17]. Hair loss in women has also been reported to be associated with iron deficiency [12–14]; however, the results of a large controlled study indicate that the incidence of iron deficiency among women with female pattern hair loss is not different than women with no hair loss [15]. Deficiencies in other minerals such as selenium may also be a factor in hair loss [18]. Biotin is a water-soluble vitamin and essential cofactor for several important enzymes [18]. Dietary deficiency of this important cofactor has also been associated with hair loss [13, 18, 19].

Currently, many medical treatments are available to men that are too dangerous for women or are unsafe for use in women of child-bearing age, such as finasteride [20]. Viviscal Extra Strength is an oral marine protein supplement (MPS) specifically designed to promote hair growth in women suffering from temporary thinning hair. MPS is a proprietary blend of shark and mollusc powder derived from sustainable marine sources which provides essential nutrients to nourish hair naturally and improve the appearance of thinning hair. It does not contain hormones or other drugs. MPS or the same ingredients contained in MPS were initially shown to have beneficial effects on hereditary androgenic alopecia in men [21] and photodamaged skin in women [22, 23]. The product has been marketed in Europe for over 15 years.

The purpose of this double-blind, placebo-controlled study was to further evaluate the ability of MPS to strengthen and promote the growth of terminal hairs in adult women with self-perceived thinning hair associated with poor diet, stress, hormonal influences, or abnormal menstrual cycles. We use the term hair loss to nonspecifically describe our study population as women who may notice their hair thinning even if it is not significantly dramatic enough for clinical diagnosis of true alopecia. True alopecia cases including alopecia areata, scarring alopecia, androgenetic alopecia, and telogen effluvium as described in our exclusion criteria were not included. Since female pattern hair loss is also characterized by changes in hair diameter associated with hair follicle miniaturization [24, 25], the effect of MPS on hair diameter will also be measured. Finally, this study also assessed the ability of MPS to decrease hair shedding.

2. Methods

2.1. Study Subjects. Women 21–65 years of age with Fitzpatrick photo skin types I–IV and self-perceived thinning hair associated with poor diet, stress, hormone influences, or abnormal menstrual cycle were eligible for enrollment. Each subject expressed her willingness to follow study procedures including maintaining their normal hair shampooing and color treatment frequency and not substantially changing their current diet, medications, or exercise routines for the duration of the study. Women of child-bearing potential were required to use a medically sound, nonhormonal form of birth control during the study.

Reasons for exclusion from study participation included a history of intolerance or allergy to fish, seafood, shellfish, or acerola; known allergy or sensitivity to any shampoo or conditioner; a stressful incident within the last 6 months, such as the death of a family member; use of hormones for birth control or hormone replacement therapy during the past 6 months; use of other therapies for hair growth such as light therapy or minoxidil within the last 3 months; use of medications known to affect the hair growth cycle

within the last 6 months such as hormone-based contraceptives, cyproterone acetate, aldactone/spironolactone, finasteride, or other 5-alpha-reductase inhibitors; self-reported active hepatitis, immune deficiency, HIV, or autoimmune disease; self-reported uncontrolled diseases such as diabetes or hypertension; an active dermatologic condition which might place the subject at risk or interfere with the objectives of the study; other hair loss disorders, such as alopecia areata, scarring alopecia, androgenetic alopecia, and telogen effluvium; participating in any clinical research study; or nursing, pregnancy, or planning to become pregnant during the study.

2.2. Test Material. Subjects were randomized in double-blind fashion to receive the oral MPS (Viviscal Extra Strength Oral Tablets; Lifes2good, Inc., Chicago, IL) or placebo. The key ingredient in MPS tablets is AminoMar marine complex, *Equisetum arvense* sp. (horsetail which contains a naturally occurring form of silica), *Malpighia glabra* (acerola cherry which provides vitamin C), biotin, and zinc. The AminoMar is composed of a proprietary blend of shark powder and mollusc powder derived from sustainable marine sources. The placebo treatment consisted of inert tablets with similar appearance.

Subjects were instructed to take one tablet of their assigned treatment twice daily in the morning and evening following a meal. They were to maintain their normal hair care routine and use the same brand/type of hair care products and maintain the same haircut, color, and style for the study duration. Subjects with color-treated hair were also instructed to have the color treatment performed at the same time interval prior to each visit (if the color treatment was done 1 week prior to Visit 1, it should be repeated 1 week prior to Visit 2). Subjects were instructed to wash their hair at home 24 hours in advance of each study visit.

2.3. Study Procedures. This study consisted of a baseline clinic visit (Visit 1) and a follow-up visit at 90 days (Visit 2). A basic physical examination was performed at both visits which included a basic body systems overview, vital signs, and scalp examination to rule out any confounding scalp conditions. Subjects were instructed to wash their hair at home 24 hours in advance of each study visit. During the clinic visit, each subject had their hair washed with a commercial shampoo (Viviscal Gentle Shampoo; Lifes2good, Inc., Chicago, IL) over a sink containing a cheesecloth positioned to collect any shed hairs which were collected and counted.

During the baseline visit, an approximately 2 cm × 2 cm (4 cm^2) area of the scalp was selected along the frontalis bone where frontal hairline and lateral hairline meet (hairline junction). A three-point location was recorded based on measurements obtained from the medial canthus, lateral canthus, and preauricular skin pit to the hairline junction. Where these three points meet (anterior lateral triangle of scalp), a target area 1 cm posterior into scalp hair was chosen. The 4 cm^2 target area was marked using a black fine-tip skin marker such that the three-point triangulation mark was in the center.

TABLE 1: Changes in hair growth and hair diameter.

MPS, $N = 30$	Baseline	Day 90	Significance[*]
Mean terminal hair count (SD)	178.3 (7.8)	235.8 (18.4)	$P < 0.0001$
Mean vellus hair count (SD)	19.6 (2.1)	21.2 (2.2)	$P < 0.0001$
Mean terminal hair diameter, mm (SD)	0.062 (0.009)	0.063 (0.009)	$P = NS$
Mean shed hair counts (SD)	27.1 (26.6)	16.5 (14.4)	$P = 0.002$
Placebo, $N = 30$	Baseline	Day 90	Significance[*]
Mean terminal hairs (SD)	178.2 (9.6)	180.9 (18.8)	$P = NS$
Mean vellus hairs (SD)	19.8 (1.7)	20.0 (1.9)	$P = NS$
Mean terminal hair diameter, mm (SD)	0.063 (0.009)	0.062 (0.008)	$P = NS$
Mean shed hair counts (SD)	23.4 (25.5)	21.9 (20.8)	$P = NS$

[*]Repeated measures ANOVA across study days contrasts per treatment group; NS, not significant. Baseline versus 90 days.

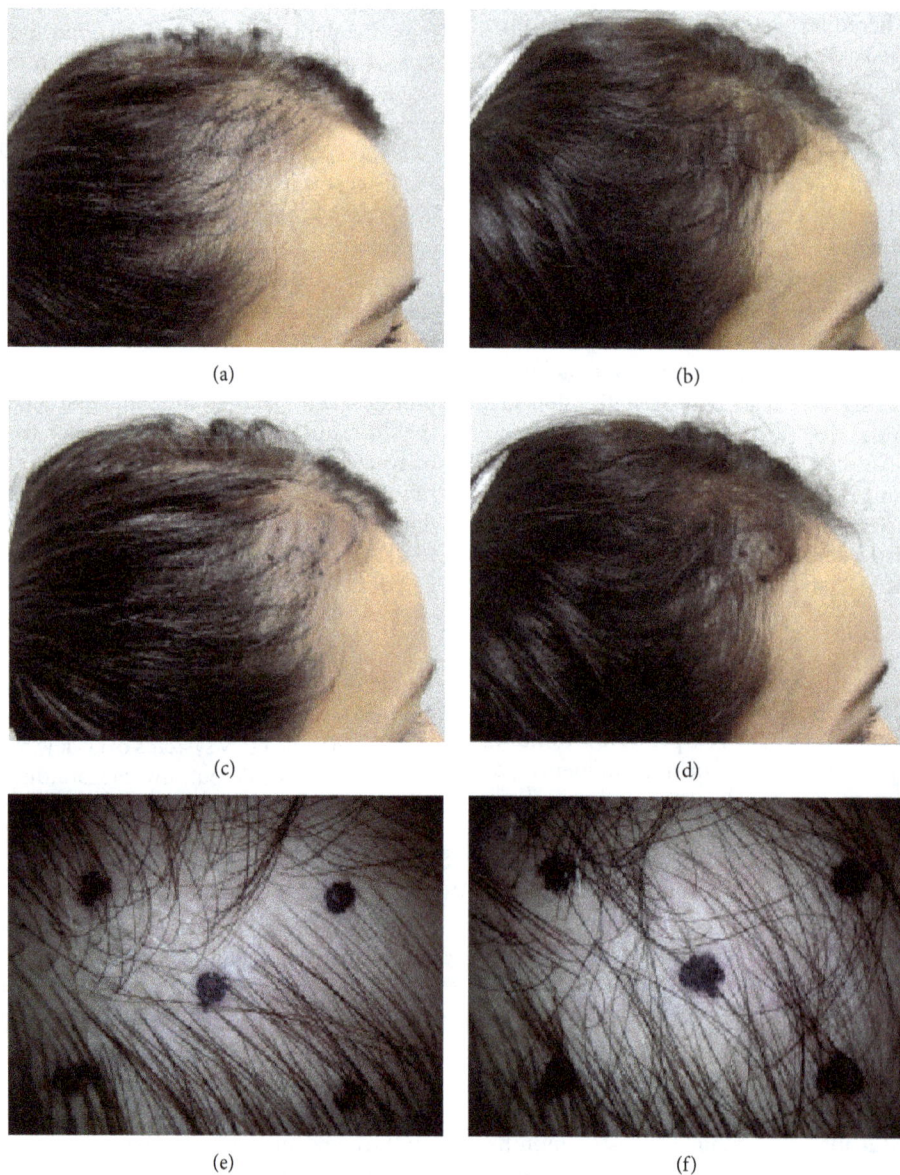

FIGURE 1: Subject 42. The number of terminal and vellus hairs at baseline (left) increased significantly after 90 days of treatment (right). The 4 cm^2 target area of the scalp is shown in the middle and bottom rows.

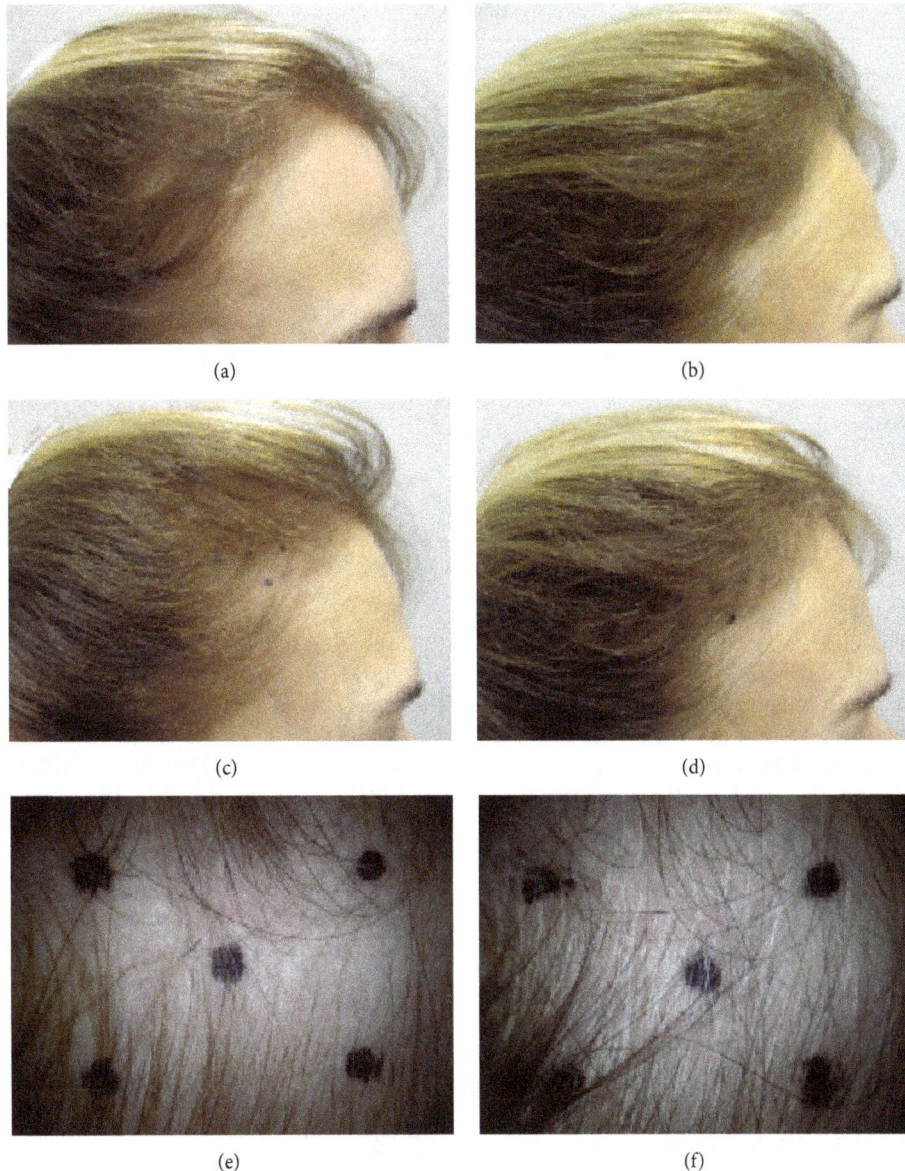

FIGURE 2: Subject 47. The number of terminal and vellus hairs at baseline (left) increased significantly after 90 days of treatment (right). The 4 cm^2 target area of the scalp is shown in the middle and bottom rows.

Phototrichograms were obtained of the scalp target area at both visits using two-dimensional digital and macrophotographs (Canon SD 4500 IS and Nikon Coolpix 4300 cameras, resp., with a 3GEN Dermlite Foto37 system). All photographs were taken by the same staff member, in the same location, and with the same lighting. Ten [10] terminal hairs in the target area were randomly chosen throughout the area and cut at the surface of the scalp. Digital photographs were obtained to measure hair diameter 1 mm from the cut end of the hair (Dino-Lite Microscope; AnMo Electronics Corp., Torrance, CA). The hair diameter was measured and used to obtain an average hair diameter for the target area.

2.4. Study Endpoints.
Using phototrichograms, the primary efficacy endpoint was the change in the number of terminal hairs and vellus hairs in the target area of the scalp at Visit 2. Terminal hairs were defined as short or long coarse hairs found on the scalp with a cross-sectional diameter of 40 μM or greater. Vellus hairs were defined as fine, short hairs with a maximum cross-sectional diameter of less than 40 μM. The secondary endpoints were changes in hair diameter, the number of shed hairs, and the responses to Quality of Life and Self-Assessment Questionnaires at Visit 2. Safety endpoints were changes in physical examinations, scalp condition, and vital signs. Subjects were queried about potential adverse events at Visit 2.

2.5. Statistical Analysis.
Descriptive statistics were obtained for all variables. Tests of normality of continuous measures were made and data were examined for homogeneity of

TABLE 2: Self-Assessment Questionnaire results.

Quality	MPS, $N = 30$ Day 90	Placebo, $N = 30$ Day 90	Significance[*]
(1) Overall hair growth	5.03 (0.85)	4.53 (0.68)	$P = 0.015$
(2) Overall hair volume	4.97 (0.72)	4.17 (0.79)	$P < 0.0001$
(3) Scalp coverage	4.70 (0.14)	4.23 (0.97)	$P = 0.042$
(4) Thickness of hair body	4.77 (0.82)	4.20 (0.89)	$P = 0.013$
(5) Softness of hair body	4.67 (0.96)	4.33 (0.84)	$P = NS$
(6) Hair shine	4.60 (1.00)	4.37 (0.77)	$P = NS$
(7) Hair strength	4.97 (1.00)	4.33 (0.92)	$P = 0.013$
(8) Nail strength	4.97 (1.03)	4.47 (1.11)	$P = NS$
(9) Nail growth rate	4.73 (0.98)	4.40 (0.89)	$P = NS$
(10) Growth of eyebrow hair	4.40 (0.86)	4.00 (0.53)	$P = 0.033$
(11) Growth of eyelashes	4.27 (0.69)	4.17 (0.59)	$P = NS$
(12) Skin smoothness	4.50 (0.82)	4.20 (0.81)	$P = NS$
(13) Overall skin health	4.63 (0.85)	4.17 (0.91)	$P = 0.045$

[*]One-way analysis of variance; NS, not significant.

variance. Changes in baseline hair growth, hair diameter, hair shedding counts with hair washing, Quality of Life responses, and Self-Assessment Questionnaire responses were tested using analyses of variance with repeated measurements. All statistical tests were two-tailed. Differences were considered statistically significant at the level of P value of ≤ 0.05 obtained.

2.6. Ethics. This study protocol and informed consent forms were approved by an institutional review board (IRB Company Inc., Buena Park, CA). Each subject provided informed consent prior to participating in any study-related activity. This study strictly adhered to all applicable guidelines for the protection of human subjects for research as outlined in the United States FDA 21 CFR Part 50, in accordance with the accepted standards for good clinical practices and the standard practices of Ablon Skin Institute Research Center.

3. Results

3.1. Subject Enrollment. The study enrolled 60 women with a mean (SD) age of 48.6 years (10.0 years) (range, 24–65 years). Subjects were randomized to receive treatment with MPS ($N = 30$) or placebo ($N = 30$) and all subjects completed the study. The race/ethnicity of subjects was Caucasian ($N = 53$; 88%), Hispanic ($N = 6$; 10%), and Asian ($N = 1$; 2%). There were no significant differences between the two groups with respect to age (MPS: 50.2 ± 12 years; placebo: 46.9 ± 9 years; $f_{1,58} = 1.58$; $P = 0.214$) or race/ethnicity (MPS: Caucasian ($N = 25$; 83.3%); placebo: Caucasian ($N = 28$; 93.3%), df = 2, $P = 0.399$).

3.2. Primary Endpoints. Among the MPS-treated subjects, there was a significant increase in the mean number of terminal hairs from 178.3 (7.8) at baseline to 235.8 (18.4) at Visit 2 ($f_{(1,29)} = 362.0$, $P < 0.0001$) but not among placebotreated subjects from 178.2 (9.6) to 180.9 (18.8) ($f_{(1,29)} = 1.25$, $P =$

0.273) (Table 1). Consequently, the number of terminal hairs among MPS-treated subjects was also significantly greater than placebo-treated subjects at Visit 2 ($f_{(1,58)} = 200.4$, $P < 0.0001$) due to the greater increase among the MPS-treated subjects (MPS: D0:178.3 ± 8; D90:235.8 ± 18; placebo: D0:178.2 ± 10, D90:180.9 ± 18). Changes in the clinical appearance of two treated subjects at baseline and after 90 days of treatment are apparent in Figures 1 and 2.

Similarly, there was a significant increase in the number of vellus hairs in MPS-treated subjects ($f_{(1,29)} = 54.1$, $P < 0.0001$) but not among the placebotreated subjects ($f_{(1,29)} = 0.67$, $P = 0.420$) (Table 1). The mean number of vellus hairs in the MPS group at Visit 2 was again significantly greater than the placebo group. The two groups were significantly different in the number of vellus hairs ($f_{(1,58)} = 24.21$, $P < 0.0001$) due to the significant increase among the MPS-treated subjects (MPS: D0:19.57 ± 2; D90:21.23 ± 2; placebo: D0:19.8 ± 2, D90:19.97 ± 2).

3.3. Secondary Endpoints. The two groups were significantly different in the hair shedding counts following hair washing ($f_{(1,58)} = 4.51$, $P = 0.038$) due to significant decrease among the MPS-treated subjects (MPS: D0: 27.13 ± 27; D90:16.47 ± 14; placebo: D0:23.4 ± 25, D90:21.87 ± 21). There was no significant increase in terminal hair diameter among MPS-treated subjects ($f_{(1,29)} = 11.42$, $P = 0.434$) or placebotreated subjects ($f_{(1,29)} = 0.29$, $P = 0.725$) and the two groups were not significantly different from one another with respect to terminal hair diameter ($f_{(1,58)} = 0.674$, $P = 0.415$).

Subjects treated with MPS obtained significantly higher total scores on the Self-Assessment Questionnaire at Visit 2 ($f_{(1,58)} = 8.27$, $P = 0.006$; MPS: 61.20 ± 7; placebo: 55.57 ± 8) with significant differences between the two groups on 7 of 13 items including overall hair growth, overall hair volume, scalp coverage, thickness of hair body, hair strength, growth of eyebrow hair, and overall skin health (Table 2).

The MPS-treated subjects also obtained significantly higher total scores on the Quality of Life Questionnaire

TABLE 3: Quality of Life Questionnaire results.

Question	MPS, $N = 30$			Placebo, $N = 30$		
	Baseline	Day 90	Significance*	Baseline	Day 90	Significance*
(1) I am embarrassed by my thinning hair.	2.70 (0.84)	2.13 (0.82)	$P < 0.0001$	2.73 (1.02)	2.47 (0.92)	$P = 0.009$
(2) Because of my thinning hair, I avoid social gatherings.	1.77 (0.68)	1.37 (0.49)	$P = 0.001$	1.67 (0.84)	1.53 (0.78)	$P = NS$
(3) I do not like meeting new people as I feel they are judging me because of my thinning hair.	2.10 (0.76)	1.63 (0.62)	$P = 0.001$	1.87 (0.94)	1.73 (0.87)	$P = NS$
(4) I avoid going out during the day because of my thinning hair.	1.77 (0.68)	1.37 (0.49)	$P = 0.001$	1.70 (0.92)	1.50 (0.78)	$P = 0.012$
(5) My condition impacts my emotional state at work.	2.10 (0.92)	1.73 (0.74)	$P = 0.005$	2.13 (0.90)	2.03 (1.03)	$P = NS$
(6) I feel my thinning hair has impacted my ability to succeed in interviews.	2.07 (0.74)	1.57 (0.94)	$P = 0.007$	1.73 (1.14)	1.60 (1.04)	$P = NS$
(7) My condition has prevented my participation in a sports activity.	2.07 (0.94)	1.57 (0.77)	$P < 0.0001$	1.83 (0.95)	1.83 (0.75)	$P = NS$
(8) My condition impacts my self-esteem.	2.87 (0.86)	2.20 (0.81)	$P < 0.0001$	2.97 (0.93)	2.53 (0.97)	$P = 0.002$
(9) My condition makes me feel self-conscious about my thinning hair.	3.03 (0.81)	2.43 (0.77)	$P < 0.0001$	3.13 (0.90)	2.80 (1.03)	$P = 0.01$
(10) Because of my thinning hair, I fear being the center of attention.	2.00 (0.91)	1.57 (0.77)	$P = 0.01$	2.37 (1.00)	2.10 (1.24)	$P = 0.043$
(11) I feel my thinning hair is affecting my personal relationships.	2.23 (0.97)	1.87 (0.86)	$P = 0.014$	2.33 (1.09)	2.03 (1.03)	$P = 0.037$
(12) Because of my thinning hair, I avoid being intimate with my partner.	1.70 (0.92)	1.37 (0.67)	$P = 0.039$	1.67 (0.92)	1.47 (0.86)	$P = NS$
(13) Because of my thinning hair, I feel less attractive to my significant other.	2.47 (1.01)	1.93 (1.05)	$P = 0.001$	2.73 (1.11)	2.47 (1.20)	$P = 0.009$
(14) Because of my thinning hair, I am less outgoing than I would like to be.	2.33 (1.03)	1.90 (0.92)	$P = 0.001$	2.27 (0.94)	2.02 (1.07)	$P = 0.032$
(15) Because of my thinning hair, I feel unattractive.	2.70 (1.02)	2.27 (0.94)	$P = 0.001$	2.87 (0.90)	2.50 (0.97)	$P = 0.001$

* Repeated measures ANOVA across study days contrasts per treatment group; NS, not significant.

($f_{(1,58)} = 4.61$, $P = 0.035$; MPS: D0:33.9 ± 10; D90:26.9 ± 8; placebo: D0:34.0 ± 11, D90:30.6 + 11). These differences were significant within each group (MPS: $f_{(1,29)} = 24.00$, $P < 0.001$; placebo: $f_{(1,29)} = 13.8$, $P < 0.001$); however, scores for MPS-treated subjects were significantly higher on all 15 questionnaire items but only 10 for the placebo-treated subjects (Table 3).

4. Discussion

The results of this study demonstrate that the use of MPS tablets for 90 days increased the number of terminal hairs and decreased hair shedding in women with self-perceived thinning hair. These changes were associated with improved hair quality including overall hair growth and increased hair strength. There were no reports of adverse events.

Other US studies have demonstrated the beneficial effects of MPS when used by women with thinning hair. In a placebo-controlled, double-blind pilot study, adult women with self-perceived thinning hair were randomized to receive MPS ($N = 10$) or placebo ($N = 5$) twice daily [26]. After 180 days, the mean (SD) number of terminal vellus hairs among placebotreated subjects at baseline was 256.0 (24.1), remaining at 245.0 (22.4) and 242.2 (26.9) after 90 and 180 days, respectively. In contrast, the mean number of baseline terminal hairs in MPS-treated subjects was 271.0

(24.2) increasing to 571 (65.7) and 609.6 (66.6) after 90 and 180 days, respectively (for each, $P < 0.001$ *versus* placebo). Subjects also reported improvements in several subjective measures of hair quality.

A randomized, double-blind, multicenter, placebo-controlled study was also designed to assess the effects of MPS on hair growth in adult women with self-perceived thinning hair (Ablon and Dayan, submitted). These subjects were randomized to receive MPS ($N = 20$) or placebo ($N = 20$) twice daily. The MPS-treated subjects achieved a significant increase in the number of baseline terminal hairs at 90 and 180 days (for each, $P < 0.0001$) and were significantly greater than placebo ($P < 0.0001$). These objective measures were correlated with numerous improvements in Self-Assessment and Quality of Life measures.

The results of this study are also in agreement with another study which showed the use of an oral supplement containing natural ingredients including marine-derived protein (shark cartilage) and fish oil (omega-3 polyunsaturated fatty acids) significantly reducing hair loss in women [27]; however, it did not promote hair growth.

5. Conclusion

Similar to previous studies, the ingredients in MPS tablets promote hair growth in women suffering from temporary thinning hair. The current study further demonstrated the ability of this product to decrease hair loss. MPS continues to demonstrate an excellent safety profile.

Conflict of Interests

The author declares that there is no conflict of interests regarding the publication of this paper.

Acknowledgments

This study was sponsored and funded by a grant from Lifes2good, Inc., Chicago, IL. The author acknowledges the editorial assistance of Dr. Carl Hornfeldt, Apothekon, Inc., and the statistical support of Dr. Shahrokh Golshan, VMRF VetStats Biostatistics Core, University of California, San Diego.

References

[1] M. E. Gonzalez, J. Cantatore-Francis, and S. J. Orlow, "Androgenetic alopecia in the paediatric population: a retrospective review of 57 patients," *British Journal of Dermatology*, vol. 163, no. 2, pp. 378–385, 2010.

[2] O. T. Norwood, "Incidence of female androgenetic alopecia (female pattern alopecia)," *Dermatologic Surgery*, vol. 27, no. 1, pp. 53–54, 2001.

[3] M. P. Birch, J. F. Messenger, and A. G. Messenger, "Hair density, hair diameter and the prevalence of female pattern hair loss," *British Journal of Dermatology*, vol. 144, no. 2, pp. 297–304, 2001.

[4] S. Harrison and W. Bergfeld, "Diffuse hair loss: its triggers and management," *Cleveland Clinic Journal of Medicine*, vol. 76, no. 6, pp. 361–367, 2009.

[5] C. C. Thiedke, "Alopecia in women," *American Family Physician*, vol. 67, no. 5, pp. 1007–1014, 2003.

[6] V. K. Jain, U. Kataria, and S. Dayal, "Study of diffuse alopecia in females," *Indian Journal of Dermatology, Venereology and Leprology*, vol. 66, pp. 65–68, 2000.

[7] J. Gatherwright, M. T. Liu, C. Gliniak, A. Totonchi, and B. Guyuron, "The contribution of endogenous and exogenous factors to female alopecia: a study of identical twins," *Plastic and Reconstructive Surgery*, vol. 130, no. 6, pp. 1219–1226, 2012.

[8] D. Williamson, M. Gonzalez, and A. Y. Finlay, "The effect of hair loss in quality of life," *Journal of the European Academy of Dermatology and Venereology*, vol. 15, no. 2, pp. 137–139, 2001.

[9] J. van der Donk, J. Passchier, C. Knegt-Junk et al., "Psychological characteristics of women with androgenetic alopecia: a controlled study," *British Journal of Dermatology*, vol. 125, no. 3, pp. 248–252, 1991.

[10] E. E. Reid, A. C. Haley, J. H. Borovicka et al., "Clinical severity does not reliably predict quality of life in women with alopecia areata, telogen effluvium, or androgenic alopecia," *Journal of the American Academy of Dermatology*, vol. 66, no. 3, pp. e97–e102, 2012.

[11] T. F. Cash, V. H. Price, and R. C. Savin, "Psychological effects of androgenetic alopecia on women: comparisons with balding men and with female control subjects," *Journal of the American Academy of Dermatology*, vol. 29, no. 4, pp. 568–575, 1993.

[12] A. M. Finner, "Nutrition and hair: deficiencies and supplements," *Dermatologic Clinics*, vol. 31, pp. 167–172, 2013.

[13] N. Yazbeck, S. Muwakkit, M. Abboud, and R. Saab, "Zinc and biotin deficiencies after pancreaticoduodenectomy," *Acta Gastro-Enterologica Belgica*, vol. 73, no. 2, pp. 283–286, 2010.

[14] E. Alhaj, N. Alhaj, and N. E. Alhaj, "Diffuse alopecia in a child due to dietary zinc deficiency," *Skinmed*, vol. 6, no. 4, pp. 199–200, 2007.

[15] M. S. Kil, C. W. Kim, and S. S. Kim, "Analysis of serum zinc and copper concentrations in hair loss," *Annals of Dermatology*, vol. 25, no. 4, pp. 405–409, 2013.

[16] T. Karashima, D. Tsuruta, T. Hamada et al., "Oral zinc therapy for zinc deficiency-related telogen effluvium," *Dermatologic Therapy*, vol. 25, no. 2, pp. 210–213, 2012.

[17] H. Park, C. W. Kim, S. S. Kim, and C. W. Park, "The therapeutic effect and the changed serum zinc level after zinc supplementation in alopecia areata patients who had a low serum zinc level," *Annals of Dermatology*, vol. 21, no. 2, pp. 142–146, 2009.

[18] S. Daniells and G. Hardy, "Hair loss in long-term or home parenteral nutrition: are micronutrient deficiencies to blame?" *Current Opinion in Clinical Nutrition & Metabolic Care*, vol. 13, no. 6, pp. 690–697, 2010.

[19] J. Zempleni, Y. I. Hassan, and S. S. K. Wijeratne, "Biotin and biotinidase deficiency," *Expert Review of Endocrinology and Metabolism*, vol. 3, no. 6, pp. 715–724, 2008.

[20] I. Herskovitz and A. Tosti, "Female pattern hair loss," *International Journal of Endocrinology and Metabolism*, vol. 11, no. 4, Article ID e9860, 2013.

[21] A. Lassus and E. Eskelinen, "A comparative study of a new food supplement, ViviScal, with fish extract for the treatment of hereditary androgenic alopecia in young males," *Journal of International Medical Research*, vol. 20, no. 6, pp. 445–453, 1992.

[22] A. Lassus, L. Jeskanen, H. P. Happonen, and J. Santalahti, "Imedeen for the treatment of degenerated skin in females," *Journal of International Medical Research*, vol. 19, no. 2, pp. 147–152, 1991.

[23] A. Eskelinin and J. Santalahti, "Special natural cartilage polysaccharides for the treatment of sun-damaged skin in females," *Journal of International Medical Research*, vol. 20, no. 2, pp. 99–105, 1992.

[24] O. de Lacharrière, C. Deloche, C. Misciali et al., "Hair diameter diversity: a clinical sign reflecting the follicle miniaturization," *Archives of Dermatology*, vol. 137, no. 5, pp. 641–646, 2001.

[25] A. Vujovic and V. del Marmol, "The female pattern hair loss: review of etiopathogenesis and diagnosis," *BioMed Research International*, vol. 2014, Article ID 767628, 8 pages, 2014.

[26] G. Ablon, "Double-blind, placebo-controlled study evaluating the efficacy of an oral supplement in women with self-perceived thinning hair," *Journal of Clinical and Aesthetic Dermatology*, vol. 5, no. 11, pp. 28–34, 2012.

[27] A. Jacquet, V. Coolen, and J. Vandermander, "Effect of dietary supplementation with INVERSION femme on slimming, hair loss, and skin and nail parameters in women," *Advances in Therapy*, vol. 24, no. 5, pp. 1154–1171, 2007.

22

Epidemiological, Clinical, and Paraclinic Aspect of Cutaneous Sarcoidosis in Black Africans

**Mamadou Kaloga,[1] Ildevert Patrice Gbéry,[1] Vagamon Bamba,[2]
Yao Isidore Kouassi,[1] Elidjé Joseph Ecra,[1] Almamy Diabate,[2]
Sarah Kourouma,[1] Kouadio Celestin Ahogo,[1] Kouassi Alexandre Kouamé,[1]
Komenan Kassi,[1] Kanga Kouame,[1] and Abdoulaye Sangaré[1]**

[1]*Department of Dermatology and Venereology, Teaching Hospital of Treichville, Abidjan, Côte d'Ivoire*
[2]*Department of Dermatology and Venereology, Teaching Hospital of Bouaké, Côte d'Ivoire*

Correspondence should be addressed to Mamadou Kaloga; kaloganas@yahoo.fr

Academic Editor: Markus Stucker

The specific objectives were to identify the epidemiology of cutaneous sarcoidosis and describe the clinical and laboratory aspects of the disease. *Materials and Methods.* We performed a descriptive cross-sectional study involving 24 referred cases of cutaneous sarcoidosis in 25 years (1990–2014) collected at Venereology Dermatology Department of the University Hospital of Treichville (Abidjan) both in consultation and in hospitalization. *Results.* The hospital frequency was one case per year. The average age was 42 years, ranging from 9 to 64. The sex ratio was 1. The shortest time interval between the appearance of the skin lesion and consultation of Dermatology Department at CHU Treichville was 3 months. The elementary lesions were represented primarily by a papule (18 cases), placard (3 cases), and nodule (2 cases) and mainly sat on the face and neck in 8 cases (38%). Extra cutaneous lesions were dominated by ganglion and respiratory involvement with 5 cases each followed by musculoskeletal damage in 3 cases. Chest radiography showed abnormality in 13 cases (54%). The pulmonary function test performed in 13 patients found 7 cases (54%) having restrictive ventilatory syndrome and 6 cases (46%) being normal. A tuberculin anergy was found in 11 cases (61%).

1. Introduction

Sarcoidosis or besnier Boeck Schaumann (BBS) disease is a chronic granulomatous skin manifestation and a multivisceral involvement [1]. Several cases have been described by Western countries in all its aspects [2–4]. In Africa a publication was made in Western Africa, South Africa, and Tunisia [5–8]. In Ivory Coast the last study of sarcoidosis dates back to 1997 [9]. However, several gray areas persist on some aspects of sarcoidosis in black Africa. We therefore decided to conduct a study of sarcoidosis whose general objective was to help improve the treatment of cutaneous sarcoidosis among the black African. The specific objectives were to identify the epidemiology of cutaneous sarcoidosis and describe the clinical and laboratory aspects of the disease.

2. Materials and Methods

Our study took place at the Dermatology Department of the University Hospital of Treichville (Abidjan) which is with the Dermatology Department of the University Hospital of Bouaké, one of two reference centers for management of dermatological diseases in Ivory Coast. This was a retrospective cross-sectional study. The period from January 1, 1990, to December 31, 2014, or 25 years was concerned. All patients of all sexes and ages observed in consultation or hospitalization meeting the clinical descriptions and having a result of the histopathological examination were included. Patients with incomplete clinical record and Caucasians were not included. The collection of information was carried out with an investigation fact sheet and the following information was collected:

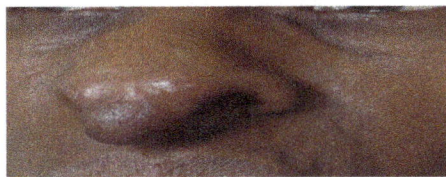

Figure 1: Nodule on the nose (Picture of Dr. Kouassi yao Isidore, CHU Treichville).

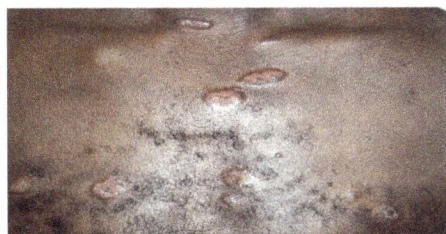

Figure 2: Papule of the chest (Picture of Dr. Kouassi yao Isidore, CHU Treichville).

the epidemiological characteristics and clinical and laboratory profiles. Data were analyzed with the EPI-DATA computer software.

3. Results

3.1. Epidemiological Characteristics. In the period of 25 years, 24 patients suffering from sarcoidosis were treated in the Dermatology Department. The average age was 42 years, ranging from 9 to 64. The age group 30 to 60 years was the most affected with 75% of cases. The sex ratio was 1. All socioprofessional categories were affected.

3.2. Clinical and Laboratory Characteristics. The shortest time interval between the appearance of the skin lesion and consultation of Dermatology Department at CHU Treichville was 3 months. The mean time to consultation was 12 months. The elementary lesions were represented essentially by a papule (18 cases), a placard (3 cases), and a nodule (2 cases with one case of erythema nodosum) (Figure 1). These elementary lesions mainly sat on the face and neck in 8 cases (38%) followed by the chest in 5 cases (24%) (Figure 2) and all the body in 4 cases (19%). Lesions out of the skin were lymph nodes in 5 patients and the lungs in 5 patients too. The bones and joints were affected in 3 cases; then it was found 1 case in the eye, 1 neurological case, 1 case of spleen, and 1 case of liver. One patient had a generalized sarcoidosis with intramedullary localization leading to a bilateral flaccid paraplegia. Chest radiography showed abnormality in 13 cases (54%). The found images are shown in Table 1. The pulmonary function test performed in 13 patients found 7 cases (54%) having restrictive ventilatory syndrome and 6 cases (46%) being normal. Hematological disturbances were marked by an accelerated sedimentation rate in 4 patients and anemia in 2 cases. The tuberculin skin test was performed in 18 patients. A tuberculin anergy was found in 11 cases (61%).

Table 1: Radiographic images of sarcoidosis.

Images	Number	Percentage (%)
Mediastinal lymphadenopathy isolated	6	46
Reaching isolated parenchymal	5	39
Mediastinal lymphadenopathy + parenchymal damage	2	15
Total	13	100

Serum calcium levels were normal in all patients in whom the examination was requested (9 cases), while a hypercalcium excretion was found in only 1 patient out of 2 examinations performed.

4. Discussion

During the study period of 25 years we have identified 24 cases. This hospital prevalence of sarcoidosis in our study is very low since 118 cases in 8 years in Spain [4], 113 cases in 13 years in Guadeloupe [3], and 118 cases in 32 years Tunisia [8] were reported. Several studies have shown that it is common in the black subject [2, 10, 11]. This low prevalence in our study could be explained by two facts. Firstly, poverty and lack of health insurance by patients limit their access to health facilities. Secondly all cases of sarcoidosis are not addressed in Dermatology Department of Treichville University Hospital because of the existence of Dermatology Department at the University Hospital of Bouaké. Young adults are the most affected with a rarity of extreme ages in our series. Our results are consistent with several African, European, American, and Asian authors [4, 7, 10, 12]. But African patients would be affected at a younger age (40 years) than patients in the Scandinavian and Asian countries with an average age of 50 years [13]. This difference could be related to life expectancy which is higher in these countries than in Africa. Sarcoidosis affects women more often than men [14]. In our series we found as many men as women with sarcoidosis. The loss and the lack of data could explain this equal frequency. Regarding history, a case of sarcoidosis was found on scarification in our study. it was a woman of thirty and she had originated in north of the Ivory Coast. Jacyk [7] also describe a similar case with a lower frequency such as a case of 54 patients with cutaneous sarcoidosis. Indeed, Olumide et al., Nigeria [6], found 43 cases of cutaneous sarcoidosis in 30 locations. These latter are all grown on cutaneous scars. These latter are all grown on cutaneous scars. The beginning of the treatment of cutaneous sarcoidosis is late. Fifty-four percent of patients said that the disease was evolving for over a year. We agree with Mahajan et al. [12] who had also found that the majority of patients present after more than one year of disease progression. Indeed the diagnosis of sarcoidosis can be difficult in forms present in early stages. Patients are then treated erroneously for other conditions such as lichen, chronic eczema, or even acne. Most often patients do not give any importance to initial lesions because there are no functional signs. The first consultation is often motivated by disfigurement. This impairs the response to therapy and therefore prognosis of the disease. No cases of sarcoidosis were discovered incidentally in our series. The diagnosis was oriented across various lesions. Among these, papules (78%) are observed and more preferably sit on the face or neck (38%). We noticed that overall general signs were almost nonexistent. In order of frequency, our results can be stacked with literature data [5, 8]. The most affected viscera during sarcoidosis in our study are the nodal unit (41.6%) and respiratory unit (33%). Niang et al. [5] and Khaled et al. [8] have made the same observation but respiratory involvement was the predominant lymph node involvement in their study. The detection of visceral involvement may be fortuitous in the paraclinical explorations. In our series, few paraclinical examinations were performed. According to data from the literature, visceral manifestations remain long asymptomatic and are discovered during diagnostic tests [15]. Erythema nodosum was found in only one patient (5%). The incidence of erythema nodosum varies across different countries and race. He found a predominance of erythema nodosum in the white matter with a frequency of 31% [16], while it is 4% among blacks [13]. Chest radiography is very important in screening for mediastinal pulmonary sarcoidosis. Some lymph nodes and miliary endothoracic origin of sarcoidosis are labeled incorrectly as a result of TB endemicity of this disease in Ivory Coast [17]. Chest radiographs were abnormal in 54% in our study and the stage I was the most common at 46%. Khaled et al. [8] found 30.1% radiographic abnormalities with a predominance of stage I or II. This high rate of pulmonary involvement could be explained in part by the poor health coverage and also by the tendency of our people to consult a doctor much later. Pathological examination was systematic in our patients. This attitude is consistent with the literature which states that the diagnosis of sarcoidosis is essentially histological [14, 18]. Laboratory tests were rarely made, which does not allow us to arrive at a judgment. Cases of anemia have no specificity. The studied immunology from the skin test revealed 61% of tuberculin anergy. Our numbers are superimposed on those in the literature [8, 19].

5. Conclusion

Cutaneous sarcoidosis is a relatively rare condition in Ivory Coast. It reached the youngest of all adult sex. The papules on the face and neck are the main physical signs. The lung and lymph nodes are the most commonly affected.

Conflict of Interests

The authors declare that there is no conflict of interests regarding the publication of this paper.

References

[1] CEDEF, "Item 207—UE 7 Sarcoïdose," *Annales de Dermatologie et de Vénéréologie*, vol. 142, supplement 2, pp. S177–S180, 2015.

[2] C. R. Heath, J. David, and S. C. Taylor, "Sarcoidosis: are there differences in your skin of color patients?" *Journal of the American Academy of Dermatology*, vol. 66, no. 1, pp. 121.e1–121.e14, 2012.

[3] G. Cadelis, N. Cordel, N. Coquart, N. Étienne, and M. Macal, "Incidence de la sarcoïdose en Guadeloupe: étude rétrospective sur 13ans (1997–2009)," *Revue des Maladies Respiratoires*, vol. 29, no. 1, pp. 13–20, 2012.

[4] G. S. Fernández and G. R. López, "Epidemiology, presentation forms, radiological stage and diagnostic methods of sarcoidosis in the area of Leon (2001–2008)," *Revista Clinica Espanola*, vol. 211, no. 6, pp. 291–297, 2011.

[5] S. O. Niang, M. T. Dieng, A. Kane, S. N. Diop, and B. Ndiaye, "Sarcoidosis in Dakar: 30 case reports," *Dakar médical*, vol. 52, no. 3, pp. 216–222, 2007.

[6] Y. M. Olumide, E. O. Bandele, and S. O. Elesha, "Cutaneous sarcoidosis in Nigeria," *Journal of the American Academy of Dermatology*, vol. 21, no. 6, pp. 1222–1224, 1989.

[7] W. K. Jacyk, "Cutaneous sarcoidosis in black South Africans," *International Journal of Dermatology*, vol. 38, no. 11, pp. 841–845, 1999.

[8] A. Khaled, A. Souissi, F. Zeglaoui et al., "Cutaneous sarcoidosis in Tunisia," *Giornale Italiano di Dermatologia e Venereologia*, vol. 143, no. 3, pp. 181–185, 2008.

[9] A. Gabla, T. Kouadio, E. Eti et al., "La sarcoïdose chez le noir africain: A propos de 30 cas," *Rhumatologie*, vol. 49, no. 2, pp. 67–69, 1997.

[10] B. A. Rybicki and M. C. Iannuzzi, "Epidemiology of sarcoidosis: recent advances and future prospects," *Seminars in Respiratory and Critical Care Medicine*, vol. 28, no. 1, pp. 22–35, 2007.

[11] S. K. Gupta, "Sarcoidosis: a journey through 50 years," *Indian Journal of Chest Diseases*, vol. 44, no. 4, pp. 247–253, 2002.

[12] V. K. Mahajan, N. L. Sharma, R. C. Sharma, and V. C. Sharma, "Cutaneous sarcoidosis: clinical profile of 23 Indian patients," *Indian Journal of Dermatology*, vol. 73, no. 1, pp. 16–21, 2007.

[13] B. A. Rybicki, M. Major, J. Popovich Jr., M. J. Maliarik, and M. C. Iannuzzi, "Racial differences in sarcoidosis incidence: a 5-year study in a health maintenance organization," *American Journal of Epidemiology*, vol. 145, no. 3, pp. 234–241, 1997.

[14] B. X. Crick, "Granulomes cutanés non infectieux," in *Dermatologie et Infections Sexuellement Transmissibles*, J. H. Saurat, J. M. Lachapelle, D. Lipsker, and L. Thomas, Eds., pp. 567–571, Masson, Paris, France, 5th edition, 2009.

[15] M. Perrin Fayolle, "Les localisations viscerale de la sarcoïdose," *La Revue du Praticien*, vol. 33, no. 39, pp. 2039–2048, 1983.

[16] G. Le Guerin, "Syndrome de LOFGREN," *La Revue du Praticien*, vol. 33, no. 39, pp. 2069–2076, 1983.

[17] M. Roudaut, H. Tiendrebeogo, B. Pigerias, D. Schmidt, N. Coulibaly, and P. Delormas, "La sarcoïdose médiastino-pulmonaire en Côte d'Ivoire. Intérêt épidémiologique et clinique de 16 nouveaux cas observés à Abidjan," *Médecine Tropicale*, vol. 40, no. 2, pp. 144–149, 1980.

[18] J. P. Battesti, "L'aide au diagnostic de sarcoïdose en 1988," *La Revue de Médecine Interne*, vol. 9, no. 4, pp. 351–353, 1988.

[19] M. H. Jouvin, D. Valeyere, and J. P. Battesti, "Immunologie de la sarcoidose," *La Revue du Praticien*, vol. 39, no. 33, pp. 2073–2076, 1983.

23

Actinic Keratosis Clinical Practice Guidelines: An Appraisal of Quality

Joslyn S. Kirby,[1] **Thomas Scharnitz,**[2] **Elizabeth V. Seiverling,**[1]
Hadjh Ahrns,[3] **and Sara Ferguson**[1]

[1]*Department of Dermatology, Penn State Milton S. Hershey Medical Center, Hershey, PA 17033, USA*
[2]*Penn State College of Medicine, Hershey, PA 17033, USA*
[3]*Department of Family and Community Medicine, Penn State Milton S. Hershey Medical Center, Hershey, PA 17033, USA*

Correspondence should be addressed to Joslyn S. Kirby; jkirby1@hmc.psu.edu

Academic Editor: Jean Kanitakis

Actinic keratosis (AK) is a common precancerous skin lesion and many AK management guidelines exist, but there has been limited investigation into the quality of these documents. The objective of this study was to assess the strengths and weaknesses of guidelines that address AK management. A systematic search for guidelines with recommendations for AK was performed. The Appraisal of Guidelines for Research and Evaluation (AGREE II) was used to appraise the quality of guidelines. Multiple raters independently reviewed each of the guidelines and applied the AGREE II tool and scores were calculated. Overall, 2,307 citations were identified and 7 fulfilled the study criteria. The Cancer Council of Australia/Australian Cancer Network guideline had the highest mean scores and was the only guideline to include a systematic review, include an evidence rating for recommendations, and report conflicts of interest and funding sources. High-quality, effective guidelines are evidence-based with recommendations that are concise and organized, so practical application is facilitated. Features such as concise tables, pictorial diagrams, and explicit links to evidence are helpful. However, the rigor and validity of some guidelines were weak. So, it is important for providers to be aware of the features that contribute to a high-quality, practical document.

1. Introduction

Actinic keratosis (AK), or solar keratosis, is a common dysplastic lesion of the keratinocyte [1, 2]. Over a 10-year period from 1990 to 1999, AK was diagnosed in more than 47 million visits and was found to occur in 14% of all patients visiting dermatologists [3]. AK may be treated due to concern for carcinogenesis, patient discomfort, or cosmesis. The most common treatment for AK is cryotherapy [4], likely due to easy access, ease of care for patients, and speed of the procedure. Other management methods include observation, alternative destructive therapies, topical chemotherapies, chemical peels, photodynamic therapy (PDT), and preventative measures such as sunscreen [5]. Given the high prevalence of AK and the variety and number of clinicians within an organization that encounter AK, CPG can serve as a resource upon which management approaches are unified.

Clinical practice guidelines (CPG) can guide clinicians' diagnostic and therapeutic decisions by succinctly reviewing the literature and proposing evidence-based management recommendations. CPG are defined by the Institute of Medicine as "statements that include recommendations intended to optimize patient care that are informed by a systematic review of evidence and an assessment of the benefits and harms of alternative care options. Rather than dictating a one-size-fits-all approach to patient care, CPG offer an evaluation of the breadth and quality of the relevant scientific literature and an assessment of the likely benefits and harms of a particular treatment" [6]. Thus, a high-quality CPG will include an extensive literature review and an evidence rating scale can help readers be aware of the potential limitations of the sources. The quality of CPG can vary for many reasons including the adequacy of the literature search, types of studies incorporated, and bias by the authors

[7, 8]. To our knowledge, there is no published assessment of AK CPG quality. We used the AGREE II instrument [9] to assess the strengths and weaknesses of CPG addressing multiple modalities of AK management for patients without immunosuppression.

2. Methods

The PRISMA checklist was used as a guide for this investigation. A medical librarian performed a systematic search of the medical literature for CPG with recommendations for AK. An extensive search of Medline/PubMed (1966–March 20, 2014) was conducted for relevant clinical practice guidelines using a combination of the key terms "actinic" and "keratosis" and "guideline" as well as "keratosis, actinic" as a major medical subject heading. Results were limited to practice guideline and guideline publication types. There were no date or language restrictions. In addition the National Guideline Clearinghouse, National Institute for Health and Clinical Excellence, European Academy of Dermatology and Venereology, Guidelines International Network, TRIP Database, Australian Government Clinical Practice Guidelines Portal, Scottish Intercollegiate Guidelines Network, Guidelines and Audit Implementation Network, Professional Organizations and Royal Colleges, Health Service Executive Guidelines and the American Academy Dermatology web sites were searched using key terms "actinic" and "keratosis."

The inclusion criteria were established *a priori* and (1) included an explicit statement identifying the document as a management guideline, (2) were written by multiple authors including at least one dermatologist, and (3) made recommendations concerning multiple options to manage AK. Exclusion criteria included (1) consensus statements or review articles that did not include identifiable management recommendations, (2) reviews of a published guideline, (3) focus on only preventative, epidemiology, or research methods, (4) focus on a limited or specific patient population, and (5) discussion of one form of management.

Two reviewers (TS and JK) independently examined the retrieved titles and abstracts to assess the articles for inclusion and exclusion criteria. The full text of these articles was retrieved and the same two reviewers (TS and JK) reviewed the selected articles again for eligibility. Disagreement was resolved through discussion by the reviewers (TS and JK). Seven of the guidelines were selected for analysis.

The AGREE II tool was used to describe the quality of the selected CPG. It was developed to evaluate the validity and feasibility of CPG as well as assess sources of bias [9]. The AGREE and AGREE II tools have been validated and widely applied, including CPG of dermatologic conditions [17, 18] as well as in other disciplines [19–21]. Four of the authors independently reviewed and scored the CPG. JK and ES are dermatologists, TS was a first-year medical student, and HA is a family practitioner. All four reviewers read the AGREE II users' manual and completed the online orientation and training.

The AGREE II instrument was used to define the assessment variables and rating system and to store data [9]. This instrument provides criteria to appraise the quality of

CPG and consists of 23 items grouped into six domains: (1) scope and purpose, (2) stakeholder involvement, (3) rigor of development, (4) clarity of presentation, (5) applicability, and (6) editorial independence. Each item is rated on a seven-point Likert scale from strongly disagree to strongly agree (1–7, resp.). The results for each domain consist of a domain score, which is the sum of the scores of the individual domain items and standardized by scaling the total as a percentage of the maximum possible score for that domain. The maximum score for each domain was the number of questions multiplied by 7 (strongly agree). The minimum score was the number of questions multiplied by number 1 (strongly disagree):

Scaled Domain Score

$$= \frac{(\text{Sum of Domain scores}) - (\text{Minimum possible score})}{(\text{Maximum possible score}) - (\text{Minimum possible score})} \quad (1)$$

$$\times\ 100\%.$$

The minimum standardized score for each domain was, therefore, 0% and the maximum was 100%. A standardized domain score above 60% has been suggested as the threshold to indicate sufficient minimum quality to consider practical use of this portion of the guideline [18]. This study was exempted from review by the Penn State Institutional Review Board.

2.1. Statistical Analysis. The scores were compiled and reviewed; upon visual inspection one investigator had scores that appeared to deviate from the other three. The Pearson correlation coefficient is very sensitive to outlying values so Spearman's Rho was used to determine interrater reliability [22]. The degree of agreement was classified as follows: poor (0.00), slight (0.00 and 0.20), fair (0.21 to 0.40), moderate (0.41 to 0.60), substantial (from 0.61 to 0.80), and very good or almost perfect (0.81 to 1.00) [23]. A descriptive statistical analysis of the scores was performed and included the mean and standard deviation. A *p* value of <.05 was considered significant. All analyses were performed using SAS 9.3 (SAS, Cary, NC).

3. Results

The search strategy identified 2,307 records and after review ultimately seven records were included in the study (Figure 1). The characteristics of the seven CPG are listed in Table 1. Of the seven CPG, one was from Australia [11], one was from Britain [12], three were from Germany [13–15], one was from Italy [16], and one was from the United States [10]. The range for interrater agreement was 0.39–0.86. Analysis showed that one appraiser had only fair agreement with other appraisers (0.39 [*p* = .38]). This rater was a first-year medical student and it was presumed that this reflected clinical experience rather than CPG quality so his scores were removed and subsequent calculations did not include these scores. The correlation coefficients among the three remaining appraisers, which included two dermatologists

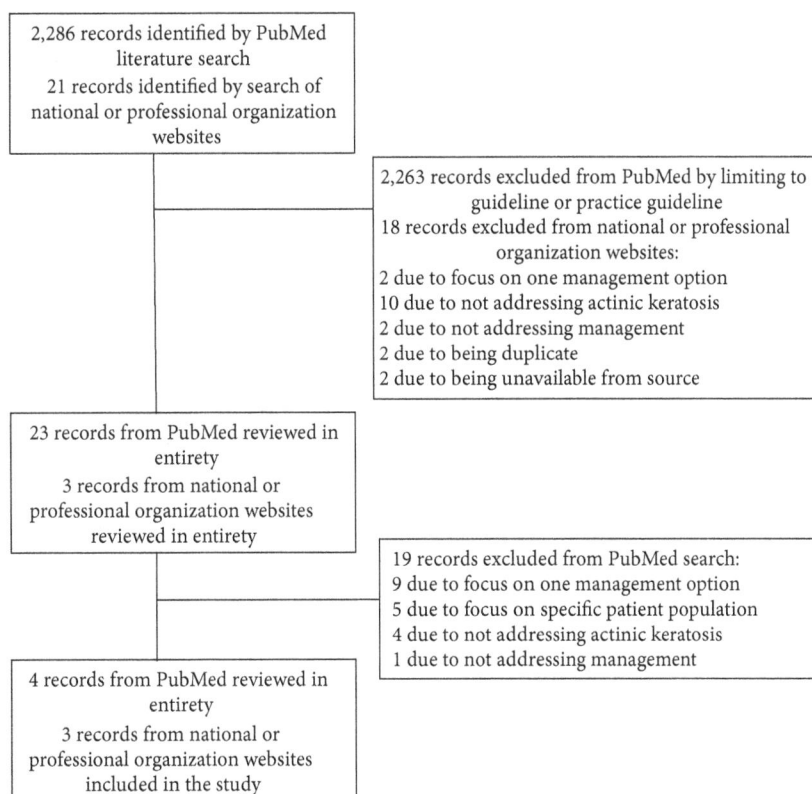

FIGURE 1: Literature search and study selection process.

TABLE 1: Characteristics of the included studies.

Guideline	Systematic review performed	Evidence grading reported	CPG funding reported	Competing interests reported
Drake et al. [10]	NR	No	NR	NR
CCA/ACN [11]	Yes	Yes	Yes	Yes
de Berker et al. [12]	No	Yes	NR	Yes
Stockfleth and Kerl (2006) [13]	NR	Yes	NR	Yes
Stockfleth et al. (2008) [14]	NR	No	Yes	Yes
Stockfleth et al. (2011) [15]	NR	Yes	NR	Yes
Rossi et al. [16]	NR	No	NR	NR

CCA/ACN: Cancer Council Australia/Australian Cancer Network. NR = not reported.

and a family practitioner, were moderate or better (0.54–0.86).

The CCA/ACN guideline [11] was the only CPG to perform a systematic review, include evidence-based ratings for recommendations, and report conflicts of interest and funding sources (Table 1). It was also the only CPG to have scores for all domains above 60% and had the highest score for each of the six domains and overall category (Table 2). The domains with the highest mean scores were domain 1 (scope and purpose) and domain 4 (clarity of presentation) with means of 50.2% and 51.1%, respectively. The domains with the lowest mean scores were domain 5 (applicability) and domain 6 (editorial independence) with means of 28.6% and 32.1%, respectively. Domain 6 (editorial independence) also had the lowest individual score of 6.3 and the greatest range

in individual scores (8.3% to 80.6%). This may reflect wide variation in disclosure of funding and conflict of interests. While five of the seven CPG included a conflict of interests statement, only two had a disclosure regarding funding sources (Table 1).

Three guidelines were recommended by at least three raters (CCA/CAN [11], de Berker et al. [12], Stockfleth and Kerl 2006 [13]). The CPG by Stockfleth et al. 2008 [14] was recommended by two of the three raters. This second article by Stockfleth et al. 2008 [14] had higher scores in domains 1 (scope and purpose), 2 (stakeholder involvement), 4 (clarity of presentation), and 5 (applicability) but lower scores in domains 3 (rigor of development) and 6 (editorial independence). Domain 3's (rigor of development) score may have been lower due to a lack of a systematic review and

TABLE 2: Clinical practice guideline scores.

| Guideline | Mean scores (% [SD]) | | | | | | Raters that would recommend, n = 3 raters | |
	(1) Scope and purpose	(2) Stakeholder involvement	(3) Rigor of development	(4) Clarity of presentation	(5) Applicability	(6) Editorial independence	Overall assessment (%, [SD])	Yes	Yes, with modifications
Drake et al. [10]	33.3 [11.1]	35.2 [8.5]	16.7 [7.3]	31.5 [8.5]	6.9 [4.8]	11.1 [12.7]	5.6 [9.6]	0	0
CCA/CAN [11]	81.5 [3.2]	96.3 [3.2]	92.6 [20.1]	75.9 [23.1]	68.1 [18.8]	80.6 [12.7]	77.8 [9.6]	2	1
de Berker et al. [12]	35.2 [21.0]	31.5 [30.6]	52.8 [11.1]	70.4 [13.9]	31.9 [23.7]	33.3 [36.3]	38.9 [25.5]	1	2
Stockfleth and Kerl (2006) [13]	53.7 [17.9]	29.6 [3.2]	69.4 [18.2]	29.6 [13.9]	20.8 [11.0]	38.9 [19.2]	27.8 [25.5]	1	2
Stockfleth et al. (2008) [14]	87.0 [8.5]	51.9 [32.6]	47.2 [12.1]	59.3 [21.0]	31.9 [8.7]	8.3 [8.3]	27.8 [9.6]	0	2
Stockfleth et al. (2011) [15]	24.1 [8.5]	16.7 [0]	35.2 [8.0]	35.2 [11.6]	13.9 [2.4]	44.4 [4.8]	33.3 [16.7]	0	2
Rossi et al. [16]	37.0 [28.0]	18.5 [17.9]	24.1 [11.2]	55.6 [30.9]	26.4 [8.7]	8.3 [14.4]	22.2 [25.5]	0	1
Mean score for domain	50.2 [27.2]	39.9 [30.3]	48.3 [27.4]	51.1 [24.1]	28.6 [21.7]	32.1 [29.1]	33.3 [26.4]		

SD = standard deviation.

TABLE 3: Samples of recommendations from the three CPG with the highest overall scores.

Guideline	Samples of CPG recommendations
CCA/ACN [11]	(i) In many cases solar keratosis [AK] regresses spontaneously and uncommonly; it evolves into squamous cell carcinoma (ii) The chances that an individual solar keratosis [AK] will develop into SCC are extremely small; however when one encounters SCC, the chance that it has arisen in association with solar keratosis is very high (iii) Thickening and tenderness on lateral palpation are signs that a solar keratosis may have developed into invasive squamous cell carcinoma
de Berker et al. [12]	(i) Studies indicate a high spontaneous regression rate in the order of 15–25% for AKs over a 1-year period and a low rate of malignant transformation, less than one in 1,000 per annum. (ii) No therapy or emollient is a reasonable option for mild AKs (iii) Sun block applied twice daily for 7 months may protect against development of AKs (iv) 5-Fluorouracil cream used twice daily for 6 weeks is effective for up to 12 months in clearance of the majority of AKs; due to side-effects of soreness, less aggressive regimens are often used, which may be effective but have not been fully evaluated (v) Cryosurgery is effective for up to 75% of lesions in trials comparing it with photodynamic therapy; it may be particularly superior for thicker lesions but may leave scars
Stockfleth and Kerl (2006) [13]	(i) Cryotherapy is often used and controlled studies are missing. Complete responses differ from 75% to 98%; the recurrence rates of AKs have been estimated from 1.2% to 12% within a 1-year follow-up period (ii) The clinical experience in AK patients receiving MAL-PDT shows complete response rate of 70–78% after a single treatment session and 90% after two treatment sessions one week apart; negative effects of PDT are local pain, risk of photosensitivity (mainly for ALA), and time delay between application of cream and treatment. Photodynamic therapy in comparison to cryotherapy shows significantly better cosmetic results

the methods which were reported as "consultation and discussion of best practice was adopted as a means of formulating a consensus of opinion." This article reported funding by a pharmaceutical company that has AK-related products in its portfolio, which may have negatively impacted the scores in domain 6 (editorial independence). The 2011 update by this group (European Dermatology Forum) was recommended by two of the three raters and compared to the CPG from 2006 and 2008; this document had lower scores than the 2006 and 2008 CPG from this group across all domains except for domain 6 (editorial independence). In contrast to the two prior versions, this CPG had a table at the beginning of the document that listed the COI for each author; however there was no explicit statement of funding.

4. Discussion

High-quality CPG can supply clinicians with succinct research findings, specific suggestions for management in particular clinical scenarios, and economic considerations for a specific condition [24]. AK is a common skin lesion and many CPG have been published. Our goal was to review the quality of CPG that are broadly applicable to AK management rather than focus on a specific population or treatment. AKs are treated by providers from multiple disciplines with an array of treatments, so it is valuable and increasingly common for CPG to be written by representatives from the stakeholder groups, including generalists, specialists, and patients [8, 25]. The CCA/ACN was the only guideline to score above 60% for the stakeholder involvement domain; it was developed by a multidisciplinary "working party" that included dermatologists, pathologists, plastic surgeons, general practitioners, health economists, epidemiologists, and patients.

The CCA/CAN was also the only CPG that utilized a systematic review and had the highest scores for the rigor of development domain. The results of this review are consistent with previous appraisals of CPG for acne, psoriasis, and pressure ulcers that showed that the rigor of development domain often had lower scores [17, 18]. This domain is important to CPG value since it supports the validity of the recommendations [8]. Other CPG had less rigorous search methods or incomplete descriptions of the methods. CPG help readers to understand the strengths and limitations of the recommendations by including a rating of the supporting evidence. The CCA/ACN, Stockfleth and Kerl 2006 [13], and Stockfleth et al. 2011 [15] CPG used a published evidence-based rating scale, while the de Berker et al. [12] CPG used a rating scale based on evaluator opinion.

CPG rigor is also supported by an evaluation of potential sources of bias, such as conflict of interests (COI). The editorial independence domain includes a rating of COI and funding sources and had the lowest mean score of all the domains. COI reporting by the CPG contributors varied greatly. The Stockfleth et al. 2008 [14] article does address COI and discloses a grant that was received but failed to divulge that the grant came from a pharmaceutical group that produces topical fluorouracil and topical diclofenac products. The CCA/ACN and Stockfleth et al. 2011 [15] CPG clearly listed COI. Other articles (Rossi et al., Drake et al.) [10, 16] lacked a COI statement. The clearly and specifically worded COI and funding statements offered in the CCA/ACN guideline likely contributed to its having the highest mean score in this domain.

One of the primary purposes of CPG is to make practical, evidence-based recommendations about management of a condition. A summary of the recommendations from the three CPG with the highest scores is presented in Table 3.

All seven CPG addressed common topical and destructive therapies. In addition, sun avoidance and sun-protection were included in all CPG as a part of AK prevention and management. Three CPG [11, 12, 16] summarized evidence that AKs have a low rate of malignant transformation, but only one [12] mentioned observation, emollients, and sunscreen as possible management options [26].

The results of this study should be considered in the context of the limitations, including CPG that were not included and the effects of score variation between raters and within raters. Since the literature search was completed in 2014, this review does not include CPG published more recently which may be valuable [27, 28]. This review included four reviewers but the scores for one reviewer were not used because they did not correlate well with the others. Also, the CPG were appraised according to the information contained within them and additional supporting documents were not evaluated. It is possible that additional information may have increased scores for some of the CPG but was simply missing from the published version of the guidelines. Also, it is important to consider that high-quality methods or well-written CPG do not necessarily produce valid recommendations.

Effective CPG are evidence-based with recommendations that are concise and organized, so practical application is facilitated [29–31]. The CCA/ACN guideline had the highest scores and included a clear, organized, and concise table at the beginning of the document with helpful evidence-linked recommendations. However, the reviewers found that the recommendations lacked sufficient detail to apply in a clinical setting. For example, the recommendations included "cryotherapy achieves consistently high cure rates for solar keratosis" but lacks details that would facilitate use, such as the duration of the freeze-thaw cycle or number of freeze-thaw cycles. Also, the CCA/ACN AK recommendations were interspersed among the recommendations for nonmelanoma skin cancer. This made identifying the AK-specific information challenging. Stockfleth et al. [14] included a pictorial algorithm and raters thought this was an effective method to present information, yet scores in other domains lagged behind the CCA/ACN CPG. In closing, CPG are useful tools to guide clinical practice based on existing evidence; however it is important for providers and guideline authors to be aware of the features that contribute to a high-quality, practical, and valuable document.

Disclosure

This study was exempted from review by the Penn State IRB. This work was presented as a poster at the Society for Investigative Dermatology Annual Meeting, May 7–10, 2015, Atlanta, Georgia.

Disclaimer

The department specifically disclaims responsibility for any analyses, interpretations, or conclusions. The sponsor was not involved in the design and conduct of the study; collection, management, analysis, and interpretation of data; preparation, review, or approval of the paper; or decision to submit the paper for publication.

Conflict of Interests

The authors have no conflict of interests related to this work.

Acknowledgments

The authors would like to thank Amy Knehans, MLS, for expertly performing the literature searches included in this study. This study was supported in part by a career development awarded to Dr. Kirby from the Dermatology Foundation and, in part, under a grant from the Pennsylvania Department of Health using Tobacco CURE Funds.

References

[1] V. J. Marks, "Actinic keratosis. A premalignant skin lesion," *Otolaryngologic Clinics of North America*, vol. 26, no. 1, pp. 23–35, 1993.

[2] R. A. Schwartz, "The actinic keratosis: a perspective and update," *Dermatologic Surgery*, vol. 23, no. 11, pp. 1009–1019, 1997.

[3] A. K. Gupta, E. A. Cooper, S. R. Feldman, and A. B. Fleischer Jr., "A survey of office visits for actinic keratosis as reported by NAMCS, 1990–1999. National Ambulatory Medical Care Survey," *Cutis*, vol. 70, no. 2, supplement, pp. 8–13, 2002.

[4] The Lewin Group, *The Burden of Skin Diseases 2004*, The Society for Investigative Dermatology and The American Academy of Dermatology Association, Washington, DC, USA, 2005.

[5] A. K. Gupta, M. Paquet, E. Villanueva, and W. Brintnell, "Interventions for actinic keratoses," *The Cochrane Database of Systematic Reviews*, vol. 12, no. 12, Article ID CD004415, 2012.

[6] IOM (Institute of Medicine), *Clinical Practice Guidelines We Can Trust*, The National Academics Press, Washington, DC, USA, 2011, http://iom.nationalacademies.org/~/media/Files/Report%20Files/2011/Clinical-Practice-Guidelines-We-Can-Trust/Clinical%20Practice%20Guidelines%202011%20Insert.pdf.

[7] P. Alonso-Coello, A. Irfan, I. Solà et al., "The quality of clinical practice guidelines over the last two decades: a systematic review of guideline appraisal studies," *Quality and Safety in Health Care*, vol. 19, no. 6, article e58, 2010.

[8] A. S. Detsky, "Sources of bias for authors of clinical practice guidelines," *Canadian Medical Association Journal*, vol. 175, no. 9, pp. 1033–1035, 2006.

[9] M. C. Brouwers, M. E. Kho, G. P. Browman et al., "AGREE II: advancing guideline development, reporting and evaluation in health care," *Canadian Medical Association Journal*, vol. 182, no. 18, pp. E839–E842, 2010.

[10] L. A. Drake, R. I. Ceilley, R. L. Cornelison et al., "Guidelines of care for actinic keratoses. Committee on Guidelines of Care," *Journal of the American Academy of Dermatology*, vol. 32, no. 1, pp. 95–98, 1995.

[11] Cancer Council Australia and Australian Cancer Network, "Basal cell carcinoma, squamous cell carcinoma (and related lesions)—a guide to clinical management in Australia," Contract, Cancer Council Australia and Australian Cancer Network, Sydney, Australia, 2014.

[12] D. de Berker, J. M. McGregor, and B. R. Hughes, "Guidelines for the management of actinic keratoses," *The British Journal of Dermatology*, vol. 156, no. 2, pp. 222–230, 2007.

[13] E. Stockfleth and H. Kerl, "Guidelines for the management of actinic keratoses," *European Journal of Dermatology*, vol. 16, no. 6, pp. 599–606, 2006.

[14] E. Stockfleth, C. Ferrandiz, J. J. Grob, I. Leigh, H. Pehamberger, and H. Kerl, "Development of a treatment algorithm for actinic keratoses: a European consensus," *European Journal of Dermatology*, vol. 18, no. 6, pp. 651–659, 2008.

[15] E. Skockfleth, D. Terhorst, L. Braathen et al., *Guidelines for the Management of Actinic Keratoses*, European Dermatology Forum, 2010.

[16] R. Rossi, P. G. Calzavara-Pinton, A. Giannetti et al., "Italian guidelines and therapeutic algorithm for actinic keratoses," *Giornale Italiano di Dermatologia e Venereologia*, vol. 144, no. 6, pp. 713–723, 2009.

[17] E. R. M. de Haas, H. C. de Vijlder, S. W. van Reesema, J. J. E. van Everdingen, and H. A. M. Neumann, "Quality of clinical practice guidelines in dermatological oncology," *Journal of the European Academy of Dermatology and Venereology*, vol. 21, no. 9, pp. 1193–1198, 2007.

[18] G. Sanclemente, J.-L. Acosta, M.-E. Tamayo, X. Bonfill, and P. Alonso-Coello, "Clinical practice guidelines for treatment of acne vulgaris: a critical appraisal using the AGREE II instrument," *Archives of Dermatological Research*, vol. 306, no. 3, pp. 269–277, 2014.

[19] A. Lo Vecchio, A. Giannattasio, C. Duggan et al., "Evaluation of the quality of guidelines for acute gastroenteritis in children with the AGREE instrument," *Journal of Pediatric Gastroenterology and Nutrition*, vol. 52, no. 2, pp. 183–189, 2011.

[20] A. Hurdowar, I. D. Graham, M. Bayley, M. Harrison, S. Wood-Dauphinee, and S. Bhogal, "Quality of stroke rehabilitation clinical practice guidelines," *Journal of Evaluation in Clinical Practice*, vol. 13, no. 4, pp. 657–664, 2007.

[21] T. Lytras, S. Bonovas, C. Chronis et al., "Occupational asthma guidelines: a systematic quality appraisal using the AGREE II instrument," *Occupational and Environmental Medicine*, vol. 71, no. 2, pp. 81–86, 2014.

[22] M. Pagano and K. Gauvreau, Eds., *Principles of Biostatistics*, Brooks/Cole, Belmont, Calif, USA, 2nd edition, 2000.

[23] M. S. Kramer and A. R. Feinstein, "Clinical biostatistics. LIV. The biostatistics of concordance," *Clinical Pharmacology and Therapeutics*, vol. 29, no. 1, pp. 111–123, 1981.

[24] M. J. Field and K. Lohr, Eds., *Clinical Practice Guidelines: Directions for a New Program*, Institute of Medicine, Washington, DC, USA, 1990.

[25] J. N. Lavis, "How can we support the use of systematic reviews in policymaking?" *PLoS Medicine*, vol. 6, no. 11, Article ID e1000141, 2009.

[26] R. N. Werner, A. Sammain, R. Erdmann, V. Hartmann, E. Stockfleth, and A. Nast, "The natural history of actinic keratosis: a systematic review," *The British Journal of Dermatology*, vol. 169, no. 3, pp. 502–518, 2013.

[27] B. Dréno, J. M. Amici, N. Basset-Seguin, B. Cribier, J. P. Claudel, and M. A. Richard, "Management of actinic keratosis: a practical report and treatment algorithm from AKTeam expert clinicians," *Journal of the European Academy of Dermatology and Venereology*, vol. 28, no. 9, pp. 1141–1149, 2014.

[28] R. N. Werner, E. Stockfleth, S. M. Connolly et al., *Evidence and Consensus Based (S3) Guidelines for the Treatment of Actinic Keratosis International League of Dermatological Societies (ILDS) in Cooperation with the European Dermatology Forum (EDF)*, 2014, http://www.euroderm.org/edf/index.php/edf-guidelines/category/5-guidelines-miscellaneous.

[29] E. C. Haagen, W. L. D. M. Nelen, R. P. M. G. Hermens, D. D. M. Braat, R. P. T. M. Grol, and J. A. M. Kremer, "Barriers to physician adherence to a subfertility guideline," *Human Reproduction*, vol. 20, no. 12, pp. 3301–3306, 2005.

[30] M. D. Cabana, C. S. Rand, N. R. Powe et al., "Why don't physicians follow clinical practice guidelines? A framework for improvement," *The Journal of the American Medical Association*, vol. 282, no. 15, pp. 1458–1465, 1999.

[31] A. L. Francke, M. C. Smit, A. J. E. De Veer, and P. Mistiaen, "Factors influencing the implementation of clinical guidelines for health care professionals: a systematic meta-review," *BMC Medical Informatics and Decision Making*, vol. 8, article 38, 2008.

24

A Comparative Study Examining the Management of Bowen's Disease in the United Kingdom and Australia

G. L. Morley,[1] J. H. Matthews,[1] I. Verpetinske,[2] and G. A. Thom[3]

[1]*College of Medical and Dental Sciences, University of Birmingham, Edgbaston, Birmingham B15 2TT, UK*
[2]*Russells Hall Hospital, Pensnett Road, Dudley, West Midlands DY1 2HQ, UK*
[3]*Royal Perth Hospital, 197 Wellington Street, Perth, WA 6000, Australia*

Correspondence should be addressed to G. L. Morley; gabriella.morley@nhs.net

Academic Editor: Lajos Kemény

Background and Aim. The optimum management of Bowen's Disease (BD) is undefined. A review of current practice is required to allow the development of best practice guidelines. *Methods.* All BD cases, diagnosed in one UK centre and one Australian centre over a year (1 July 2012–30 June 2013), were analysed retrospectively. Patients with BD were identified from histopathology reports and their medical records were analysed to collect demographic data, site of lesion, and treatment used. *Results.* The treatment of 155 lesions from the UK centre and 151 lesions from the Australian centre was analysed. At both centres BD was most frequently observed on the face: UK had 70 (45%) lesions and Australia had 83 (55%) lesions ($P = 0.08$). The greatest number of lesions was managed by the plastic surgery department in the UK centre, 72 (46%), and the dermatology department in the Australian centre, 121 (80%). The most common therapy was surgical excision at both centres. *Conclusions.* In both UK and Australia, BD arises on sun-exposed sites and was most commonly treated with surgical excision despite a lack of robust evidence-based guidelines.

1. Introduction

Bowen's Disease (BD) is an intraepidermal precancerous lesion. Clinically, it appears as a well-defined erythematous plaque with a scaly or crusted surface, but variants include verrucous and pigmented BD [1]. Histopathology shows full-thickness epidermal dysplasia without dermal invasion [2]. BD is usually indolent and slow-growing; however, there is a small risk of progression to invasive SCC, estimated at 3–5% [3].

BD affects predominantly older individuals, with a peak incidence in the seventh decade [1]. The most commonly affected sites are the face [4], neck, and lower limbs [3, 5].

The strongest risk factor for the development of BD is long-term sun exposure [2]. Further risk factors include fair skin, increased longevity, genetics, and immunosuppression [4, 6].

There are numerous treatment options for BD which can be broadly categorized as surgical or nonsurgical. Surgical treatments include excision, curettage, and Mohs micrographic surgery [4]. Nonsurgical treatments include topical 5-fluorouracil (5-FU), topical Imiquimod, cryotherapy, photodynamic therapy (PDT), ablative laser, and radiotherapy. Observation without active treatment is also a reasonable option in select cases [1, 3].

The British Association of Dermatologists (BAD) in the UK [1] and the Cancer Council in Australia [7] have each produced national guidelines to aid their respective clinicians' therapy choices for the treatment of BD. Both guidelines allow for much clinical interpretation because there is no single modality that can be regarded as optimum for BD management [3]. There are many variables which affect the optimum choice of treatment in an individual patient, including patient age, body site, number of lesions, size of lesions, presence of adnexal extension, failure of previous treatments, cosmesis, cost, local availability, and patient preference [1, 3]. There is a paucity of prospective trials and head-to-head comparisons of the various treatment modalities, and hence literature reviews on this topic [5, 8] have been unable to reach firm conclusions about the comparative effectiveness of treatments.

This study aims to describe and compare current clinical practice for the treatment of BD between one centre in the UK and one centre in Australia.

2. Methods

This retrospective comparison study selected patients from centre 1, a public district general hospital in the West Midlands, UK, and centre 2, a tertiary referral public hospital in Perth, Western Australia. All cases of BD of the skin diagnosed in each centre's histopathology department over a 12-month period (1 July 2012 to 30 June 2013) were identified from the histopathology departmental databases. This included both partial biopsy specimens and full excisional specimens, collected by any department within the hospital. The patients' medical records were retrieved, and the following information was collected for each lesion: patient age, gender, site of lesion, dermoscopy use, whether the specimen was a definitive excision versus diagnostic biopsy, treatment modality used, and specialty managing the lesion. Data was recorded in two Microsoft Excel spreadsheets, one for each centre. The results from each centre were compared using frequency tables, and statistical analysis was conducted including Student's t-test and the chi-squared test.

Ethical approval was granted for this study by the Audit and Research Department at both centres.

3. Results

In the UK centre, there were 193 lesions among 185 patients during the study period. Of those, medical records were available for 149 patients (81%), allowing data collection on 155 lesions (80%). In the Australian centre, there were 200 lesions among 124 patients, and medical records were available for 98 patients (79%), allowing data collection on 151 lesions (76%) (Table 1).

3.1. Demographics. In both cohorts, there was a small majority of males: 83 (56%) in the UK and 58 (59%) in Australia ($P = 0.58$). The mean age in the UK was 79 ($\pm$9), and the range was 40–97 years, while in Australia the mean age was 76 ($\pm$12), and the range was 36–99 years ($P = 0.03$) (Table 1).

3.2. Lesion Site. In both the UK and Australia, the most common site for a BD lesion was the face: 70 (45%) lesions and 83 (55%) lesions, respectively ($P = 0.08$). The second most frequent lesion site for both centres was the lower leg: 41 (26%) lesions in the UK cohort and 21 (14%) lesions in the Australian cohort ($P = 0.006$) (Table 2).

3.3. Specialty Managing the BD Lesions. The majority of lesions (80%) in the Australian centre were managed by the dermatology department, compared with only 42% of lesions managed by the dermatology department in the UK centre ($P = 0.001$). In the UK centre, the greatest number of lesions (46%) was managed by the plastic surgery department, compared with only 17% of lesions managed by the plastic surgery department in the Australian centre ($P = 0.001$). In the UK centre, a number of BD lesions, 15 (10%), were managed in the community by general practitioners (GP) using the hospital

TABLE 1: Patient demographics.

	UK	Australia
Number of patients included	149	98
Number of patients not included	36	26
Total patients	185	124
Number of BD lesions	155	151
Number of BD lesions not included	38	49
Total lesions	193	200
Number of males	83	58
Number of females	66	40
Mean age in years (SD)	79 ($\pm$9)	76 ($\pm$12)
Age range in years	40–97	36–99

pathology lab for diagnostic purposes. Finally, 1 lesion was managed by the maxillofacial department.

Dermoscopic examination was recorded for 107 (69%) lesions in the UK and 124 (82%) lesions in Australia. For those lesions with no record of dermatoscopic observation in the notes, it was deemed unknown as to whether it was carried out. The treatment choice of lesions did not appear to be associated with dermatoscopy examination which may be due to the majority of lesions being completely excised at biopsy.

3.4. Biopsy Types and Treatment Modalities Used. The lesions captured in the data collection included both outright excisions, curetting specimens, and partial (diagnostic) biopsies. The excisional specimens accounted for 103 lesions (66%) in the UK cohort and 102 lesions (68%) in the Australian cohort (Table 2). By definition, surgical excision was the treatment modality used for these lesions, and this was the most common treatment modality used in both centres. The majority of the excisions (70%) were performed by the plastic surgery department in the UK centre and by the dermatology department (75%) in the Australian centre. Curettage was used for 8 lesions (5%) in the UK centre but was not used in any cases in the Australian centre.

Partial (diagnostic) biopsies accounted for 52 specimens (34%) in the UK group and 49 specimens (32%) in the Australian group. The subsequent choices for management of these lesions are shown in Table 2. The commonest nonsurgical modality used for biopsy-proven BD was topical 5-FU in both centres: 20 lesions (48%) in the UK centre and 31 lesions (69%) in the Australian centre ($P = 0.039$). Cryotherapy was the next most frequently used nonsurgical therapy for 14 (33%) lesions in the UK and 7 (16%) lesions in Australia ($P = 0.047$). Imiquimod was less commonly used: 5 lesions (12%) in the UK centre and 3 lesions (7%) in the Australian centre ($P = 0.36$).

3.5. Lesion Primaries and Recurrences. In the UK, 13 (8.4%) lesions were recurrences and 142 (91.6%) lesions were primaries. There were 17 lesions in Australia which were recurrences (11.3%) and 134 (88.7%) which were primary presentations. During the year of data collection there was 1 facial lesion recurrence in the UK (0.7%) which was initially

TABLE 2: Frequency of treatment modality usage at each lesion site.

Lesion site	Surgical excision*		Curettage		5-FU		Imiquimod		Cryotherapy		PDT		Radiotherapy		No treatment**		Total BD lesions	
	UK	Aus.	UK	Aus.	UK	Aus.	UK	Aus.	UK	Aus.	UK	Aus.	UK	Aus.	UK	Aus.	UK	Aus.
Abdomen	1	1	0	0	0	0	0	0	0	0	0	0	0	0	0	0	1	1
Arm	2	1	0	0	1	0	0	0	1	1	0	0	0	0	0	0	4	2
Face	44	53	3	0	9	20	4	2	8	2	2	3	0	1	0	2	70	83
Foot	2	2	0	0	1	1	0	1	0	1	0	0	0	0	0	0	3	5
Forearm and wrist	4	9	0	0	0	4	0	0	1	1	0	0	0	0	0	0	5	14
Hand	10	8	0	0	0	1	0	0	0	0	0	0	0	0	0	1	10	10
Thigh	2	1	1	0	0	1	0	0	0	0	0	0	0	0	0	0	3	2
Lower leg	26	15	3	0	8	3	0	0	3	2	1	0	0	0	0	1	41	21
Neck and chest	9	8	0	0	1	1	1	0	0	0	0	0	0	0	0	0	11	9
Shoulder and back	3	4	1	0	0	0	0	0	1	0	0	0	0	0	2	0	7	4
Total treatment modality	103	102	8	0	20	31	5	3	14	7	3	3	0	1	2	4	155	151

*Surgical excision includes all lesions excised by the plastic surgery department, dermatology department, general practitioners, and maxillofacial department.
**No treatment; observation follow-up/did not attend/deceased.
Aus. = Australia; UK = United Kingdom.

treated by dermatological excision. On recurrence this lesion was referred to the plastic surgery department for further excision and grafting. In Australia during the year of data collection 3 lesions recurred (2%), 2 facial lesions and 1 foot lesion. The foot lesion was initially treated with Imiquimod; on recurrence this lesion was then treated by excision in the plastic surgery department. One facial lesion was treated with 5-FU and the other with dermatological excision. On recurrence the latter lesion was referred to plastic surgery for a wider resection and the former was treated by PDT under patient request.

4. Discussion

This is the first study to compare the current clinical practice for BD management in the UK and Australia. The study assessed a similar population at each site and found that surgical excision was the most frequent treatment. There was a significant difference between the UK and Australia with regard to which specialist was responsible for the therapy.

4.1. Limitations of the Study. This study utilized histopathology reports as a basis for case identification and data collection; therefore our data was only able to capture those cases of BD undergoing histopathologic analysis in each centre. It is recognized that additional cases of BD will have been diagnosed and managed on clinical grounds in both centres during the study period, and these cases will not have been captured by our data collection. Our data included a significant number of excisional procedures performed in hospital-based dermatologic surgery and plastic surgery settings, which may lead to an overestimation of the utilization of surgical excision for BD, given that all excision specimens are sent for histopathology and would therefore be captured in our data. In addition, the hospital-based population in both centres may be skewed towards more complex cases rather than being treated in the community by general practitioners. Nevertheless, our data provides useful information in relation to the incidence and management of BD in both centres.

4.2. Incidence of BD. In both centres, the patient populations had a mean age in the eighth decade. This is slightly older than the peak incidence of 60–69 years commonly cited in the literature [1, 4]. The Australian cohort differed from the UK cohort with a wider age range and BD occurring in patients as young as 36 years. This is unsurprising given climatic differences and the higher incidence of skin cancer in Australia generally compared with the UK [9]. In both centres, there was a slight predominance of male patients, which is in contrast to the female predominance commonly cited in the literature [1, 4].

The most common site for BD in both centres was the face, which is consistent with chronic UV exposure at this body site and consistent with the findings of other studies [4, 8, 10]. The lower leg is commonly reported as a frequent site for BD [3], particularly in women [5], but this site was slightly less represented by our data, particularly in the Australian cohort (14% of lesions). However, it is possible that clinically typical BD lesions on the lower leg may be treated on clinical

grounds, without a biopsy, and such cases would not have been captured by our data.

4.3. Surgical Treatment of BD. In both centres, surgical excision was the most commonly used treatment modality for BD, although we recognize that our study design may have led to an overestimation of the use of surgical excision for BD. Nevertheless, surgical excision is accepted as the gold standard for the treatment of BD, particularly in recurrent or resistant lesions or those with adnexal extension [11]. Interestingly, there was a significant disparity between the two centres with regard to the specialist involved in performing surgery: in Australia the majority of excisions were performed by dermatologists, whilst in the UK the majority of excisions were performed by plastic surgeons. This may reflect differences in local practices and referral patterns. Due to the very high incidence of skin cancer in Australia, it is possible that dermatologists in Australia routinely perform a greater number of surgical procedures for skin cancer compared with their counterparts in the UK.

Curettage was utilized less commonly than might have been expected, particularly in the Australian cohort, in which it was not utilized in any cases during the study period. Mohs micrographic surgery was not utilized in either centre during the study period, which likely reflects lack of local availability in the study centres.

4.4. Nonsurgical Treatment of BD. The commonest nonsurgical treatments used in this study were (in descending order) 5-fluorouracil, cryotherapy, Imiquimod, and photodynamic therapy. The patterns of usage of these modalities were similar between the two centres.

5-Fluorouracil is typically applied bd for 3–8 weeks with published clearance rates, after 3 months, ranging from 67% to 83% [12, 13]. A longer duration of treatment and application under occlusion [14] appears to be associated with improved cure rates. Imiquimod has been described in a variety of treatment regimens varying from 3 times per week to daily application, with treatment durations up to 16 weeks. Published cure rates for Imiquimod are in the range of 73%–93% [15, 16]. Studies have identified that one cycle of photodynamic therapy can establish complete clearance for up to 93% of lesions after three months [13, 17, 18]. While there is literature to support the use of each of these modalities in BD, there is a paucity of robust comparative literature to support preference for one modality over another. Other factors which may influence the choice of nonsurgical modality include local availability, cost, and patient adherence to treatment.

4.5. Conclusions. Although the limitations of this study are recognized, its results have revealed significant points which enhance our understanding of BD in clinical practice. In both the UK and Australia BD arises in the older population on sun-exposed sites, with particular predilection to the face and lower limbs. Surgical excision was the commonest treatment modality used in this study, although we recognize that the study design may have led to an overestimation of the utilization of surgery for BD overall. A variety of nonsurgical treatments were used, and the lack of strong preference for one modality over another reflects the lack of a clearly defined optimum treatment in the published literature and guidelines. A large prospective randomized study comparing treatment modalities would help to provide greater clarity regarding the optimal management of BD.

Conflict of Interests

The authors declare that there is no conflict of interests regarding the publication of this paper.

Acknowledgments

Thanks are due to the institutions involved with collection of the study data.

References

[1] C. A. Morton, A. J. Birnie, and D. J. Eedy, "British Association of Dermatologists' guidelines for the management of squamous cell carcinoma in situ (Bowen's disease) 2014," *British Journal of Dermatology*, vol. 170, no. 2, pp. 245–260, 2014.

[2] A. Westers-Attema, F. Van Den Heijkant, B. G. P. M. Lohman et al., "Bowen's disease: a six-year retrospective study of treatment with emphasis on resection margins," *Acta Dermato-Venereologica*, vol. 94, no. 4, pp. 431–435, 2014.

[3] T. Neubert and P. Lehmann, "Bowen's disease—a review of newer treatment options," *Therapeutics and Clinical Risk Management*, vol. 4, no. 5, pp. 1085–1095, 2008.

[4] J. P. Hansen, A. L. Drake, and H. W. Walling, "Bowen's disease: a four-year retrospective review of epidemiology and treatment at a university center," *Dermatologic Surgery*, vol. 34, no. 7, pp. 878–883, 2008.

[5] F. J. Bath-Hextall, R. N. Matin, D. Wilkinson, and J. Leonardi-Bee, "Interventions for cutaneous Bowen's disease," *The Cochrane Database of Systematic Reviews*, vol. 6, Article ID CD007281, 2013.

[6] C. Garbe and U. Leiter, "Epidemiology of melanoma and non-melanoma skin cancer-the role of sunlight," *Advances in Experimental Medicine and Biology*, vol. 624, pp. 89–103, 2008.

[7] Cancer Council Australia and Australian Cancer Network, *Basal Cell Carcinoma, Squamous Cell Carcinoma (and Related Lesions)—A Guide to Clinical Management in Australia*, Cancer Council Australia and Australian Cancer Network, Sydney, Australia, 2008.

[8] S. Kossard and R. Rosen, "Cutaneous Bowen's disease: an analysis of 1001 cases according to age, sex, and site," *Journal of the American Academy of Dermatology*, vol. 27, no. 3, pp. 406–410, 1992.

[9] Australian Institute of Health and Welfare (AIHW) and Australasian Association of Cancer Registries (AACR), "Cancer in Australia; an overview 2006," AIHW Cat. No. CAN 232, Australian Institute of Health and Welfare, Canberra, Australia, 2007.

[10] C. C. I. Foo, J. S. S. Lee, V. Guilanno, X. Yan, S.-H. Tan, and Y.-C. Giam, "Squamous cell carcinoma and Bowen's disease of the skin in Singapore," *Annals of the Academy of Medicine Singapore*, vol. 36, no. 3, pp. 189–193, 2007.

[11] G. Moreno, A. L. Chia, A. Lim, and S. Shumack, "Therapeutic options for Bowen's disease," *Australasian Journal of Dermatology*, vol. 48, no. 1, pp. 1–10, 2007.

[12] A. Salim, J. A. Leman, J. H. McColl, R. Chapman, and C. A. Morton, "Randomized comparison of photodynamic therapy with topical 5-fluorouracil in Bowen's disease," *British Journal of Dermatology*, vol. 148, no. 3, pp. 539–543, 2003.

[13] C. Morton, M. Horn, J. Leman et al., "Comparison of topical methyl aminolevulinate photodynamic therapy with cryotherapy or fluorouracil for treatment of squamous cell carcinoma in situ: results of a multicenter randomized trial," *Archives of Dermatology*, vol. 142, no. 6, pp. 729–735, 2006.

[14] H. M. Strurm, "Bowen's disease and 5-flurouracil," *Journal of the American Academy of Dermatology*, vol. 1, pp. 513–522, 1979.

[15] G. K. Patel, R. Goodwin, M. Chawla et al., "Imiquimod 5% cream monotherapy for cutaneous squamous cell carcinoma in situ (Bowen's disease): a randomized, double-blind, placebo-controlled trial," *Journal of the American Academy of Dermatology*, vol. 54, no. 6, pp. 1025–1032, 2006.

[16] A. Mackenzie-Wood, S. Kossard, J. de Launey, B. Wilkinson, and M. L. Owens, "Imiquimod 5% cream in the treatment of Bowen's disease," *Journal of the American Academy of Dermatology*, vol. 44, no. 3, pp. 462–470, 2001.

[17] P. G. Calzavara-Pinton, M. Venturini, R. Sala et al., "Methyl-aminolaevulinate-based photodynamic therapy of Bowen's disease and squamous cell carcinoma," *British Journal of Dermatology*, vol. 159, no. 1, pp. 137–144, 2008.

[18] P. Lehmann, "Methyl aminolaevulinate-photodynamic therapy: a review of clinical trials in the treatment of actinic keratoses and nonmelanoma skin cancer," *British Journal of Dermatology*, vol. 156, no. 5, pp. 793–801, 2007.

25

Evaluation of Subcision for the Correction of the Prominent Nasolabial Folds

R. M. Robati,[1] F. Abdollahimajd,[1] and A. M. Robati[2]

[1]Skin Research Center, Shahid Beheshti University of Medical Sciences, Shohada-e Tajrish Hospital, Shahrdari Sreet,
Tehran 1989934148, Iran
[2]Department of Surgery, Bam University of Medical Sciences, Bam, Iran

Correspondence should be addressed to R. M. Robati; rezarobati@sbmu.ac.ir

Academic Editor: Iris Zalaudek

Background. A prominent nasolabial fold (NLF) is a cosmetic problem. Currently, numerous therapeutic modalities are available for pronounced NLFs with variable efficacy. *Objective.* To determine the efficacy and safety of subcision using a hypodermic needle for the correction of the prominent NLFs and its effect on skin elasticity. *Methods.* Sixteen patients with prominent NLFs underwent subcision. The investigators' assessment of improvement and the patients' satisfaction were both recorded 1 and 6 months after the procedure. Also, we evaluate the skin elasticity of NLFs before and after the treatment using a sensitive biometrologic device with the measurement of cutaneous resonance running time (CRRT). *Results.* Thirteen (81.25%) patients showed a moderate improvement at 1st month and 13 (81.25%) patients had at least a mild improvement at 6th month. There was no persistent side effect lasting more than a few days. Mean CRRT at 1 and 6 months after the treatment was significantly higher compared to the baseline. *Conclusion.* Subcision may be considered effective for the correction of pronounced NLFs. However, further controlled studies with larger sample size are necessary to assess the efficacy of this technique in particular with use of more objective assessment of skin biometric characteristics. This trial is registered with IRCT201108097270N1 (registered on January 27, 2012).

1. Introduction

The nasolabial fold (NLF) is a unique boundary between the cheek, mouth, and chin [1, 2]. Its shape can be concave, convex, or straight. It is generally imperceptible in children, in part, due to their skin elasticity [1]. The NLF often becomes apparent around the age of 25 years and then becomes more obvious with aging as a combination of thinning and relaxation of the skin [3, 4]; also other factors can be effective on this process such as ultraviolet radiation [1]. A prominent nasolabial crease is a cosmetic problem. Currently, numerous therapeutic options such as synthetic dermal fillers [1], fat grafts [4], Nd:YAG laser [5], radiofrequency device [6], direct excision or rhytidectomy [7, 8], and intense focused ultrasound [9] are available for improvement of a pronounced NLF with variable outcomes.

Subcision or subcutaneous incisionless surgery was first described by D. S. Orentreich and N. Orentreich in 1995. It is a surgical modality for the treatment of wrinkles and depressed scars with a tribeveled hypodermic needle inserted under the depressed area [10]. The releasing action of this procedure separates the fibrotic attachment. Moreover, the connective tissue forms during the wound-healing process, so the depression is raised [11]. Subsequently, several reports introduced that subcision with various types of needles or blades is effective for wrinkles, depressed scars, and prominent NLFs, as well as for acne scars [12–16]. The NLF is often a function of dermal atrophy. Therefore, subcision may be a useful option for the treatment of NLF not only due to its releasing action but also due to its induction of connective tissue formation.

In general, few studies have assessed the efficacy and safety of subcision in the treatment of prominent NLFs. In this study, we assess the efficacy and safety of subcision for the correction of pronounced NLFs. Also, we quantitatively evaluate the efficacy of this technique on skin elasticity using a sensitive biometrologic device (Reviscometer RVM 600) before and after the treatment. Reviscometer RVM 600 is useful in evaluating the skin elasticity and the direction of skin tension lines based on resonance running time [17].

2. Patients and Methods

2.1. Patients. This study is an open-label clinical trial. Sixteen patients with prominent NLFs were recruited to the study; all of them were female in the age group from 33 to 60 years. This study was approved by the ethical committee of Shahid Beheshti University of Medical Sciences and was performed according to the principles of the Declaration of Helsinki. All of the subjects signed a written informed consent after explanation of the procedure. Exclusion criteria included those who had connective tissue disorders (acquired or inherited), had a bleeding diathesis or a history of coagulation disorders in which anticoagulation therapies or medications such as aspirin and vitamin E prolonged the bleeding time, had susceptibility to keloid formation, were of age less than 30 years, were pregnant or lactating females, had active infection or history of cutaneous malignancy on the face, were on topical treatment (except for sunscreen agents) for the last 4 weeks, had isotretinoin therapy in the last 12 months, and had inability to attend follow-up visits. Cosmetic procedures such as laser or neurotoxin injection anywhere on the face in 12 months and filler injection anywhere on the face in 5 years before the study were also regarded as exclusion criteria.

2.2. Methods. Baseline demographic data of all patients were recorded at the start of the study. Photographs of the affected anatomic sites were taken before subcision as well as 1 and 6 months after the treatment with the same digital camera. The grade of wrinkles (in NLF) was evaluated by a wrinkle severity rating scale (WSRS) [18] before the treatment and at 1 and 6 months after the treatment as follows:

> 1 = absent (no visible fold), 2 = mild (shallow fold), 3 = moderate (not visible when stretched), 4 = severe (prominent, long, and deep fold), and 5 = extreme (extremely deep and long folds detrimental to facial appearance).

Outcomes and side effects of subcision procedure were evaluated by investigators at 1 and 6 months after the treatment. Moreover, another dermatologist who was blinded to the clinical data performed these evaluations. The degree of improvement was scored as follows:

> No response is <10%; mild response is 10–25%; moderate response is 26–75%; and excellent response is >75%.

The patients were asked to complete a questionnaire to determine their satisfaction (no, relative, or absolute satisfaction) and treatment complications (bruising, hematoma, hemorrhage, and keloid) during each follow-up visit.

2.3. Skin Elasticity. The loss of elasticity is one of the important characteristics of skin aging. Reviscometer RVM 600 is a sensitive biometrologic device used to measure

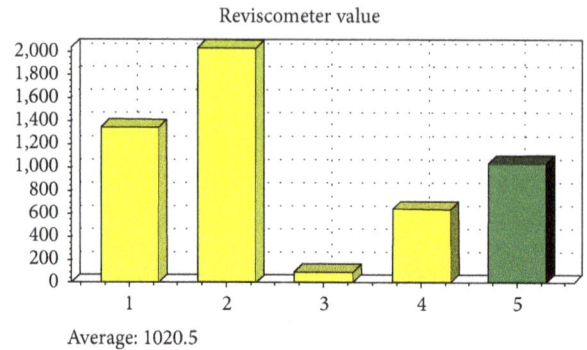

FIGURE 1: The diagrams provided by Reviscometer RVM 600 probe after measurement of CRRT.

the skin elasticity. The measurement is based on cutaneous resonance running time (CRRT) of an acoustical shockwave. It determines the mechanical properties of the skin and the direction of collagen and elastic fibers. The CRRT is expressed in arbitrary units (AU) [19]. Two sensors are applied to the skin surface in supine position. The mean CRRT over the four axes (0°, 180°, 90°, and 270°) was calculated for the NLFs. These measurements were conducted at room temperature 24–26°C with a relative humidity of 50 ± 3%. These measurements were recorded for each patient before the treatment and also repeated at each visit (Figure 1).

2.4. Subcision Procedure. The procedures were performed by the same dermatologist under constant conditions using a substantially identical method. The subcision was performed with the use of an 18-gauge hypodermic needle (Nokor Admix, Becton Dickinson Co.). First, the subcutaneous anesthesia (lidocaine 1% without epinephrine) was performed and then the needle was inserted, with blade facing upward, through a tiny incision in the middle of each NLF. Afterward, it was turned so that the tip was in a horizontal orientation (parallel to skin surface) just below the dermal-subcutaneous junction plane and a gentle fanning motion (side-to-side needle motion) was performed. The needle passed along these folds parallel to the skin surface. In addition, a gentle piston-like motion was used to advance the needle just below the dermal-subcutaneous junction plane. The width of the subcised area was approximately 7 mm around each NLF. We performed the procedure until the fold was effaced. We did subcision in upward direction to the proximal NLF. Afterward, the needle was inserted downward into the previous entry site and the mentioned procedure was repeated for distal portion of the NLF. We performed subcision just below the dermal-subcutaneous junction plane with no vigorous motion avoiding deeper structure to protect vessels especially facial artery branches. After the procedure, a piece of gauze without pressure was applied on the entry site for 24 h; also topical and oral antibiotics were prescribed.

2.5. Statistical Analysis. All descriptive statistics are summarized as mean + SD or frequency (%). Comparison of outcome variables between any two time points was done by Wilcoxon Signed Ranks Test. Trend of measures for grade

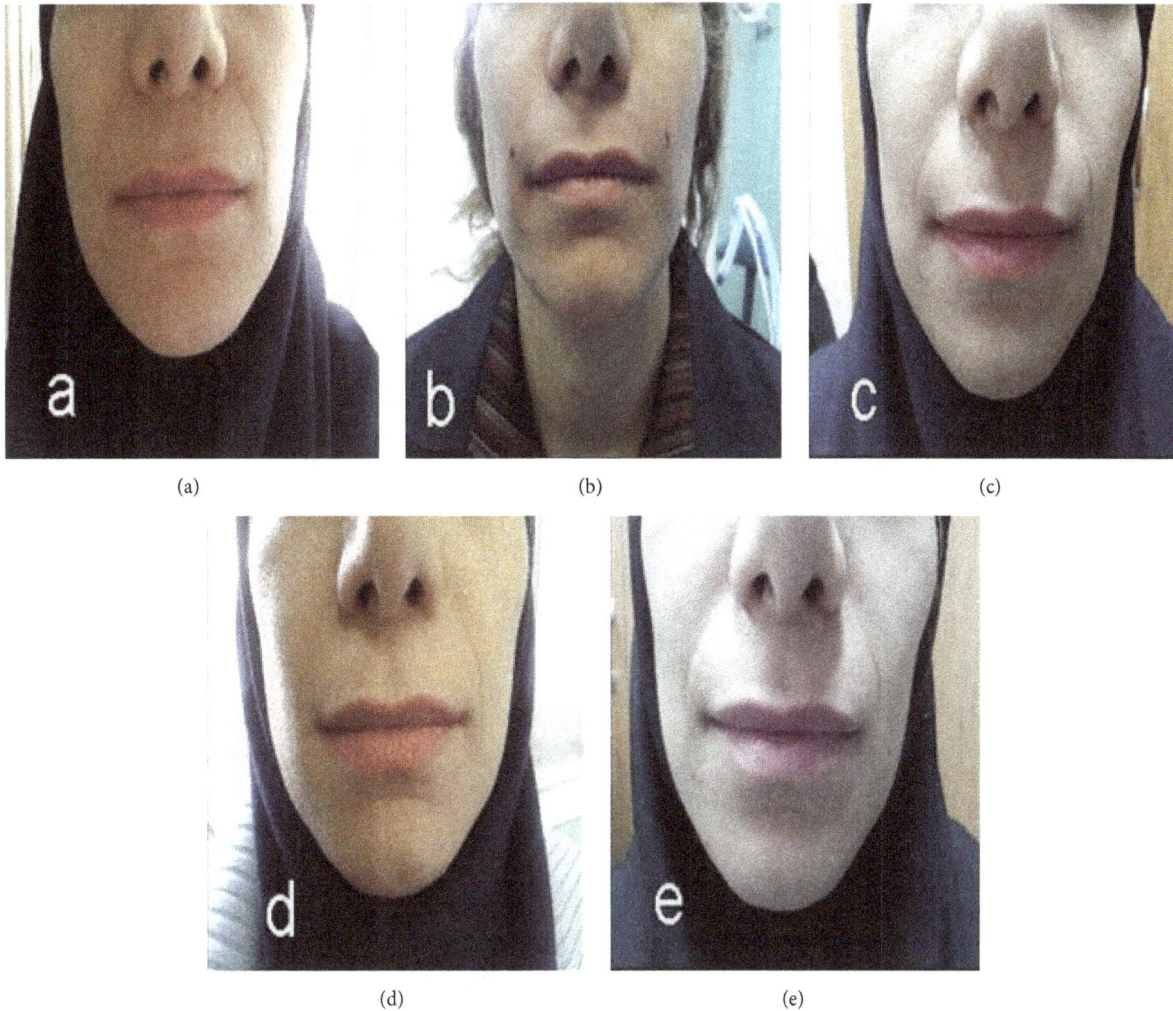

FIGURE 2: The considerable improvement of nasolabial folds after subcision; (a) before and (b) immediately after treatment (>75% improvement), (c) one month (50–75% improvement) and (d) three months after subcision (25–50% improvement), and (e) six months after treatment (≈25% improvement especially in upper portion of NLFs). No depression at the needle insertion points was seen.

of wrinkles as an ordinal variable was investigated using Friedman's test statistic. For skin elasticity, the trend of measurement was assessed by repeated measures ANOVA test.

3. Results

3.1. Baseline Data. Sixteen female patients were included in this study. Mean age of patients was 45.1 years (SD = 9.8). Most of the patients (62.5%) had a moderate grade of wrinkles at the beginning of the study followed by four patients in the severe grade, one in mild grade, and one in extreme grade. Mean skin CRRT was 1007.5 ± 494.2 (AU) before the treatment. Baseline demographics and outcomes of the subcision procedure are presented in Table 1.

3.2. After Treatment. The grades of improvement in WSRS (compared to baseline) in different time points of the study are shown in Table 2. Comparison of the grade of wrinkles at 1 and 6 months after the treatment with baseline data showed

a significant difference (1 month versus baseline: test statistic = -3.69, $p < 0.001$; 6 months versus baseline: test statistic = -3.00, $p = 0.003$). Trend of measurement in different time points was also statistically significant (Friedman's test statistics = 23.5, $p < 0.001$). Mean degree of improvement was $42.8 \pm 18.7\%$ at 1 month and $18.8 \pm 10.8\%$ at 6 months after the treatment. The improvement degrees (compared to baseline) at one and 6 months after procedure are shown in Table 3. Patients showed less improvement after 6 months compared to 1 month after the treatment (Wilcoxon Signed Ranks Test statistic: -3.05, $p = 0.002$) (Figures 2 and 3).

One month after the treatment, patients had higher satisfaction. We found that 4 (25%) patients had moderate satisfaction and 12 (75%) patients were fully satisfied. Six months after the treatment, 3 (18.75%) patients had no satisfaction, 9 (56.25%) patients had moderate satisfaction, and 4 (25%) patients were fully satisfied. Satisfaction after 6 months was significantly lower than 1 month after the intervention (Wilcoxon Signed Ranks Test statistic: -3.05,

TABLE 1: Baseline demographics and outcomes of the subcision procedure in patients.

N	Sex/age	Dx. duration (year)	WSRS (0)	WSRS 1 m	WSRS 6 m	CRRT 0	CRRT 1 m	CRRT 6 m	Complication 1 wk	Complication 1, 6 m	Satis. 1 m	Satis. 6 m	Improve. % 1 m	Improve. degree 1 m	Improve. % 6 m	Improve. degree 6 m
1	f/42	10	3	2	3	1328	1835.2	1799	Bruising	No	Full	Relative	20	2	10	2
2	f/56	25	4	3	3	1427	1983	1891	Bruising	No	Full	Relative	70	3	30	3
3	f/59	30	4	3	3	460	657.25	623.2	Bruising	No	Full	Relative	60	3	30	3
4	f/38	10	3	2	2	589	949	846.5	No	No	Full	Relative	40	3	20	2
5	f/33	2	3	2	3	920	950	895.5	No	No	Relative	No	20	2	5	1
6	f/36	3	2	1	2	2141.2	2200	2481.5	Bruising	No	Full	Full	50	3	20	2
7	f/60	25	5	3	4	949.3	958.75	952.25	No	No	Full	Relative	40	3	20	2
8	f/35	6	3	2	3	1406.8	1561.8	1410	No	No	Relative	Relative	50	3	20	2
9	f/52	20	4	3	3	560	890	818	Bruising	No	Full	Relative	50	3	30	3
10	f/36	6	3	2	2	194.2	2677	2594	No	No	Full	Full	30	3	15	2
11	f/35	5	3	2	3	1206	1430	1291	No	No	Full	No	25	3	5	1
12	f/60	34	4	3	4	460	589	480	Bruising	No	Relative	Relative	30	3	10	2
13	f/51	20	3	2	2	949	1251	1631	No	No	Full	Full	70	3	40	3
14	f/42	10	3	2	2	1305	1480	1447	No	No	Full	Relative	40	3	10	2
15	f/41	5	3	1	2	1376	1510	1626.2	No	No	Full	Full	70	3	30	3
16	f/46	8	3	3	3	849	983.75	972.5	No	No	Relative	No	20	2	5	1

N, number; Dx, disease; WSRS (0), Wrinkle Severity Rating Scale (base); m, month; CRRT, cutaneous resonance running time; wk, week; satis., satisfaction; improve, improvement.

WSRS: 1 = absent (no visible fold), 2 = mild (shallow fold), 3 = moderate (not visible when stretched), 4 = severe (prominent, long, and deep fold), and 5 = extreme (extremely deep and long folds detrimental to facial appearance).

Improvement degree (evaluated by investigators and also one dermatologist): 1 = no response: <10%; 2 = mild response: 10–25%; 3 = moderate response: 26–75%; and 4 = excellent response: >75%.

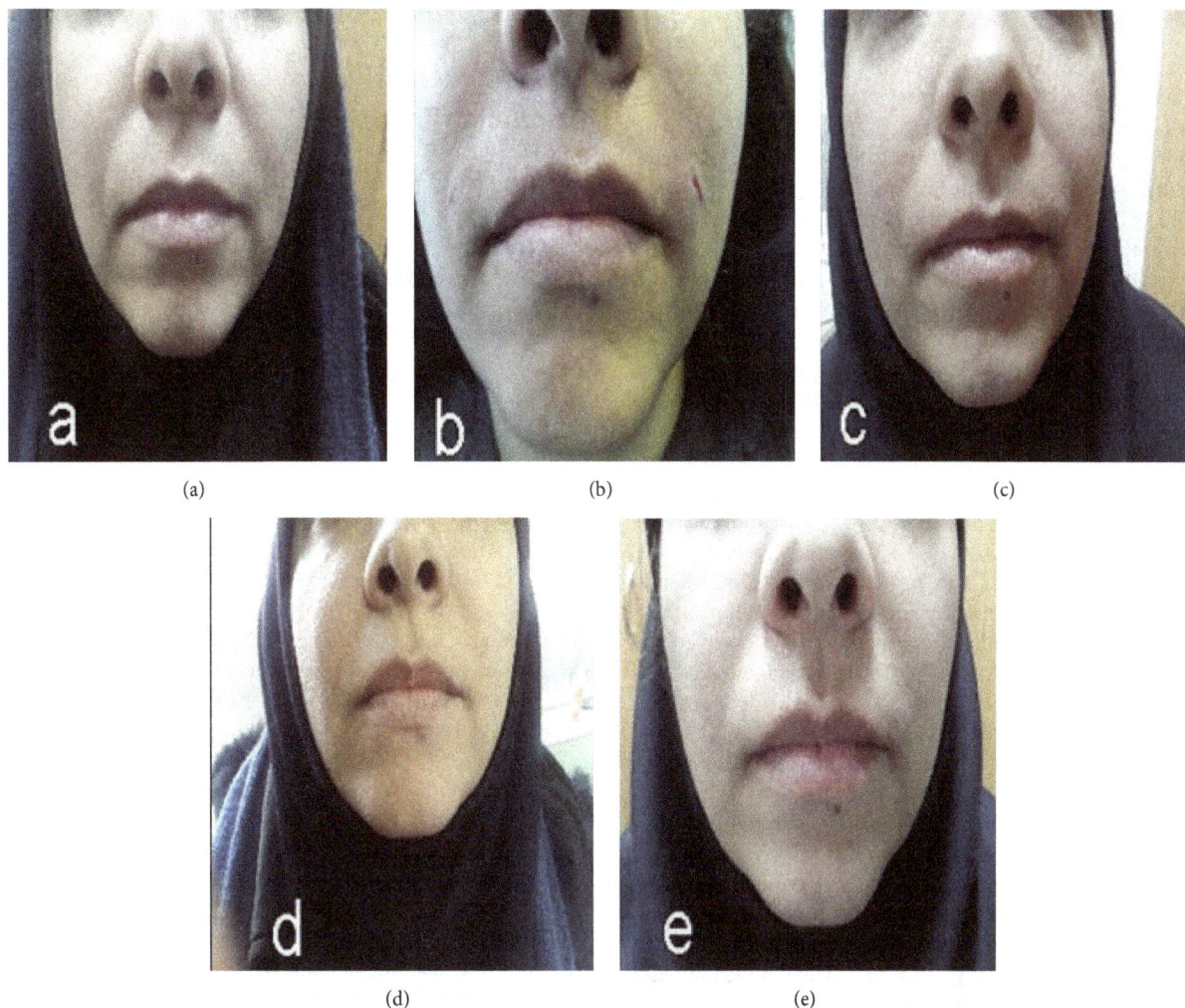

FIGURE 3: Marked improvement of nasolabial folds after subcision: (a) before and (b) immediately after treatment (>75% improvement), (c) one month (50–75% improvement) and (d) three months after subcision (25–50% improvement), and (e) six months after procedure (≈25% improvement). No depression at the needle insertion points was seen.

TABLE 2: The grades of improvement in WSRS (compared to baseline) at one month and 6 months after the beginning of the procedure.

WSRS improvement (compare to baseline)	After 1 month	After 6 months
No change	1 (6.25%)	7 (43.75%)
At least 1 grade	15 (93.75%)	9 (56.25%)
2 grades or greater	2 (12.5%)	0

WSRS, Wrinkle Severity Rating Scale.
WSRS: 1 = absent (no visible fold), 2 = mild (shallow fold), 3 = moderate (not visible when stretched), 4 = severe (prominent, long, and deep fold), and 5 = extreme (extremely deep and long folds detrimental to facial appearance).

TABLE 3: Improvement degree (compared to baseline) at one month and 6 months after the beginning of the procedure.

Improvement degree (compared to baseline)	After 1 month	After 6 months
No response	0 (0)	3 (18.75%)
At least a mild response	3 (18.75%)	8 (50%)
A moderate response or greater	13 (81.25%)	5 (31.25%)

Improvement degree (evaluated by investigators and also one dermatologist): 1 = no response: <10%; 2 = mild response: 10–25%; 3 = moderate response: 26–75%; and 4 = excellent response: >75%.

$p = 0.002$). Also, 5 (31.25%) patients had only mild bruising that resolved after 2-3 days in all of them. One and 6 months after the treatment, there was no complication.

Mean CRRT was 1007.5 ± 494.2 (AU) before the treatment. It was 1369.1 ± 582.9 (AU) and 1359.9 ± 622.9 (AU) 1 and six months after the treatment, respectively. Comparison of mean CRRT at 1 and 6 months after the treatment to baseline data showed a significant difference (1 month versus baseline: t-test statistic $= -2.46$, $p = 0.02$; 6 months versus baseline: t-test statistic $= -2.42$, $p = 0.03$). Trend of measurement in different time points was also statistically significant (repeated measures test statistics $= 1239408$, $p = 0.02$).

4. Discussion

The treatment plan for prominent NLFs should be individualized according to some factors such as aesthetic needs, the patient's age, and economic burden [20]. Several modified subcision techniques were introduced for depressed scars and wrinkles and also for prominent NLFs [3, 12–15]. In our study, 13 (81.25%) patients showed moderate improvement at 1st month and 13 (81.25%) patients had at least mild improvement at 6th month. One month after the treatment, 75% of patients were fully satisfied and 6 months after the treatment, 81.25% of them had at least moderate satisfaction. There was no persistent side effect lasting more than a few days. No contracture in lower portion of NLF was observed.

The CRRT is influenced by collagen fibers in the upper dermis. As aging progresses, defragmentation of elastin network occurs and configuration of dermal collagen network changes, which could increase skin stiffness and decrease skin elasticity and CRRT [21]. In our study, mean CRRT at 1 and 6 months after the procedure was significantly higher compared to the baseline. The releasing action of this procedure separates the fibrotic attachments. Moreover, the new connective tissue with new elastin and collagen networks forms during the wound-healing process, so the depression is raised [11] and CRRT increased.

The immediate improvement after subcision seems to be the result of edema or mild bleeding under the NLFs. However, we followed the participants 1 and 6 months after the procedure to assess the persistence of improvement. The continued improvement may be due to the connective tissue formation after subcision. It would be better if we could perform a biopsy of NLF 6 months after the procedure to assess the histopathological pattern of possible neocollagenesis. Unfortunately, none of the participants agreed to undergo skin biopsy of NLFs after the procedure in this study.

To achieve the best results, it may be important to induce the formation of adequate amounts of scar tissue in the subcision area [3]. Although this is usually not complete with a single procedure, we can repeat this procedure at regular intervals to achieve more favorable and persistent results [3]. Moreover, it might be better to perform this study in a split-face design and do subcision only for right or left NLF to achieve a comparison of its efficacy. But the ethic committee of our center did not allow us to perform this pilot study in a split-face design with no treatment on a NLF. Unfortunately, we faced some restrictions of facilities to perform filler injection or fat graft for one side and subcision for the other side to compare them in a more controlled manner.

In conclusion, our study shows that subcision is an easy, safe, and inexpensive technique, with minimal complication and considerable rate of improvement for correction of prominent NSFs. It improves both the clinical appearance and skin elasticity of NLFs. However, we planned this study as a preliminary assay to evaluate the possible efficacy of subcision on the prominent NFLs. Therefore, we entered limited participants in this study with limited follow-up periods. So, further controlled studies with larger sample size and longer follow-up and use of more objective assessment of skin biometric or histopathologic characteristics are beneficial to elucidate the efficacy of subcision in improving NLFs more definitely.

Conflict of Interests

The authors declare that they have no conflict of interests regarding the publication of this paper.

Acknowledgment

Skin Research Center of Shahid Beheshti University of Medical Sciences funded this study.

References

[1] Y. Ducic and P. A. Hilger, "The aesthetic challenges of the nasolabial fold," *FACE*, vol. 5, no. 2, pp. 103–108, 1997.

[2] F. Flowers and J. R. T. Breza, "Surgical anatomy of the head and neck," in *Dermatology*, J. Bolognia, J. Jorrizzo, and J. Schaffer, Eds., pp. 23–34, Mosby Elsevier, 3rd edition, 2012.

[3] S.-Y. Lee and K.-Y. Sung, "Subcision using a spinal needle cannula and a thread for prominent nasolabial fold correction," *Archives of Plastic Surgery*, vol. 40, no. 3, pp. 256–258, 2013.

[4] B. Guyuron and B. Michelow, "The nasolabial fold: a challenge, a solution," *Plastic and Reconstructive Surgery*, vol. 93, no. 3, pp. 522–532, 1994.

[5] S. H. Lee, M. R. Roh, J. Y. Jung, H. Jee, K. A. Nam, and K. Y. Chung, "Effect of subdermal 1,444-nm pulsed neodymium-doped yttrium aluminum garnet laser on the nasolabial folds and cheek laxity," *Dermatologic Surgery*, vol. 39, no. 7, pp. 1067–1078, 2013.

[6] N. Kushikata, K. Negishi, Y. Tezuka, K. Takeuchi, and S. Wakamatsu, "Non-ablative skin tightening with radiofrequency in Asian skin," *Lasers in Surgery and Medicine*, vol. 36, no. 2, pp. 92–97, 2005.

[7] C. Rouveroux, J. P. Binder, M. Revol, and J. M. Servant, "Direct excision of the deep nasolabial fold: a logical and easy surgical management," *Annales de Chirurgie Plastique et Esthetique*, vol. 51, no. 3, pp. 211–216, 2006.

[8] C. Sen, D. I. Cek, and M. Reis, "Direct skin excision fat reshaping and repositioning for correction of prominent nasolabial fold," *Aesthetic Plastic Surgery*, vol. 28, no. 5, pp. 307–311, 2004.

[9] D. H. Suh, M. K. Shin, S. J. Lee et al., "Intense focused ultrasound tightening in asian skin: clinical and pathologic results: clinical," *Dermatologic Surgery*, vol. 37, no. 11, pp. 1595–1602, 2011.

[10] D. S. Orentreich and N. Orentreich, "Subcutaneous incisionless (Subcision) surgery for the correction of depressed scars and wrinkles," *Dermatologic Surgery*, vol. 21, no. 6, pp. 543–549, 1995.

[11] B. S. Chandrashekar and A. S. Nandini, "Acne scar subcision," *Journal of Cutaneous and Aesthetic Surgery*, vol. 3, no. 2, pp. 125–126, 2010.

[12] G. H. Sasaki, "Comparison of results of wire subcision performed alone, with fills, and/or with adjacent surgical procedures," *Aesthetic Surgery Journal*, vol. 28, no. 6, pp. 619–626, 2008.

[13] B. Kotlus and R. Dryden, "Modification of the nasolabial crease with wire scalpel and autologous fat transfer," *American Journal of Cosmetic Surgery*, vol. 23, pp. 75–78, 2006.

[14] M. Graivier, "Wire subcision for complete release of depressions, subdermal attachments, and scars," *Aesthetic Surgery Journal*, vol. 26, no. 4, pp. 387–394, 2006.

[15] M. A. Sulamanidze, G. Salti, M. Mascetti, and G. M. Sulamanidze, "Wire scalpel for surgical correction of soft tissue contour defects by subcutaneous dissection," *Dermatologic Surgery*, vol. 26, no. 2, pp. 146–151, 2000.

[16] K. Balighi, R. M. Robati, H. Moslehi, and A. M. Robati, "Subcision in acne scar with and without subdermal implant: a clinical trial," *Journal of the European Academy of Dermatology and Venereology*, vol. 22, no. 6, pp. 707–711, 2008.

[17] Y. J. Hwang, Y. N. Lee, Y. W. Lee, Y. B. Choe, and K. J. Ahn, "Treatment of acne scars and wrinkles in asian patients using carbon-dioxide fractional laser resurfacing: its effects on skin biophysical profiles," *Annals of Dermatology*, vol. 25, no. 4, pp. 445–453, 2013.

[18] D. J. Day, C. M. Littler, R. W. Swift, and S. Gottlieb, "The wrinkle severity rating scale: a validation study," *American Journal of Clinical Dermatology*, vol. 5, no. 1, pp. 49–52, 2004.

[19] F. Fanian, S. Mac-Mary, A. Jeudy et al., "Efficacy of micronutrient supplementation on skin aging and seasonal variation: a randomized, placebo-controlled, double-blind study," *Clinical Interventions in Aging*, vol. 8, pp. 1527–1537, 2013.

[20] S. Y. Lee, "Prominent nasolabial fold: an overview of treatments," *Archives of Aesthetic Plastic Surgery*, vol. 17, no. 3, pp. 143–152, 2011.

[21] S. Xin, W. Man, J. W. Fluhr, S. Song, P. M. Elias, and M.-Q. Man, "Cutaneous resonance running time varies with age, body site and gender in a normal Chinese population," *Skin Research and Technology*, vol. 16, no. 4, pp. 413–421, 2010.

26

Botanical Agents for the Treatment of Nonmelanoma Skin Cancer

Jillian W. Millsop,[1] **Raja K. Sivamani,**[2] **and Nasim Fazel**[2]

[1] *University of Utah, School of Medicine, 30 N 1900 E, Salt Lake City, UT 84132, USA*
[2] *University of California, Davis, Department of Dermatology, 3301 C Street, Sacramento, CA 95816, USA*

Correspondence should be addressed to Nasim Fazel; nasim.fazel@ucdmc.ucdavis.edu

Academic Editor: H. Peter Soyer

Nonmelanoma skin cancers, including basal cell carcinoma and squamous cell carcinoma, are common neoplasms worldwide and are the most common cancers in the United States. Standard therapy for cutaneous neoplasms typically involves surgical removal. However, there is increasing interest in the use of topical alternatives for the prevention and treatment of nonmelanoma skin cancer, particularly superficial variants. Botanicals are compounds derived from herbs, spices, stems, roots, and other substances of plant origin and may be used in the form of dried or fresh plants, extracted plant material, or specific plant-derived chemicals. They possess multiple properties including antioxidant, anti-inflammatory, and immunomodulatory properties and are, therefore, believed to be possible chemopreventive agents or substances that may suppress or reverse the process of carcinogenesis. Here, we provide a review of botanical agents studied for the treatment and prevention of nonmelanoma skin cancers.

1. Introduction

Nonmelanoma skin cancer (NMSC) is common worldwide and includes basal cell carcinoma (BCC) and squamous cell carcinoma (SCC). Approximately two to three million NMSCs occur globally each year [1]. In the United States (U.S.), BCC is the most common form of malignancy [2, 3]. In 2012, two million new cases of NMSCs were estimated to occur in the U.S., with delays in treatment leading to significant morbidity [4] and deaths occurring in less than 1,000 [5]. Delay in treatment of NMSCs can lead to significant morbidity as well. Extrinsic and intrinsic risk factors contribute to skin cancer development including fair skin color, red and blond hair, and high susceptibility to sunburn [6]. Chronic sun exposure is also associated with skin cancer risk, especially for SCC [7]. Furthermore, chronically immunocompromised organ transplant patients have a higher risk of developing SCCs [8, 9].

Traditional recommendations for prevention of NMSC include generous use of sunscreens and avoidance of chronic or intense ultraviolet (UV) exposure. Conventional therapy for NMSCs involves surgical removal or directed topical therapies in the most superficial subtypes of NMSC. However, there is increasing interest in alternative, noninvasive treatments and preventative measures in recent years, specifically in the use of naturally occurring botanicals. Botanicals are a group of compounds derived from herbs, spices, stems, roots, and other substances of plant origin and may be used in the form of dried or fresh plants or extracted plant material [10]. They possess multiple properties including antioxidant, anti-inflammatory, and immunomodulatory properties, and, therefore, they are believed to be possible chemopreventive agents or substances that may suppress or reverse the process of carcinogenesis [7]. For example, topical ingenol mebutate, extracted from *Euphorbia*, was recently approved by the U.S. Food and Drug Administration (FDA) for treatment of actinic keratosis [11]. There is perceived safety and efficacy with botanicals despite a lack of controlled clinical trials and scientific data [10]. Furthermore, botanical extracts are often distributed as dietary supplements in the United States with little regulation [12]. Therefore, there is need for controlled studies that evaluate both of their efficacy and side effects.

Here, we review botanical agents that have been used for the treatment and prevention of NMSCs. Botanical agents studied in humans as well as agents investigated in preclinical trials are reviewed.

2. Methods

We conducted a search of the PubMed and Embase databases of articles published from 1990 to 2013 to include the most recent literature. Articles containing combinations of MeSH terms "nonmelanoma skin cancer," "basal cell carcinoma," "squamous cell carcinoma," "complementary therapies," "plant preparations," "edible plants," "herbal medicine," "antineoplastic agents," "phytogenic," and "botanical" were reviewed. Based on the initial review using these terms, botanical agents and extracts identified as having possible effects on NMSC treatment and prevention through studies, reviews, and case reports, were reviewed. The search was limited to articles in English and initially resulted in 91 articles. The article abstracts were reviewed for relevance to the subject matter of treatment and prevention of UV light-induced NMSCs, BCCs, and SCCs, using botanical agents. We examined reference lists to identify any missing articles, and a total of 74 articles were included in this review. We included only botanical agents that have been investigated in more than one study and/or have been reported in more than one case.

3. Botanical Agents Studied in Humans and Animals (Tables 1 and 2)

3.1. Ingenol Mebutate. Ingenol mebutate is an extract from the *Euphorbia peplus* (*E. peplus*) plant that has been identified for its chemotherapeutic potential, and, more recently, approved by the U.S. FDA for the treatment of actinic keratoses. Preclinical studies in murine models have shown that ingenol mebutate causes mitochondrial swelling of the dysplastic keratinocytes and apoptosis by primary necrosis [48]. In a phase I/II clinical study to determine the efficacy of the *E. peplus* sap, for which the main ingredient was ingenol mebutate, on the treatment of BCCs, SCCs, and intraepidermal carcinomas, Ramsay et al. enrolled 36 patients with a total of 48 lesions who had failed past treatments, refused surgical treatment, or were found unfit for surgical therapy due to anticoagulant use, age, site, or nature of the lesion [13]. Patients were treated once daily for three consecutive days. Complete clinical response (tumor absence after clinical examination) following treatment was 82% ($n =$ 28) for BCCs, 75% ($n = 4$) for SCCs, and 94% ($n = 16$) for intraepidermal carcinomas at 1 month [13]. However, partial responses were noted in five of the BCCs treated. Although the authors note that 6 of the treated BCCs were of the nodular subtype while the rest were of the superficial subtype, they do not mention if it was the nodular subtypes that were the partially responding tumors. Also, a full histopathological examination of the treatment sites was not performed as the subjects were not suitable surgical candidates. Instead, 2–4 millimeter (mm) biopsy samplings were obtained but this was only partial sampling as the average size of the NMSC was

noted to be 16 mm. The most common side effects included dry skin, erythema, and patchy moist desquamation. After a mean of 15 months for followup, the complete clinical response rates were 57% for BCCs, 50% for SCCs, and 75% for intraepidermal carcinomas [13]. For superficial carcinomas that were less than 16 mm, the complete clinical response rates were 78% ($n = 9$) for BCCs and 100% ($n = 10$) for intraepidermal carcinomas [13].

Furthermore, a phase IIa randomized, vehicle-controlled study of 60 patients evaluated the safety (primary endpoint) and efficacy (secondary endpoint) of ingenol mebutate gel for superficial basal cell carcinoma, with a lesion size of 4–15 mm. In this study, Siller et al. randomized patients to Arm A, treatment on days 1 and 2, or Arm B, treatment on days 1 and 8 [14]. Within each arm, patients were also randomized to application of ingenol mebutate gel 0.0025%, 0.01%, or 0.05%, or a matching vehicle gel [14]. No severe adverse events were reported. In four patients, severe local skin reactions occurred. The most common side effects were erythema, flaking, scaling, and dryness. The histopathological clearance rate was 71% (5/7) in the treatment group of Arm A that received 0.05% ingenol mebutate gel, and 86% (6/7) showed marked or complete clearance (50–90%) on clinical examination [14].

3.2. Hypericin. *Hypericum perforatum*, St. John's wort, contains the photoactive compound, hypericin, which is a potent photosensitizer in photodynamic therapy. It is activated by visible (400–700 nm) or UVA (320–400 nm) light [49]. Hypericin has demonstrated cytotoxic and antiproliferative properties against cancer cells. Although an early study by Alecu et al. reported that hypericin was effective for treatment of BCCs and SCCs without necrosis of the surrounding tissue when injecting hypericin solution intralesionally and then irradiating the site with visible light [15], subsequent studies did not demonstrate efficacy of hypericin in skin cancer treatment.

A prospective pilot study by Kacerovská et al. investigated the use of an extract of *H. perforatum* in combination with photodynamic therapy for BCCs, actinic keratoses, and Bowens disease (carcinoma in situ) [16]. A total of 34 patients were enrolled, 21 of which had BCCs. The extract was applied under occlusion to the skin lesions, followed two hours later by irradiation with 75 Joules per square centimeter (J/cm^2) of red light. Patients underwent treatment for six weeks on average. They found complete clinical response for 28% of superficial BCC patients, and only partial remission was seen in nodular BCC patients [16]. By histology, a complete disappearance of cancer cells was found in 11% of the superficial BCCs [16]. All patients in the study complained of pain and burning during irradiation. The authors concluded that the results of this clinical trial showed that this combination therapy was not effective and that further studies are needed to examine the enhancement of hypericin delivery. Furthermore, a recent study by Boiy et al. demonstrated that topical hypericin with photodynamic therapy was less effective in clearance of UV light-induced tumors in mouse skin as compared to methylaminolevulinic acid with photodynamic therapy (44% clearance of skin tumors as compared to 80% clearance, resp.) [30].

TABLE 1: Summary of the effects of botanical agents studied in humans.

Botanical agent	Source	Efficacy	Histopathological assessment of efficacy	References
Ingenol mebutate	*Euphorbia peplus*	Demonstrated clinical response (tumor clearance) for BCCs and SCCs.	No	[13, 14]
Hypericin	*Hypericum perforatum*	Reported clinical response for BCCs and SCCs to hypericin and photodynamic therapy in one study [15], but found the combination to be less effective in another human study [16].	Yes	[15, 16]
Coffee	*Coffea* plant	Coffee consumption was related to decreased prevalence of NMSC in two studies [17, 18]. No association between coffee consumption and NMSC in one study [19].	No	[17–19]
Tea	*Camellia sinensis*	Inconsistent results in human studies. Regular tea consumption was associated with reduced risk of SCC and BCC incidence in one study [20], but no reduction in SCC risk in another study [21]. Case reported efficacy for basal cell nevus syndrome with green tea body wrap [22].	No	[20–22]
Escharotic botanical agents	Black salve (containing bloodroot, galangal, sheep sorrel, and red clover) Bloodroot (*Sanguinaria canadensis*)	Cases reported no improvement of BCC and extensive skin necrosis with black salve application [23, 24]. Case reported metastasis of BCC with bloodroot [25].	No	[23–25]
Paclitaxel	*Taxus brevifolia*	In vitro study demonstrated topical paclitaxel increased antiproliferative activity in a squamous cell carcinoma model [26]. Demonstrated clinical response to recurrent BCC cases [27].	No	[26, 27]
Beta-carotene	*Various plants with rich hues*	No efficacy for NMSCs.	No	[28, 29]

TABLE 2: Summary of the effects of botanical agents studied in mice that have also been studied in humans.

Botanical agent	Source	Efficacy	References
Hypericin	*Hypericum perforatum*	The combination of hypericin and photodynamic therapy had poor efficacy in one mouse model [30].	[30]
Tea	*Camellia sinensis*	Animal studies demonstrate catechins have antitumor effects in mice [31–34].	[31–34]

3.3. Coffee. Coffee derives from seeds of the *Coffea* plant. Inconsistent results have been found for the association between coffee and various cancers. A prospective study by Jacobsen et al. in Norway of 13,664 men and 2,891 women demonstrated a strong inverse association between coffee drinking and NMSC [17]. Furthermore, a hospital-based case control study by Corona et al. of 166 case patients with histopathologically confirmed BCC and 158 control patients found that there was no statistically significant association between coffee consumption and BCC risk in a Mediterranean population from central-southern Italy [19].

More recently, Abel et al. performed a cross-sectional analysis of 93,676 Caucasian women in the Women's Health Initiative Observational Study to determine the relationship between consumption of coffee on a daily basis with the prevalence of NMSCs [18]. They found that women who

drank caffeinated coffee daily had a 10.8% lower occurrence of NMSCs compared to women who did not drink coffee. After adjusting for lifestyle and demographic variables, they found that daily consumption of six or more cups of coffee had a 30% reduction in occurrence of NMSC [18]. Consumption of decaffeinated coffee was not related to a significant change in rate of NMSCs. The authors concluded that, in Caucasian women, daily consumption of caffeinated coffee had a dose-related association with decreased occurrence of NMSC.

3.4. Tea. Dried and unfermented *Camellia sinensis* leaves are often used primarily for green and black tea and have anti-inflammatory and anticarcinogenic properties. Previous mouse models demonstrated that green tea catechins or polyphenols, such as the major catechin (-)-epigallocatechin and (-)-epigallocatechin-3-gallate (EGCG), may protect against UVB radiation-induced NMSC [50, 51]. EGCG is believed to act as a scavenger of reactive oxygen species [52] and may augment the native antioxidant defense mechanisms of the cell.

A study by Lu et al. demonstrated that when hairless mice were irradiated with UVB light twice weekly for a total of 20 weeks followed three weeks later by treatment with topical caffeine or EGCG once daily for five days over 18 weeks, the number of cutaneous tumors decreased [31]. Application of caffeine reduced the number of malignant and nonmalignant skin tumors by 72% and 44%, respectively, and EGCG reduced the number of malignant and nonmalignant tumors by 66% and 55% [31]. Further immunohistochemical analysis demonstrated that EGCG and caffeine augmented apoptosis in nonmalignant cutaneous tumors and in squamous cell carcinomas, but did not affect the epidermis lacking tumor cells. Wang et al. demonstrated that oral consumption of leaf extracts from caffeinated black and green tea and decaffeinated black and green tea, similar to the composition of tea beverages for humans, decreased the risk of UVB-induced skin tumor formation in hairless mice [32].

Expanding on the animal studies, the use of green tea and its ingredients have been studied in humans. Asgari et al. performed a case-control study of 415 cases from the Kaiser Permanente Northern California database with pathology-verified SCC in 2004 to determine the association between tea consumption, containing C. sinensis, and SCC risk [21]. Controls were matched based on age, gender, and race and had no previous history of skin cancer. Asgari et al. demonstrated no reduction in SCC risk with regular consumption of tea, defined as consumption at least once per week (OR = 1.11, 95% confidence interval (CI): 0.81–1.54) [21]. There was no association between SCC risk and the dose or amount of tea consumed, duration or years of use, nor the "cup-years" measurement, which accounts for dose and duration simultaneously.

Rees et al. performed a case control study to determine the relationship between regular tea consumption, defined as one cup daily for one month, and the incidence of BCCs and SCCs [20]. The type of tea consumed, such as black or green tea, was not specified. Among the subjects, they had 770 people with BCC, 696 with SCC, and 715 sex- and age-matched controls. They found that regular tea consumption significantly lowered the risk of SCC (odds ratio, OR = 0.70, 95% confidence interval, CI = 0.53–0.92) [20]. This reduction was most noticeable in long-term tea drinkers and people who drank two cups daily. Similarly, the study demonstrated that tea consumption had an inverse relationship with the development of BCC risk (OR = 0.79; 95% CI = 0.63–0.98) [20]. However, this relationship was weaker with regards to SCCs. The authors report that there may be a possible effect of citrus peel used in tea associated with the decreased SCC risk, however, they did not investigate this possible association further. Furthermore, it is unclear the reason for the differences in risk for BCCs and SCCs with tea consumption.

In addition to oral consumption of tea, topical tea application was reported in a 47-year-old female with basal cell nevus syndrome. She used green tea body wraps once per month for a year without any new BCCs developing in that time. The ingredients in the gel wrap included green tea primarily, as well as other plant extracts—ginger oil, algae, calendula oil, and mustard oil [22].

3.5. Escharotic Agents. Black salve, a combination of botanical agents, and bloodroot are two escharotic botanical agents that have been described in isolated case reports for their use in NMSCs. One case reported a 63-year-old male with a BCC confirmed by histopathology and located below the right eye [23]. Though Mohs micrographic surgery was recommended, the patient chose to self-treat the BCC with black salve ointment containing 300 mg of bloodroot, galangal, sheep sorrel, and red clover. However, he had no improvement and, ultimately, underwent Mohs surgery. Ten years prior to developing the BCC, he had a suspected melanoma on the left naris, which he treated with black salve. Although the lesion resolved, he had extensive tissue damage at the site of application and was left with an absent left naris [23]. Another case report of an 87-year-old male with a biopsy-proven BCC treated with black salve resulted in complete loss of the nasal ala at the site of application [24]. With regards to bloodroot, a 52-year-old man with recurrent BCC on the nose treated with Sanguinaria canadensis, bloodroot, instead of surgery resulted in metastasis of the BCC to the distal bones and death of the patient [25].

3.6. Paclitaxel. Paclitaxel is a plant alkaloid derived from the bark of the Pacific yew tree Taxus brevifolia. It is known as a chemotherapy agent. Paclitaxel binds tubulin of microtubules and stabilizes the microtubule structure to block its breakdown and, therefore, inhibits cell division leading to apoptosis of the cancer cells [53, 54]. It is more commonly used to treat Kaposis sarcoma, nonsmall cell lung cancer, breast cancer, and ovarian cancer. However, there are many side effects with the intravenous administration of paclitaxel. Therefore, Paolino et al. studied the use of a topical colloid formulation for paclitaxel, paclitaxel-loaded ethosomes, a vehicle devised to decrease systemic side effects and improve patient compliance [26]. In their in vitro study, Paolino et al. demonstrated that the paclitaxel-loaded ethosomes increased the antiproliferative activity of paclitaxel in an SCC model.

Paclitaxel has also been reported in two cases for the treatment of BCC. A 60-year-old male with a sclerosing BCC on the right eyelid refractory to local therapy, surgery, radiation, and six cycles of cisplatin and capecitabine was subsequently treated with paclitaxel 175 milligrams per square meter (mg/m^2) intravenously every 21 days for a total of 15 cycles. Complete response with elimination of the BCC was achieved after 12 cycles. The patient tolerated the treatment well and remained in complete remission documented clinically 13 months from his first cycle of treatment [27]. In another case report, a 74-year-old male with right scapular and nodal axillary relapse of BCC after surgical excision was treated with cisplatin 75 mg/m^2 intravenously and paclitaxel 75 mg/m^2 intravenously every 21 days. Partial response was noted after five cycles including elimination of pleural effusion, nodal and skin involvement. However, the patient died following

TABLE 3: Summary of the effects of botanical agents investigated only in preclinical studies.

Botanical agent	Source	Efficacy	References
Curcumin	*Curcuma longa* Linn	Curcumin inhibits skin tumor carcinogenesis in mice.	[35–41]
Genistein	Soy, Greek sage, Greek oregano, and gingko biloba extract	Genistein inhibits skin tumor carcinogenesis in mice.	[42, 43]
Proanthocyanidin	Grape seed	Grape seed proanthocyanidins demonstrated anticarcinogenic effects against ultraviolet B-induced skin tumors in mice.	[44, 45]
Lycopene	Various plants with red pigment	Lycopene prevents photodamage in mice and humans, suggesting potential for possible prevention of NMSC.	[46, 47]

neurotoxicity and complications of deep venous thrombosis and lung thromboembolism induced by chemotherapy [27].

3.7. Beta-Carotene. Beta carotene is a pigment found in a variety of plants, including carrots and richly hued vegetables. Many studies have demonstrated that a high consumption of vegetables and fruits with a high concentration of beta carotene has an inverse association with the risk of cancer [55–59]. Greenberg et al. randomly assigned 1,805 patients with a recent diagnosis of NMSC either 50 mg of beta carotene or placebo daily [28]. They followed the patients with annual skin examinations up to five years. At the five year endpoint, they found that there was no difference between the experimental and placebo groups in the rate of occurrence of the first new NMSC (relative rate, RR = 1.05; 95% CI = 0.91–1.22) [28]. In the U.S. Physicians' Health Study, a randomized, double-blind, placebo-controlled clinical trial, Frieling et al. randomized 22,071 male participants to take beta-carotene 50 mg every other day or placebo for 12 years [29]. They found that beta carotene supplementation did not affect the incidence of the first NMSC (RR = 0.98, 95% CI = 0.92–1.05), including BCCs (RR = 0.99, 95% CI = 0.92–1.06) and SCCs (RR = 0.97, 95% CI = 0.84–1.13) [29].

4. Botanical Agents Studied Only in Preclinical Studies (Table 3)

4.1. Curcumin. Curcumin is a spice that originates from the root of the *Curcuma longa* Linn plant and is the major contributor to the yellow pigment in turmeric and curry. It has been shown to have an anticarcinogenic effect; its proposed mechanisms of action are that it either induces apoptosis by augmenting the level of p53 [60] or it activates caspase-8, induced by the Fas receptor [61]. Topical curcumin was found to have inhibitory activity against skin tumor promotion in mice through mouse models [35–38, 58]. Furthermore, these studies demonstrated skin tumor chemoprevention through inhibition of arachidonic acid induced inflammation in vivo [37], inhibition of epidermal cyclooxygenase and lipoxygenase activity in vitro [37, 39], and suppression of oxidative stress through inhibition of leukocyte infiltration into inflammatory regions [38]. Limtrakul et al. found that Swiss albino mice given a diet containing 1% curcumin had significantly suppressed the

number of dimethylbenz[α]anthracene (DMBA) and 12-O-tetradecanoylphorbol-13-acetate (TPA) induced skin tumors per mouse ($P < 0.05$) and the tumor volume ($P < 0.01$) as compared to mice on the standard diet [40]. Skin tumor formation was initiated by 7,12-dimethylbenz[a]anthracene (DMBA) and promoted with 12-O-tetradecanoylphorbol-13-acetate (TPA). Furthermore, in a mouse skin cancer model, Sonavane et al. found that curcumin at 15 mg applied topically had a similar effect as oral curcumin at 15 mg for inhibiting tumor growth [41]. However, no reports have been published to assess the use of curcumin in human clinical trials.

4.2. Genistein. Genistein is a flavonoid found in soy, Greek sage, Greek oregano, and ginkgo biloba extract and is specifically a major isoflavone in soybeans. Studies have shown that genistein have antioxidant and anticarcinogenic activity in the skin [42, 62] as well as protection against photodamage in mice [63]. Studies in mice have demonstrated that genistein inhibits skin carcinogenesis. Wei et al. demonstrated that genistein inhibited DMBA-initiated and TPA-promoted skin carcinogenesis by treating SENCAR (sensitive to carcinogenesis) mice with 10 micromoles of topical genistein for one week [43]. A later study by Wei et al. found that topical genistein also reduced ultraviolet B-induced skin tumor multiplicity and incidence in hairless mice [42]. Although there are no reported studies assessing the effect of genistein on human skin cancer development, genistein was found to inhibit UVB-induced photodamage in a small study of six men [42]. Genistein was topically applied to the six participants one hour prior to and five minutes after they were UVB irradiated. The study demonstrated that genistein applied to human skin inhibited UVB-induced erythema. More specifically, topical application of genistein prior to UVB irradiation inhibited erythema and cutaneous discomfort while application after UVB irradiation improved discomfort but had a weaker effect on erythema.

4.3. Grape Seed. Grape seeds contain proanthocyanidins, a group of polyphenols that have been found to possess anti-inflammatory and antioxidant properties [64, 65]. Although not extensively studied nor investigated in clinical trials, the proanthocyanidins have demonstrated possible anticarcinogenic effects to ultraviolet-induced cutaneous tumors in mice. Zhao et al. extracted proanthocyanidins in grape seeds after grape seeds were air-dried and made into a powder. They demonstrated that proanthocyanidins in grape seeds had a strong inhibitory effect for UVB-induced skin tumor development in SENCAR mice [44]. Mittal et al. found that dietary feeding of proanthocyanidins from grape seeds prevented photocarcinogenesis in hairless mice as compared to mice on the control diet [45]. Mice that consumed proanthocyanidins had reduced tumor size (29%–94%), tumor incidence (20%–95%), and tumor multiplicity (46%–95%) for UVB-induced stages of photocarcinogenesis [45]. Furthermore, they found that through in vivo and in vitro systems, photoprotection was a result of antioxidant mechanisms.

4.4. Lycopene. Lycopene is a carotenoid that provides the red pigmentation found in tomatoes, guava, watermelon, pink grapefruit, papaya, rosehips, and other vegetables and fruits. Though it is a phytochemical that lacks provitamin A activity, lycopene has been studied for its anticarcinogenic and antioxidant activity for breast [66], prostate [67], lung [68], and colon cancer [69]. Fazekas et al. demonstrated that topical lycopene application inhibited UVB-induced skin damage in mice [46]. Although a randomized controlled trial by Rizwan et al. found that tomato paste containing a high concentration of lycopene reduced ultraviolet-induced skin erythema and markers of ultraviolet-induced DNA damage (matrix metalloproteinase-1 and mitochondrial DNA 3895 bp) [47], there are no reports assessing lycopene effects on skin cancer in humans.

4.5. Silymarin. Silymarin is a flavonoid derived from *Silybum marianum*, a milk thistle plant. It is known to have antioxidant and anti-inflammatory properties [70, 71]. The primary component in silymarin is silybin, which has demonstrated to have anticarcinogenic properties for the cervix, breast, and prostate [72]. Due to its antioxidant activity, silymarin has been studied in mouse models for its effects on tumorigenesis. Katiyar et al. found that silymarin inhibited UVB-induced NMSC in hairless mice with topical silymarin in three different protocols to assess the effects of silymarin at various tumor stages [73]. Subsequently, Lahiri-Chatterjee et al. demonstrated that application of silymarin to SENCAR mice, in doses of 3, 6, and 12 mg reduced tumor incidence (by 25%, 40%, and 75%, $P < 0.001$), tumor multiplicity (76%, 84%, 97%, $P < 0.001$), and tumor volume (76%, 94%, 96%, $P < 0.001$) [74]. Silymarin has not yet been investigated in human clinical trials.

5. Utility against Nonmelanoma Skin Cancer

Ingenol mebutate, hypericin, coffee, tea, black salve, bloodroot, paclitaxel, and beta-carotene have been studied for their effects on NMSC in humans or have been reported to be used in humans with BCCs and SCCs. Clinical trials assessing the effectiveness of ingenol mebutate on BCCs and SCCs and case reports with patients using paclitaxel for BCCs suggest efficacy of these agents for treating NMSCs in humans. Despite favorable results, more human studies are needed to assess the chemopreventive and therapeutic effects of these botanical agents. In particular, prospective trials with efficacy as the primary outcome are still needed.

Furthermore, black salve and bloodroot were reported to be more harmful than therapeutic. Participants taking beta carotene showed no difference in skin cancer rate compared to the control groups. Although clinical response has been reported using hypericin with photodynamic therapy, coffee, and tea in humans with NMSCs, there is no consensus as to the effectiveness of these agents based on the results of the studies. Finally, it is important to note that in short studies, such as the study of ingenol mebutate by Siller et al. that lasted only 12 weeks [14], histopathological examination for clearance is more appropriate rather than clinical observation for clearance. In this regard, this study was a phase IIa study with the intent to assess side effects, and the primary intent was not to assess treatment efficacy. Topical ingenol appears to be well-tolerated overall. Although it is tempting to speculate that application on sequential days may be better than spacing the applications by a week, a study specifically designed to assess efficacy is awaited before any conclusions regarding the treatment of superficial BCCs can be drawn.

Although histopathological evaluation of clearance is the gold standard, future studies should consider additional incorporation of confocal microscopy. Confocal microscopy may have a role in noninvasively assessing superficial BCC recurrence [75–77]. Further studies will be needed to assess its efficacy in delineating recurrences in studies with botanical agents that may have a significant component of inflammation in addition to wound healing.

Five botanical agents appear to have potential for anticarcinogenesis based on preclinical studies. Curcumin, genistein, grape seed proanthocyanidin, and silymarin have demonstrated reduction in UV-induced skin cancers in mice, and lycopene has been shown to prevent photodamage in mice and humans. However, one botanical agent that has been studied for its effects on NMSCs, beta carotene, does not appear to be effective against skin cancer. Curcumin, genistein, grape seed, lycopene, and silymarin have not yet been studied in humans for the treatment or prevention of NMSC.

6. Role of Lipophilicity and Hydrophilicity

An important characteristic that is highly important for topical delivery of botanical agents is their hydrophilicity and lipophilicity. Phytochemical subgroups that tend to be more hydrophilic, such as polyphenol, may not penetrate the stratum corneum well. This may explain why topical polyphenols do not seem to be as efficacious as oral/systemic delivery. On the other hand, topical delivery of more lipophilic phytochemicals, such as ingenol or silymarin, will be able to penetrate the stratum corneum more effectively. One option in conducting studies with agents that have a lower partition coefficient will be to facilitate their transit through the stratum corneum through penetration enhancers such as liposomes, iontophoresis, sonophoresis, or microneedle technology. Our suggestion for future evaluation of topical botanicals is that investigators take the octanol-water partition coefficient or the mode of extraction of the extract into account in designing future studies. For example, a nonaqueous extract or a phytochemical with a high partition coefficient may not require a penetration enhancer; on the other hand, it would be prudent to consider the use of penetration enhancers when studying aqueous extracts or phytochemicals with low partition coefficients.

7. Conclusions

In vitro and in vivo models have been developed with the hypothesis that natural products rich in complex chemicals that have been shown to induce apoptosis in animal models of chemoprevention may therefore possess the ability to arrest the cell cycle at different stages and, therefore, control the proliferation of cancer cells. Botanical agents have been studied, and some have been reported to have favorable effects against NMSC.

In this review, we have included a variety of botanical agents that have been studied or reported for the treatment of NMSCs. A limitation of this review is that we did not include botanical agents that were reported in a single case or a single preclinical study. However, we have provided an up-to-date and concise review of botanical agents used in NMSC that is currently found in the literature. Although the limited preclinical data and clinical data available in the literature demonstrate favorable effects of some botanical agents on NMSC, for now, surgical therapy is the preferred mode of treatment for high-risk NMSCs. Botanical agents may have a preventive role in the development of cutaneous malignancies and a potentially therapeutic role for carefully chosen localized NMSCs of an appropriate subtype. The topical use of some botanical extracts and phytochemicals in the treatment of NMSC is promising. However, more studies, both preclinical and clinical, are needed to make more definitive conclusions regarding safety and efficacy.

Conflict of Interests

Ms. Wong, Dr. Sivamani, and Dr. Fazel have no conflict of interests to report.

References

[1] World Health Organization, *Skin Cancers*, World Health Organization, Geneva, Switzerland, 2012.

[2] Division of Cancer Prevention and Control NCfCDPaHP, *Skin Cancer*, Centers for Disease Control and Prevention, Atlanta, Ga, USA, 2012.

[3] R. V. Patel, A. Frankel, and G. Goldenberg, "An update on nonmelanoma skin cancer," *Journal of Clinical and Aesthetic Dermatology*, vol. 4, no. 2, pp. 20–27, 2011.

[4] L. E. Dubas and A. Ingraffea, "Nonmelanoma skin cancer," *Facial Plastic Surgery Clinics of North America*, vol. 21, pp. 43–53, 2013.

[5] United States National Institutes of Health, *Skin Cancer*, United States National Institutes of Health, Institute, NC, USA, 2012.

[6] D. N. Syed and H. Mukhtar, "Botanicals for the prevention and treatment of cutaneous melanoma," *Pigment Cell and Melanoma Research*, vol. 24, no. 4, pp. 688–702, 2011.

[7] M. S. Baliga and S. K. Katiyar, "Chemoprevention of photocarcinogenesis by selected dietary botanicals," *Photochemical and Photobiological Sciences*, vol. 5, no. 2, pp. 243–253, 2006.

[8] E. W. Cowen and E. M. Billingsley, "Awareness of skin cancer by kidney transplant patients," *Journal of the American Academy of Dermatology*, vol. 40, no. 5, pp. 697–701, 1999.

[9] C. C. Otley and M. R. Pittelkow, "Skin cancer in liver transplant recipients," *Liver Transplantation*, vol. 6, no. 3, pp. 253–262, 2000.

[10] J. Reuter, I. Merfort, and C. M. Schempp, "Botanicals in dermatology: an evidence-based review," *American Journal of Clinical Dermatology*, vol. 11, no. 4, pp. 247–267, 2010.

[11] M. Lebwohl, N. Swanson, L. L. Anderson, A. Melgaard, Z. Xu, and B. Berman, "Ingenol mebutate gel for actinic keratosis," *New England Journal of Medicine*, vol. 366, no. 11, pp. 1010–1019, 2012.

[12] C. Thornfeldt, "Cosmeceuticals containing herbs: fact, fiction, and future," *Dermatologic Surgery*, vol. 31, no. 7, pp. 873–880, 2005.

[13] J. R. Ramsay, A. Suhrbier, J. H. Aylward et al., "The sap from Euphorbia peplus is effective against human nonmelanoma skin cancers," *British Journal of Dermatology*, vol. 164, no. 3, pp. 633–636, 2011.

[14] G. Siller, R. Rosen, M. Freeman, P. Welburn, J. Katsamas, and S. M. Ogbourne, "PEP005 (ingenol mebutate) gel for the topical treatment of superficial basal cell carcinoma: results of a randomized phase IIa trial," *Australasian Journal of Dermatology*, vol. 51, no. 2, pp. 99–105, 2010.

[15] M. Alecu, C. Ursaciuc, F. Hălălău et al., "Photodynamic treatment of basal cell carcinoma and squamous cell carcinoma with hypericin," *Anticancer Research B*, vol. 18, no. 6, pp. 4651–4654, 1998.

[16] D. Kacerovská, K. Pizinger, F. Majer, and F. Šmíd, "Photodynamic therapy of nonmelanoma skin cancer with topical Hypericum perforatum extract—a pilot study," *Photochemistry and Photobiology*, vol. 84, no. 3, pp. 779–785, 2008.

[17] B. K. Jacobsen, E. Bjelke, G. Kvale, and I. Heuch, "Coffee drinking, mortality, and cancer incidence: results from a Norwegian prospective study," *Journal of the National Cancer Institute*, vol. 76, no. 5, pp. 823–831, 1986.

[18] E. L. Abel, S. O. Hendrix, S. G. McNeeley et al., "Daily coffee consumption and prevalence of nonmelanoma skin cancer in Caucasian women," *European Journal of Cancer Prevention*, vol. 16, no. 5, pp. 446–452, 2007.

[19] R. Corona, E. Dogliotti, M. D'Errico et al., "Risk factors for basal cell carcinoma in a Mediterranean population: role of recreational sun exposure early in life," *Archives of Dermatology*, vol. 137, no. 9, pp. 1162–1168, 2001.

[20] J. R. Rees, T. A. Stukel, A. E. Perry, M. S. Zens, S. K. Spencer, and M. R. Karagas, "Tea consumption and basal cell and squamous cell skin cancer: results of a case-control study," *Journal of the American Academy of Dermatology*, vol. 56, no. 5, pp. 781–785, 2007.

[21] M. M. Asgari, E. White, E. M. Warton, M. K. Hararah, G. D. Friedman, and M. Chren, "Association of tea consumption and cutaneous squamous cell carcinoma," *Nutrition and Cancer*, vol. 63, no. 2, pp. 314–318, 2011.

[22] F. Tjeerdsma, M. F. Jonkman, and J. R. Spoo, "Temporary arrest of basal cell carcinoma formation in a patient with basal cell naevus syndrome (BCNS) since treatment with a gel containing various plant extracts," *Journal of the European Academy of Dermatology and Venereology*, vol. 25, no. 2, pp. 244–245, 2011.

[23] K. L. Eastman, L. V. McFarland, and G. J. Raugi, "Buyer beware: a black salve caution," *Journal of the American Academy of Dermatology*, vol. 65, no. 5, pp. e154–e155, 2011.

[24] F. Saltzberg, G. Barron, and N. Fenske, "Deforming self-treatment with herbal "black salve"," *Dermatologic Surgery*, vol. 35, no. 7, pp. 1152–1154, 2009.

[25] D. R. Laub Jr., "Death from metastatic basal cell carcinoma: herbal remedy or just unlucky?" *Journal of Plastic, Reconstructive and Aesthetic Surgery*, vol. 61, no. 7, pp. 846–848, 2008.

[26] D. Paolino, C. Celia, E. Trapasso, F. Cilurzo, and M. Fresta, "Paclitaxel-loaded ethosomes: potential treatment of squamous cell carcinoma, a malignant transformation of actinic keratoses," *European Journal of Pharmaceutics and Biopharmaceutics*, vol. 81, no. 1, pp. 102–112, 2012.

[27] R. Barceló, A. Viteri, A. Muñoz, A. Gil-Negrete, I. Rubio, and G. López-Vivanco, "Paclitaxel for progressive basal cell carcinoma," *Journal of the American Academy of Dermatology*, vol. 54, supplement 2, pp. S50–S52, 2006.

[28] E. R. Greenberg, J. A. Baron, T. A. Stukel et al., "A clinical trial of beta carotene to prevent basal-cell and squamous-cell cancers of the skin," *New England Journal of Medicine*, vol. 323, no. 12, pp. 789–795, 1990.

[29] U. M. Frieling, D. A. Schaumberg, T. S. Kupper, J. Muntwyler, and C. H. Hennekens, "A randomized, 12-year primary-prevention trial of beta carotene supplementation for non-melanoma skin cancer in the physicians' health study," *Archives of Dermatology*, vol. 136, no. 2, pp. 179–184, 2000.

[30] A. Boiy, R. Roelandts, and P. A. M. De Witte, "Photodynamic therapy using topically applied hypericin: comparative effect with methyl-aminolevulinic acid on UV induced skin tumours," *Journal of Photochemistry and Photobiology B*, vol. 102, no. 2, pp. 123–131, 2011.

[31] Y. Lu, Y. Lou, J. Xie et al., "Topical applications of caffeine or (-)-epigallocatechin gallate (EGCG) inhibit carcinogenesis and selectively increase apoptosis in UVB-induced skin tumors in mice," *Proceedings of the National Academy of Sciences of the United States of America*, vol. 99, no. 19, pp. 12455–12460, 2002.

[32] Z. Y. Wang, M.-T. Huang, Y.-R. Lou et al., "Inhibitory effects of black tea, green tea, decaffeinated black tea, and decaffeinated green tea on ultraviolet B light-induced skin carcinogenesis in 7,12-dimethylbenz[a]anthracene-initiated SKH-1 mice," *Cancer Research*, vol. 54, no. 13, pp. 3428–3435, 1994.

[33] Z.-Y. Wang, M.-T. Huang, T. Ferraro et al., "Inhibitory effect of green tea in the drinking water on tumorigenesis by ultraviolet light and 12-O-tetradecanoylphorbol-13-acetate in the skin of SKH-1 mice," *Cancer Research*, vol. 52, no. 5, pp. 1162–1170, 1992.

[34] Z. Y. Wang, R. Agarwal, D. R. Bickers, and H. Mukhtar, "Protection against ultraviolet B radiation-induced photocarcinogenesis in hairless mice by green tea polyphenols," *Carcinogenesis*, vol. 12, no. 8, pp. 1527–1530, 1991.

[35] M. Huang, W. Ma, P. Yen et al., "Inhibitory effects of topical application of low doses of curcumin on 12-O-tetradecanoylphorbol-13-acetate-induced tumor promotion and oxidized DNA bases in mouse epidermis," *Carcinogenesis*, vol. 18, no. 1, pp. 83–88, 1997.

[36] M.-T. Huang, N. Ma, Y.-P. Lu et al., "Effects of curcumin, demethoxycurcumin, bisdemethoxycurcumin and tetrahydrocurcumin on 12-O-tetradecanoylphorbol-13-acetate-induced tumor promotion," *Carcinogenesis*, vol. 16, no. 10, pp. 2493–2497, 1995.

[37] A. H. Conney, T. Lysz, T. Ferraro et al., "Inhibitory effect of curcumin and some related dietary compounds on tumor promotion and arachidonic acid metabolism in mouse skin," *Advances in Enzyme Regulation*, vol. 31, pp. 385–396, 1991.

[38] Y. Nakamura, Y. Ohto, A. Murakami, T. Osawa, and H. Ohigashi, "Inhibitory effects of curcumin and tetrahydrocurcuminoids on the tumor promoter-induced reactive oxygen species generation in leukocytes in vitro and in vivo," *Japanese Journal of Cancer Research*, vol. 89, no. 4, pp. 361–370, 1998.

[39] M.-T. Huang, T. Lysz, T. Ferraro, T. F. Abidi, J. D. Laskin, and A. H. Conney, "Inhibitory effects of curcumin on in vitro lipoxygenase and cyclooxygenase activities in mouse epidermis," *Cancer Research*, vol. 51, no. 3, pp. 813–819, 1991.

[40] P. Limtrakul, S. Lipigorngoson, O. Namwong, A. Apisariyakul, and F. W. Dunn, "Inhibitory effect of dietary curcumin on skin carcinogenesis in mice," *Cancer Letters*, vol. 116, no. 2, pp. 197–203, 1997.

[41] K. Sonavane, J. Phillips, O. Ekshyyan, T. Moore-Medlin, J. Roberts Gill et al., "Topical curcumin-based cream is equivalent to dietary curcumin in a skin cancer model," *Journal of Skin Cancer*, vol. 2012, Article ID 147863, 9 pages, 2012.

[42] H. Wei, R. Saladi, Y. Lu et al., "Isoflavone genistein: photoprotection and clinical implications in dermatology," *Journal of Nutrition*, vol. 133, no. 11, 2003.

[43] H. Wei, R. Bowen, X. Zhang, and M. Lebwohl, "Isoflavone genistein inhibits the initiation and promotion of two-stage skin carcinogenesis in mice," *Carcinogenesis*, vol. 19, no. 8, pp. 1509–1514, 1998.

[44] J. Zhao, J. Wang, Y. Chen, and R. Agarwal, "Anti-tumor-promoting activity of a polyphenolic fraction isolated from grape seeds in the mouse skin two-stage initiation-promotion protocol and identification of procyanidin B5-3'-gallate as the most effective antioxidant constituent," *Carcinogenesis*, vol. 20, no. 9, pp. 1737–1745, 1999.

[45] A. Mittal, C. A. Elmets, and S. K. Katiyar, "Dietary feeding of proanthocyanidins from grape seeds prevents photocarcinogenesis in SKH-1 hairless mice: relationship to decreased fat and lipid peroxidation," *Carcinogenesis*, vol. 24, no. 8, pp. 1379–1388, 2003.

[46] Z. Fazekas, D. Gao, R. N. Saladi, Y. Lu, M. Lebwohl, and H. Wei, "Protective effects of lycopene against ultraviolet B-induced photodamage," *Nutrition and Cancer*, vol. 47, no. 2, pp. 181–187, 2003.

[47] M. Rizwan, I. Rodriguez-Blanco, A. Harbottle, M. A. Birch-Machin, R. E. B. Watson, and L. E. Rhodes, "Tomato paste rich in lycopene protects against cutaneous photodamage in humans in vivo: a randomized controlled trial," *British Journal of Dermatology*, vol. 164, no. 1, pp. 154–162, 2011.

[48] S. M. Ogbourne, A. Suhrbier, B. Jones et al., "Antitumor activity of 3-ingenyl angelate: plasma membrane and mitochondrial disruption and necrotic cell death," *Cancer Research*, vol. 64, no. 8, pp. 2833–2839, 2004.

[49] F. E. Fox, Z. Niu, A. Tobia, and A. H. Rook, "Photoactivated hypericin is an anti-proliferative agent that induces a high rate of apoptotic death of normal, transformed, and malignant T lymphocytes: implications for the treatment of cutaneous lymphoprohferatlve and inflammatory disorders," *Journal of Investigative Dermatology*, vol. 111, no. 2, pp. 327–332, 1998.

[50] I. R. Record and I. E. Dreosti, "Protection by tea against UV-A + B-induced skin cancers in hairless mice," *Nutrition and Cancer*, vol. 32, no. 2, pp. 71–75, 1998.

[51] S. K. Katiyar, "Green tea prevents non-melanoma skin cancer by enhancing DNA repair," *Archives of Biochemistry and Biophysics*, vol. 508, no. 2, pp. 152–158, 2011.

[52] H. Mukhtar and N. Ahmad, "Cancer chemoprevention: future holds in multiple agents," *Toxicology and Applied Pharmacology*, vol. 158, no. 3, pp. 207–210, 1999.

[53] M. C. Wani, H. L. Taylor, M. E. Wall, P. Coggon, and A. T. McPhail, "Plant antitumor agents. VI. The isolation and structure of taxol, a novel antileukemic and antitumor agent from Taxus brevifolia," *Journal of the American Chemical Society*, vol. 93, no. 9, pp. 2325–2327, 1971.

[54] P. B. Schiff and S. B. Horwitz, "Taxol stabilizes microtubules in mouse fibroblast cells," *Proceedings of the National Academy of Sciences of the United States of America*, vol. 77, no. 3, pp. 1561–1565, 1980.

[55] R. G. Ziegler, "A review of epidemiologic evidence that carotenoids reduce the risk of cancer," *Journal of Nutrition*, vol. 119, no. 1, pp. 116–122, 1989.

[56] T. Hirayama, "Epidemiology of prostate cancer with special reference to the role of diet," *National Cancer Institute Monograph*, vol. 53, pp. 149–155, 1979.

[57] T. Hirayama, "A large scale cohort study on cancer risks by diet—with special reference to the risk reducing effects of green-yellow vegetable consumption," *Princess Takamatsu Symposia*, vol. 16, pp. 41–53, 1985.

[58] G. A. Colditz, L. G. Branch, and R. J. Lipnick, "Increased green and yellow vegetable intake and lowered cancer deaths in an elderly population," *American Journal of Clinical Nutrition*, vol. 41, no. 1, pp. 32–36, 1985.

[59] A. Paganini-Hill, A. Chao, R. K. Ross, and B. E. Henderson, "Vitamin A, β-carotene, and the risk of cancer: a prospective study," *Journal of the National Cancer Institute*, vol. 79, no. 3, pp. 443–448, 1987.

[60] S. H. Jee, S. C. Shen, C. R. Tseng, H. C. Chiu, and M. L. Kuo, "Curcumin induces a p53-dependent apoptosis in human basal cell carcinoma cells," *Journal of Investigative Dermatology*, vol. 111, no. 4, pp. 656–661, 1998.

[61] J. A. Bush, K. J. Cheung Jr., and G. Li, "Curcumin induces apoptosis in human melanoma cells through a Fas receptor/caspase-8 pathway independent of p53," *Experimental Cell Research*, vol. 271, no. 2, pp. 305–314, 2001.

[62] H. Wei, R. Bowen, Q. Cai, S. Barnes, and Y. Wang, "Antioxidant and antipromotional effects of the soybean isoflavone genistein," *Proceedings of the Society for Experimental Biology and Medicine*, vol. 208, no. 1, pp. 124–130, 1995.

[63] E. Q. Shyong, Y. Lu, A. Lazinsky et al., "Effects of the isoflavone 4′,5,7,-trihydroxyisoflavone (genistein) on psoralen plus ultraviolet A radiation (PUVA)-induced photodamage," *Carcinogenesis*, vol. 23, no. 2, pp. 317–321, 2002.

[64] P. Cos, T. de Bruyne, N. Hermans, S. Apers, D. Vanden Berghe, and A. J. Vlietinck, "Proanthocyanidins in health care: current and new trends," *Current Medicinal Chemistry*, vol. 11, no. 10, pp. 1345–1359, 2004.

[65] L. Wen-Guang, Z. Xiao-Yu, W. Yong-Jie, and T. Xuan, "Anti-inflammatory effect and mechanism of proanthocyanidins from grape seeds," *Acta Pharmacologica Sinica*, vol. 22, no. 12, pp. 1117–1120, 2001.

[66] A. Nahum, K. Hirsch, M. Danilenko et al., "Lycopene inhibition of cell cycle progression in breast and endometrial cancer cells is associated with reduction in cyclin D levels and retention of p27Kip1 in the cyclin E-cdk2 complexes," *Oncogene*, vol. 20, no. 26, pp. 3428–3436, 2001.

[67] S. K. Clinton, C. Emenhiser, S. J. Schwartz et al., "cis-trans lycopene isomers, carotenoids, and retinol in the human prostate," *Cancer Epidemiology Biomarkers and Prevention*, vol. 5, no. 10, pp. 823–833, 1996.

[68] D. J. Kim, N. Takasuka, H. Nishino, and H. Tsuda, "Chemoprevention of lung cancer by lycopene," *BioFactors*, vol. 13, no. 1–4, pp. 95–102, 2000.

[69] T. Narisawa, Y. Fukaura, M. Hasebe et al., "Prevention of N-methylnitrosourea-induced colon carcinogenesis in F344 rats by lycopene and tomato juice rich in lycopene," *Japanese Journal of Cancer Research*, vol. 89, no. 10, pp. 1003–1008, 1998.

[70] H. Wagner, P. Diesel, and M. Seitz, "The chemistry and analysis of silymarin from Silybum marianum Gaertn," *Arzneimittel-Forschung*, vol. 24, no. 4, pp. 466–471, 1974.

[71] A. Comoglio, G. Leonarduzzi, R. Carini et al., "Studies on the antioxidant and free radical scavenging properties of IdB 1016 a new flavanolignan complex," *Free Radical Research Communications*, vol. 11, no. 1–3, pp. 109–115, 1990.

[72] T. I. Wright, J. M. Spencer, and F. P. Flowers, "Chemoprevention of nonmelanoma skin cancer," *Journal of the American Academy of Dermatology*, vol. 54, no. 6, pp. 933–946, 2006.

[73] S. K. Katiyar, N. J. Korman, H. Mukhtar, and R. Agarwal, "Protective effects of silymarin against photocarcinogenesis in a mouse skin model," *Journal of the National Cancer Institute*, vol. 89, no. 8, pp. 556–566, 1997.

[74] M. Lahiri-Chatterjee, S. K. Katiyar, R. R. Mohan, and R. Agarwal, "A flavonoid antioxidant, silymarin, affords exceptionally high protection against tumor promotion in the SENCAR mouse skin tumorigenesis model," *Cancer Research*, vol. 59, no. 3, pp. 622–632, 1999.

[75] S. A. Webber, E. M. T. Wurm, N. C. Douglas et al., "Effectiveness and limitations of reflectance confocal microscopy in detecting persistence of basal cell carcinomas: a preliminary study," *Australasian Journal of Dermatology*, vol. 52, no. 3, pp. 179–185, 2011.

[76] V. Ahlgrimm-Siess, M. Horn, S. Koller, R. Ludwig, A. Gerger, and R. Hofmann-Wellenhof, "Monitoring efficacy of cryotherapy for superficial basal cell carcinomas with in vivo reflectance confocal microscopy: a preliminary study," *Journal of Dermatological Science*, vol. 53, no. 1, pp. 60–64, 2009.

[77] M. Goldgeier, C. A. Fox, J. M. Zavislan, D. Harris, and S. Gonzalez, "Noninvasive imaging, treatment, and microscopic confirmation of clearance of basal cell carcinoma," *Dermatologic Surgery*, vol. 29, no. 3, pp. 205–210, 2003.

27

The Effect of Q-Switched Nd:YAG 1064 nm/532 nm Laser in the Treatment of Onychomycosis In Vivo

Kostas Kalokasidis,[1] **Meltem Onder,**[2,3] **Myrto-Georgia Trakatelli,**[4]
Bertrand Richert,[5] **and Klaus Fritz**[2,6,7,8]

[1] *Dermatology and Laser Clinic, 88 Tsimiski Street, 54622 Thessaloniki, Greece*

[2] *Dermatology and Laser Center, Reduitstrare 13, 76829 Landau, Germany*

[3] *Gazi University Medical Faculty, Department of Dermatology, 06510 Ankara, Turkey*

[4] *Aristotle University School of Medicine, Second Department of Dermatology and Venereology, 54622 Thessaloniki, Greece*

[5] *Université Libre de Bruxelles, Department CHU Brugmann-Saint Pierre, 1050 Brussels, Belgium*

[6] *Carol Davila University of Medicine, Dionisie Lupu Street, 020021 Bucharest, Romania*

[7] *Osnabrueck University, Sedanstraße 115, 49090 Osnabrueck, Germany*

[8] *Bern University, Department of Dermatology, 117 Inselspital, 3010 Bern, Switzerland*

Correspondence should be addressed to Klaus Fritz; drklausfritz@t-online.de

Academic Editor: Craig G. Burkhart

In this prospective clinical study, the Q-Switched Nd:YAG 1064 nm/532 nm laser (Light Age, Inc., Somerset, NJ, USA) was used on 131 onychomycosis subjects (94 females, 37 males; ages 18 to 68 years). Mycotic cultures were taken and fungus types were detected. The laser protocol included two sessions with a one-month interval. Treatment duration was approximately 15 minutes per session and patients were observed over a 3-month time period. Laser fluencies of 14 J/cm^2 were applied at 9 billionths of a second pulse duration and at 5 Hz frequency. Follow-up was performed at 3 months with mycological cultures. Before and after digital photographs were taken. Adverse effects were recorded and all participants completed "self-evaluation questionnaires" rating their level of satisfaction. All subjects were well satisfied with the treatments, there were no noticeable side effects, and no significant differences were found treating men versus women. At the 3-month follow-up 95.42% of the patients were laboratory mycologically cured of fungal infection. This clinical study demonstrates that fungal nail infections can be effectively and safely treated with Q-Switched Nd:YAG 1064 nm/532 nm laser. It can also be combined with systemic oral antifungals providing more limited treatment time.

1. Introduction

Onychomycosis is defined as a fungal infection of the nail that expands slowly and if left untreated leads to complete destruction of the nail plate. Onychomycosis can be dermatophytic (99%) and/or nondermatophytic (1%) (including yeasts) infections of the nail plate.

The dermatophytes *Trichophyton rubrum* and *Trichophyton mentagrophytes* are the most common causative pathogens responsible for up to 90% of all cases [1]. Onychomycosis represents about 30% of all dermatophyte infections and accounts for 18%–40% of all nail disorders. The prevalence of onychomycosis ranges between 2% and 28% of the general population and it is estimated to be significantly higher in specific populations such as in diabetes mellitus, the immunosuppressed, and elderly [2, 3].

Among the nondermatophytes, the yeast *Candida albicans*, *Candida tropicalis*, *aspergillus*, and other molds may be responsible. It usually represents contamination and is an emerging problem in HIV patients.

Toenails are far more likely to be involved than fingernails. Initially solitary nails are involved; later, many may be infected, but often one or more can stay disease-free. Onychomycosis has no tendency for spontaneous remission and should be considered as a problem with serious medical, social, and emotional extensions, not solely a cosmetic problem. The primary concerns of the patients are the risk of spread to other nails or to people in their environment. Others consider their deformed nails as unattractive to other people, which may lead to lower self-esteem, a sense of inadequacy, and even depression [4, 5]. In addition to these social and emotional problems, onychomycosis is a serious medical problem that can be the source of further fungal infections to surrounding tissues. Also, it may predispose patients to secondary bacterial infections leading to localized paronychia and perhaps worse and deeper infections such as erysipelas-cellulitis, especially in the high-risk groups such as diabetics [6, 7]. Clinically it can cause varying degrees of pain or discomfort (especially in walking) and problems in cutting nails.

Classical treatment options include mechanical and chemical debridement, topical antifungal lacquers, systemic antifungal drugs, and finally various combinations of the above. The most effective mono-therapies for onychomycosis are antifungal agents which have been the gold standard and mainstay of therapy for years. The downside of the antifungals are that they require blood testing to monitor the liver because they are systemic and also that they require long treatment courses (approximately 6 months for toenails and 4 months for fingernails). This requires liver function-transaminases and kidney function blot test control. Patients may also receive concomitant medications for comorbidities, so there is also the issue of drug interactions. Additionally, long lasting treatment means high treatment costs for both the patient and health insurers. Finally, high recurrence rates have been described, 22% three years after completion of treatment and higher recurrence rates at five years follow-up [8–10].

Recently, lasers have emerged as potential new treatment modalities. These treatments offer the advantage of having few contraindications and minimal side effects [11–13]. Laser energy has the potential to eliminate microorganisms. Vural et al. recently demonstrated direct inhibitory activity of laser energy on *T. rubrum* isolates in vitro [14]. Manevitch et al. recently published the direct antifungal effect of the femtosecond laser on *T. rubrum* onychomycosis as well [7]. The laser must have the ability to penetrate under the nail plate in order to reach the fungi colonies of the nail bed and nail matrix. When it gets to that point it should selectively deliver laser energy to fungi while respecting the surrounding healthy tissues.

In this study we planned to evaluate the effect of the neodymium: yttrium-aluminum-garnet (Nd:YAG) 1064 nm/ 532 nm laser in the treatment of onychomycosis in vivo.

2. Material and Methods

2.1. Nail Sampling and Fungal Cultures. Nail cuttings sized 2 × 3 mm were obtained from patients with clinical suspicion of onychomycosis. After direct microscopy to observe spores, hyphae, mycelia, and colonies of the latter, samples were plated on *Sabouraud glucose agars* with *cyclohexamide* to select for dermatophytes, in order to verify fungal infection.

Cultures were incubated at 28°C for 3 weeks until fungal colonies developed.

2.2. Evaluation of Fungal Elimination. Before the treatment culture was performed and 4 weeks after the second treatment session (8 weeks after the first positive culture), culture was repeated. Mycological cure is defined as negative microscopy and culture. Clinical cure is associated with the alteration of the percentages of disease-free nails. Complete cure is accepted as the combination of mycological and clinical cure. Three months after the first treatment session, laser treatment was evaluated [15, 16].

2.3. Inclusion Criteria. To take part in the study each patient had to have one or more toenail and/or fingernail fungal infections of the following types: distal subungual onychomycosis, proximal subungual onychomycosis, superficial white onychomycosis, or total dystrophic type onychomycosis. Patients with diabetes mellitus, immunocompromised patients, and organ transplant patients were also included, although we considered that these patient groups success rates could be considerably less.

2.4. Exclusion Criteria. Patients who used systemic antifungal or isoretinoin within 6 months of the first scheduled laser session were excluded. The following conditions, which can cause various physiological changes to the nail plate, were also excluded: subungual hematoma, nevoid subungual formation, bacterial nail infections, concomitant nail disorders due to psoriasis, atopic dermatitis, lichen planus, and pregnant women were not included.

2.5. Pretreatment. As onychomycosis causes significant thickening (hyperkeratosis) of the nail plate, before starting our laser sessions we performed the mechanical debridement of any excessive nail thickness. This procedure was conducted with a file by a trained podiatrist. This mechanical debridement alone does not constitute an effective treatment, but it helps the laser penetrate under the nail plate to reach the fungal colonies of the nail bed and nail matrix.

2.6. Grading the Severity of Onychomycosis: Onychomycosis Severity Index. The Onychomycosis Severity Index (OSI) score is obtained by multiplying the score for the area of involvement with a range of 0–5 (1–10% is rated with 1, 11–25% with 2, 26–50% with 3, 51–75% with 4, and finally 76–100% with 5) by the score for the proximity of disease to the matrix with also a range of 1–5. Ten points are added for the presence of a longitudinal streak or a patch (dermatophytoma) or for greater than 2 mm of subungual hyperkeratosis. Mild onychomycosis corresponds to a score of 1 through 5; moderate, 6 through 15; and severe, 16 through 35. All patients were examined monthly for the evidence of proximal extension of the nail bed lesion. Any proximal extension of the lesion during treatment was a treatment failure [17, 18].

2.7. Laser Irradiation. The irradiation was performed with a Q-Switched Nd:YAG 1064 nm (Q-Clear, Light Age, Somerset, New Jersey, USA). Laser protocol was performed with 2.5 mm spot size and a power level of 4 which delivers 14 joules/cm^2, 9 billionths of a second pulse duration, and a 5 Hz frequency.

The second pass was done with the same laser operating at 532 nm Nd:YAG with the following parameters: 2.5 mm spot size and a power level of 4 which delivers 14 joules/cm^2, 9 billionths of a second pulse duration, and a 5 Hz frequency. No local anesthesia was applied preoperatively.

In one session two passes across each nail plate were performed with two minutes pauses between each pass. The first pass was performed with the 1064 nm Nd:YAG laser. Each nail was fully covered with a laser beam, including the areas of the hyponychium and the proximal and lateral nail folds. After a two minute intermission the second pass was performed with the 532 nm Nd:YAG, fully covering the nail plate but not the hyponychium and nail folds. All patients were also evaluated with posttreatment fungal cultures.

Postoperative analgesic treatment was not required. No prophylactic antibiotics or antivirals were given to any patient.

The full treatment consisted of two sessions executed on days 0 and 30. Nails were photographed with a high-resolution digital camera before treatment at day 0 (pretreatment photograph). Follow-up visits were done at day 30 (before the second session). Photographs were taken again using the same camera settings, with lighting and nail position at baseline and day 60.

3. Results

3.1. Clinical Onychomycosis Types. Patients had all four major clinical types of onychomycosis: distal subungual onychomycosis, proximal subungual onychomycosis, superficial white onychomycosis, or dystrophic type onychomycosis. Another group is onychomycosis that affects only the lateral edge. The clinical onychomycosis types separated by gender and age group are given in Table 1.

Distal subungual is the most common clinical type of onychomycosis among both genders and all age groups since it appears in 123 (93.9%) of the total patients, followed by lateral edge (in 47 patients (35.9%)), dystrophic type (in 13 or 9.9%), superficial white (in 2 patients or 1.5%), and, last, proximal subungual (in only 1 patient or 0.8%). Moreover, 94.7% of female patients, 91.9% of the males, 95% of patients under 30 years old, 93% between 30 and 60 years old, and 95.8% over 60 suffer from distal subungual. The corresponding counts and percents for the rest of the clinical types of onychomycosis may be seen in Table 1.

3.2. Fungus Types. The most frequent fungus found among treated patients was *T. rubrum* (in 108 patients or 82.3%), followed by *Candida* (in 19 patients 14.6%) and then *Trichophyton mentagrophytes* (in 4 patients 3.1%). Table 2 presents the types of fungi found in patient populations and their percentages. The fungus types can also be seen by patient's ages and genders.

3.3. Severity of Onychomycosis. Table 3 shows all patients according to onychomycosis severity.

Regarding the severity of onychomycosis, severe onychomycosis seems to be more frequent in men (78.4% versus 62.8%). A chi-square test for the differences between genders suggested that those differences are not statistically significant at any significance level ($\chi^2 = 3.681$, $P = 0.159$). We draw the same conclusions from a chi-square test for the differences in age ($\chi^2 = 3.002$, $P = 0.557$).

We also evaluated our patients according to great nail and/or multiple nail involvement (Table 4).

3.4. Mycologic Cure of Nail Fungal Infections. At 3-month follow-up 125 patients (95.42%) showed mycological cure (negative microscopy and culture). There was no treatment failure (proximal extension of the lesion during treatment). Clinical cure is associated with the alteration of percentages of disease-free nail. We find a change of >76% as excellent response, 51–75% as very good response, 26–50 as good response, 6–25% as moderate response, and >5% as low response to treatment.

It can be seen in Table 5 that the clinical type of onychomycosis seems to have an important influence on response: "distal subungual" had the best response followed by "lateral edge, dystrophic type, and superficial white"; however "proximal subungual" type showed the lowest response.

Dermatophytes (*T. rubrum*) seem to have the best response rate followed by *Trichophyton mentagrophytes* and *Candida* comes last. Paradoxically, *moderate* onychomycosis showed the best results, while *mild* is next and *severe* last.

The age group under 30 revealed the best results, additionally women showed the best response (Figures 1(a), 1(b), 2(a), 2(b), 3(a), 3(b), 4(a), 4(b), 5(a), 5(b), 6(a), 6(b), 7(a), and 7(b)).

Among the above differences, only three are statistically significant.

The following are the differences.

(i) Genders: women seem to be cured more effectively than men do at a 5% significance level ($f = 5.237$ and P-value = 0.024).

(ii) Severity of onychomycosis: mild severity patients are cured most effectively, followed by moderate severity and lastly severe severity patients at a 1% significance level ($f = 9.963$ and P-value = 0.00).

(iii) The responsible nail fungi: *T. rubrum* recedes more quickly after the cure, followed by *trichophyton mentagrophytes* and *Candida* at a 1% significance level ($f = 15.347$ and P-value = 0.00).

3.5. Adverse Event Evaluation. Most patients, 94 (83.21%), reported mild pain; 22 patients (16.79%) reported no pain. This "pain" sensation was described as "a stinging" during the 1064 nm pass and as "burning" during the 532 nm pass. None of the patients treated had severe or intolerable pain. No postoperative analgesic treatment was required. Interestingly many of patients developed a kind of pain resistance during the therapy, meaning they reported the highest level of pain

TABLE 1: Clinical onychomycosis types.

| Patients | Total | Distal subungual | Proximal subungual | Superficial white | Dystrophic type | Lateral edge |
	131 (100.0%)	123 (93.9%)	1 (0.8%)	2 (1.5%)	13 (9.9%)	47 (35.9%)
Gender						
Female	94 (71.8%)	89 (94.7%)	0 (0.0%)	2 (2.1%)	9 (9.6%)	26 (27.7%)
Male	37 (28.2%)	34 (91.9%)	1 (2.7%)	0 (0.0%)	4 (10.8%)	24 (56.8%)
Age group						
<30	20 (15.3%)	19 (95.0%)	0 (0.0%)	1 (5.0%)	4 (20.0%)	1 (5.0%)
30–60	86 (65.6%)	80 (93.0%)	0 (0.0%)	1 (1.2%)	7 (8.1%)	31 (36.0%)
>60	25 (18.3%)	23 (95.8%)	1 (2.7%)	0 (0.0%)	2 (8.3%)	14 (58.3%)

TABLE 2: Fungal culture results and distribution according to age and gender.

| Patients | Fungus type | | | |
| | Trichophyton rubrum | Candida | Trichophyton mentagrophytes | All types of onychomycosis |
	108 (82.3%)	19 (14.6%)	4 (3.1%)	131 (100.0%)
Gender				
Female	79 (84.0%)	12 (12.8%)	3 (3.2%)	94 (100.0%)
Male	29 (78.4%)	7 (18.9%)	1 (2.7%)	37 (100.0%)
Age Group				
<30	19 (95.0%)	1 (5.0%)	0 (0.0%)	20 (100.0%)
30–60	71 (82.6%)	12 (14.0%)	3 (3.5%)	86 (100.0%)
>60	17 (70.8%)	6 (25%)	1 (4.2%)	24 (100.0%)

TABLE 3: Onychomycosis severity index [15, 17] with age and gender relation.

| Patients | Mild (1–5) | Moderate (6–15) | Severe (16–30) |
	6 (4.6%)	37 (28.2%)	88 (67.2%)
Gender			
Female	4 (4.3%)	31 (33.0%)	59 (62.8%)
Male	2 (5.4%)	6 (16.2%)	29 (78.4%)
Age group			
<30	1 (5.0%)	5 (25.0%)	14 (70.0%)
30–60	5 (5.8%)	27 (31.4%)	54 (62.8%)
>60	0 (0.0%)	5 (20.8%)	19 (79.2%)

TABLE 4: Evaluation of patients to multiple nail involvements.

| Patients | Great nail involvement | Multiple nail involvement |
	74 (56.5%)	33 (25.2%)
Gender		
Female	58 (61.7%)	27 (28.7%)
Male	16 (43.2%)	6 (16.2%)
Age group		
<30 y.o	7 (35%)	5 (25.0%)
30–60	54 (62.8%)	23 (26.7%)
>60	12 (50%)	5 (20.8%)

during the first session. We believe this suggests the patients knew what to expect or that the fear of an unknown treatment no longer existed.

Patients were also asked to report all possible adverse events that could be related to our treatment. There were no reports of any other side effects.

4. Discussion

Treatment of onychomycosis is difficult. Laser treatment is considered by some authors to be a promising new method. Our study population comprised of 131 individuals. 15.3% of the participants in the study were below 30 years of age, 65.6% between 30 and 60 years, and finally 18.3%, were over 60 years old. These groups allowed us to maintain a large enough sample within each group to compare the effectiveness of the laser treatment on different age groups. Women were the 71.8% of our patient sample. This does not mean that onychomycosis occurs more frequently in women but that men may be more negligent in matters relating to the cosmetic appearance and hygiene of their feet.

In a recent paper Vural et al. showed that 1064 nm and 532 nm Q-Switched Nd:YAG laser systems had significant inhibitory effect upon *T. rubrum* isolates and caused colony growth inhibition in vitro [14]. It is well known that the efficacy of laser energy depends on the light-tissue interaction which is a function of wavelength, fluence, and tissue optics [7]. We have used various spot sizes in all power levels with our system. This can provide combinations which deliver different energy fluence. We found that the most powerful treatment was 14 joules/cm^2; additionally, the 7.5 joules/cm^2 (3.5 mm spot size and a power level of 4) was also effective. Since the treatment session is very well tolerated in the maximum energy fluence, we used these settings. We have noticed a significant improvement in the proximal

TABLE 5: Laser treatment response according to age, gender, type of fungi, clinical type of onychomycosis, and location.

Patients	Excellent response (>75%)	Very good response (50–74)	Good response (25–49)	Moderate response (10–24%)	Low response (>9%)	No response (0%)
Gender						
Female	10 (10.6%)	44 (46.8%)	25 (26.6%)	10 (10.6%)	0 (0.0%)	5 (5.3%)
Male	2 (5.4%)	9 (24.3%)	16 (43.2%)	9 (24.3%)	0 (0.0%)	1 (2.7%)
Age						
<30 y.o	3 (15.0%)	4 (20.0%)	10 (50.0%)	2 (10.0%)	0 (0.0%)	1 (5.0%)
30–60	9 (10.5%)	37 (43.0%)	24 (27.9%)	13 (15.1%)	0 (0.0%)	3 (3.5%)
>60	0 (0.0%)	12 (50.0%)	6 (25.0%)	4 (16.7%)	0 (0.0%)	2 (8.3%)
Onychomycosis severity						
Mild	3 (50.0%)	2 (33.3%)	1 (16.7%)	0 (0.0%)	0 (0.0%)	0 (0.0%)
Moderate	5 (13.5%)	23 (62.2%)	9 (24.3%)	0 (0.0%)	0 (0.0%)	0 (0.0%)
Severe	4 (4.5%)	28 (31.8%)	31 (35.2%)	19 (21.6%)	0 (0.0%)	6 (6.8%)
Types of fungi						
T. rubrum	10 (9.3%)	51 (47.2%)	38 (35.2%)	8 (7.4%)	0 (0.0%)	1 (0.9%)
Candida	1 (5.3%)	1 (5.3%)	3 (15.8%)	10 (52.6%)	0 (0.0%)	4 (21.1%)
Non dermatophytes	1 (25.0%)	1 (25.0%)	0 (0.0%)	1	0 (0.0%)	1 (25.0%)
T. mentographytes	9 (9.4%)	48 (50.0%)	35 (36.5%)	4 (4.2%)	0 (0.0%)	0 (0.0%)
Clinical type of onychomycosis						
Distal subungual	9 (7.3%)	50 (40.7%)	40 (32.5%)	18 (14.6%)	0 (0.0%)	6 (4.9%)
Proximal subungual	0 (0.0%)	1 (100.0%)	0 (0.0%)	0 (0.0%)	0 (0.0%)	0 (0.0%)
Superficial white	1 (50.0%)	0 (0.0%)	0 (0.0%)	1 (50.0%)	0 (0.0%)	0 (0.0%)
Dystrophic	2 (4.3%)	14 (29.8%)	17 (36.2%)	11 (23.4%)	0 (0.0%)	3 (6.4%)
Lateral edge	2 (4.3%)	5 (38.5%)	5 (38.5%)	0 (0.0%)	0 (0.0%)	1 (7.7%)
Location						
Hand	0 (0.0%)	1 (9.1%)	3 (27.3%)	6 (54.5%)	0 (0.0%)	1 (9.1%)
Feet	9 (9.9%)	38 (41.8%)	27 (29.7%)	14 (15.4%)	0 (0.0%)	3 (3.3%)

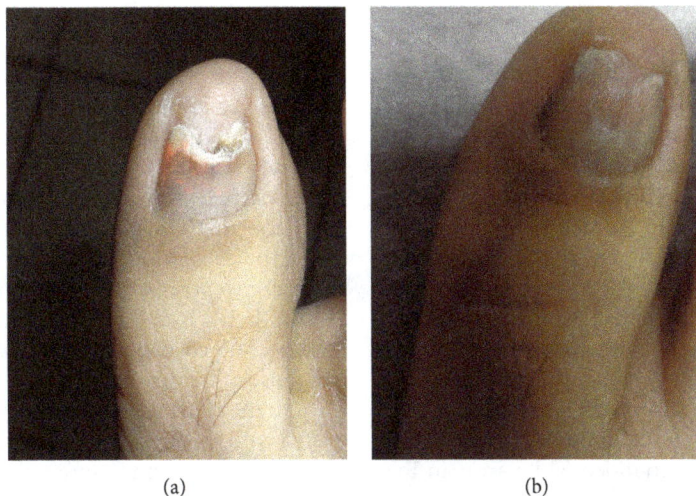

(a)   (b)

FIGURE 1: (a) 68-year-old female patient, before treatment. *Trichophyton rubrum* was isolated on mycological testing. Onychomycosis severity index (OSI) was 16. (b) After treatment with good improvement. OSI is 6 showing 69.5% improvement.

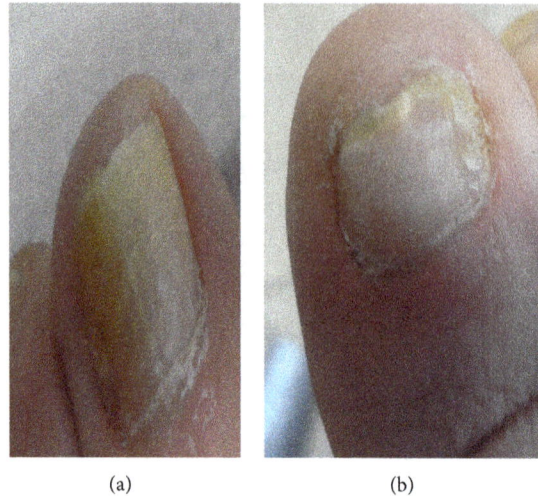

FIGURE 2: (a) 64-year-old female patient before treatment. *Trichophyton rubrum* was isolated on mycological testing. OSI is 26. (b) After treatment with great improvement. OSI is 9 showing 65.38% improvement.

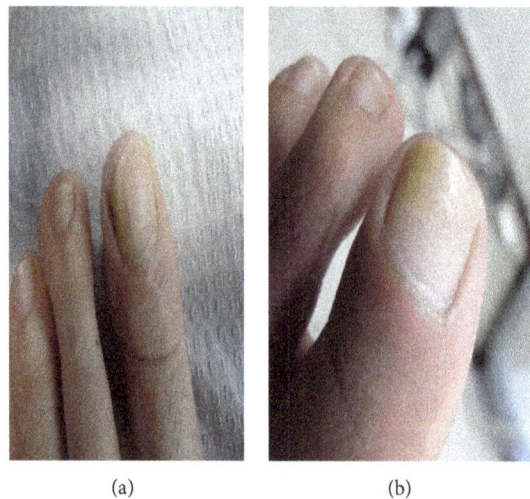

FIGURE 3: (a) 48-year-old female patient before treatment. *Trichophyton rubrum* was isolated on mycological testing. OSI was 9. (b) After treatment with great improvement. OSI is 2, showing 77.78% improvement.

portion of the nail where there was mild initial mycotic involvement. Our results were better especially in moderate severity patients. That seems reasonable as severe cases are accompanied by dermatophytoma or significant subungual hyperkeratosis, which require more time for the nail plate to restore. Poor prognostic indicators are the total dystrophic onychomycosis, the involvement of the lateral edge of the nail plate, and the involvement of the matrix [18–21]. The thick plate or subungual hyperkeratosis >2 mm histologically contains numerous air-filled spaces in which fungal spores can survive for weeks or months. These resting arthrospores do not form hyphae, so various antifungal agents have proven ineffective. This phenomenon, termed as dermatophytoma, can be seen as linear streaks or rounded white areas in the nail plate. The fungal elements are believed to be forming a biofilm, making them refractory to therapy [15, 22, 23]. Laser therapy seems not to be affected of this biofilm formation;

this may explain why we achieved very good and good response in 67% of our severe cases. Moreover, old age, presence of immunosuppression, poor peripheral circulation and nonresponsive organisms (nondermatophyte molds), other dermatoses (e.g., nail psoriasis), and drug resistance are poor prognostic indicators [15, 23, 24]. With the laser we solve the problem of resistance. We suggest that we do not have nonresponsive cases but some poor responding fungi. As another example, occupational factors, as well as occlusive and prolonged contact with water, can contribute to poor response of treatment [21].

On the contrary, superficial white onychomycosis is associated with the best therapeutic response to antifungal drugs, and our results seem to agree with this [16, 19]. Our distal subungual clinical cases had good results as well. Even dystrophic types showed a very good and good response in 66% of the cases. This supports laser treatment efficacy. Laser treatment

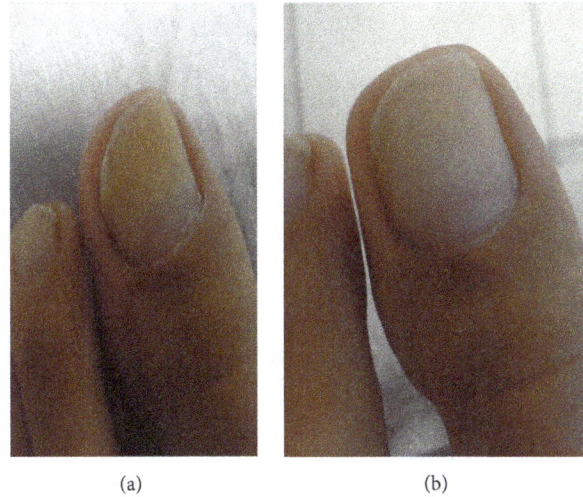

FIGURE 4: (a) 28-year-old female patient before treatment. *Trichophyton rubrum* was isolated on mycological testing. OSI was 12. (b) After treatment with great improvement. OSI is 1, showing 91.67% improvement.

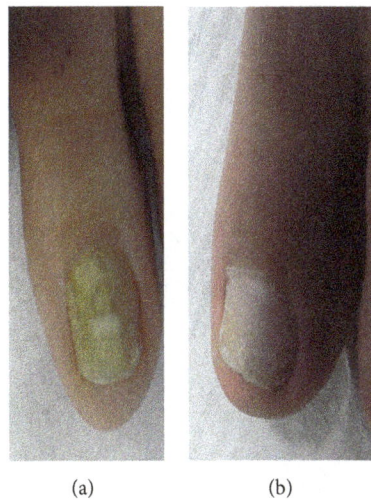

FIGURE 5: (a) 60-year-old female patient, before treatment. *Verticillium sp.* was isolated on mycological testing. OSI was 30. (b) After treatment with great improvement. OSI is 4 showing 86.67% improvement.

seems to outweigh classical treatments where involvement of the matrix, a thick plate, or subungual hyperkeratosis >2 mm are factors associated with poor outcome [15, 21].

The Q-Clear Laser System, in differentiation to other laser treatments, provides a selective, both thermal (photothermolytic) and mechanical (photomechanical), effect on the fungi. The mechanism of this fungal destruction may offer some differences. The inhibitory effect is likely due to more than simple nonspecific thermal damage. Denaturing one or more of the molecules within the pathogen may deactivate the fungi. Vural et al. discusses that 532 nm setting, which is well absorbed by red pigment in canthomegnin in *T. rubrum*, this wavelength generates mechanical damage in the irradiated fungal colony [14].

The 1064 nm setting is beyond the absorption spectrum of xanthomegnin, but its effectiveness is due to another absorbing chromophore, perhaps melanin, which is present in the fungal cell wall [14]. Melanin is an essential inhabitant of the fungal cell wall and has been described in many pathogenic species. The type of melanin varies, although it is commonly Dopa or pentaketide melanin. Moreover, the laser beam may initiate a photobiological or photochemical reaction that attacks the pathogen cell. We can also suggest a multiphoton dielectric breakdown at the fungal target as the cause of their destruction, while depth-selective thermal effects by the laser could also be occurring [7].

Another possible scenario is by inducing an immune response that attacks the organism. All of the above hypotheses explain how the surrounding host tissue cells are protected from this attack, with little or no collateral damage. The amount of energy delivered by our treatment session may serve as a deactivating dose. That amount of energy can

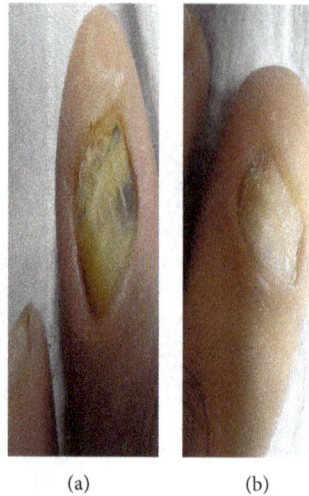

FIGURE 6: (a) 32-year-old male patient, before treatment. *Trichophyton rubrum* was isolated on mycological testing. OSI was 35. (b) After treatment with great improvement. OSI is 12 showing 65.71% improvement.

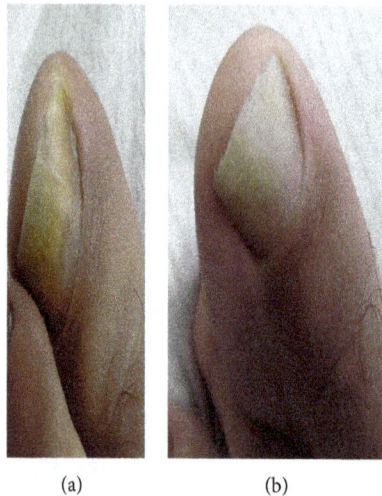

FIGURE 7: (a) 58-year-old male patient, before treatment. *Trichophyton rubrum* was isolated on mycological testing. OSI was 30. (b) After treatment with great improvement. OSI is 9 showing 70.00% improvement.

deactivate 80–99% of the organisms present in an affected nail without instantly killing the fungal colonies but it can disable their ability to replicate or survive according to an apoptotic mechanism. Apoptosis, a physiological type of cell death, plays an important role in the selective deletion of cells in divergent situations of various tissues [25]. Induced apoptosis may cause direct DNA damage, for example, strand breaks, chromosomal aberrations, induction by transduced signals, for example, FAS/APO-1 transmembrane signals, and stress (heat) mediated death. Hyperthermia, a typical environmental stress, has long been known as toxic to cells. It has been recognized the mode of cell killing to be influenced by the severity of the heat treatment [26]. A number of reports have been published to demonstrate the induction of apoptosis by mild hyperthermia [27, 28].

We are waiting to assess our results following twelve months since the completion of treatment, which is the time required for complete regeneration of the nail plate.

Additionally, we will follow the patients at greater time intervals to assess the occurrence of relapse. Zaias et al. recommended that the treatment of onychomycosis with oral antifungals should be continued until the mycotic nail bed had been completely replaced by a new mycotic bed (that requires about 12 months for toenails). With this treatment the authors achieved significantly better cure rates [18]. It may be that this maintenance therapy will provide a safety net for those at risk of relapse after the discontinuation of laser treatments.

In contrast to our results, recently Carney et al. evaluated thermal response and optical effects of a submillisecond neodymium: yttrium-aluminum-garnet (Nd:YAG) 1064 nm laser on common fungal nail pathogens and the clinical efficacy and safety laser of onychomycotic toenails. A fungicidal effect for *T. rubrum* was seen at 50°C after 15 minutes and for Epidermophyton floccosum at 50°C after 10 minutes. No inhibition was observed after laser treatment of fungal colonies or suspensions. In vivo treatment of toenails showed no improvement in Onychomycosis Severity Index score. They discussed that laser treatment of onychomycosis was not related to thermal damage or direct laser effects [29].

Similarly Hees et al. were also unable to show the effect of Nd:YAG laser on *T. rubrum* colonies. They assumed that the effect could be due to unspecific tissue heating with a subsequent increase in circulation and stimulation of immunologic process. They also discussed the associated risks of laser treatment with the use of higher densities [30]. Laser systems vary widely and it is understandable that there are differing results. The Q-Clear's 1064/532 nm wavelengths and unique time-structured pulse profile specifically target the fungal elements, inducing a progressive and eventually lethal temperature increase. At the same time the low-absorption, high water content tissues (dermal), and vascular flow, allow rapid dissipation of absorbed energy, thus "antitargeting" the nail bed and other dermal tissues.

Competing "long pulse" systems presumably relay on bulk heating of fungal colonies in situ on the nail bed with the associated discomfort which necessitate multiple treatments and a high treatment failure rate. Some of the papers in the literature calling laser a failure were also only Petri dish studies which cannot replicate these in vitro applications.

Although some studies have yielded conflicting results, other studies like ours have shown some promise [31–34].

Zhang et al. had satisfactory results with the Nd:YAG without significant complications. They discussed that the thicker the nail plates the higher the laser energy needed to be. Different fungal strains may also have different sensitivities [32]. Hochman [33] and Bornstein et al. [34] described the formation of free radicals as well as the influence of the laser on cellular reaction. These results support our study.

Finally, we find the treatment of onychomycosis with this specific Q-Switched Nd:YAG, 1064 nm/532 nm laser in vivo as extremely promising and efficient. In addition, laser-based treatments have the advantage of a regimen that is devoid of mutagenic and genotoxic effects. They could be combined with systemic oral antifungals providing the benefit of limiting treatment time.

4.1. Weaknesses of the Research. Whereas the present study demonstrates the efficacy of the specific laser in the treatment of onychomycosis, we should keep in mind that negative cultures, that is, mycological cure, do not always constitute proof of clinical cure due to the well-known high rate of false-negative culture results.

Conflict of Interests

The authors declare that they have no conflict of interests.

Authors' Contribution

Kostas Kalokasidis, Myrto-Georgia Trakatelli, and Bertrand Richert performed this clinical trial. Meltem Onder and Klaus Fritz did scientific evaluation.

References

[1] M. A. Ghannoum, R. A. Hajjeh, R. Scher et al., "A large-scale North American study of fungal isolates from nails: the frequency of onychomycosis, fungal distribution, and antifungal susceptibility patterns," *Journal of the American Academy of Dermatology*, vol. 43, no. 4, pp. 641–648, 2000.

[2] A. K. Gupta and S. Humke, "The prevalence and management of onychomycosis in diabetic patients," *European Journal of Dermatology*, vol. 10, no. 5, pp. 379–384, 2000.

[3] D. T. Roberts, "Prevalence of dermatophyte onychomycosis in the United Kingdom: results of an omnibus survey," *British Journal of Dermatology, Supplement*, vol. 126, supplement 39, pp. 23–27, 1992.

[4] B. S. Schlefman, "Onychomycosis: a compendium of facts and a clinical experience," *Journal of Foot and Ankle Surgery*, vol. 38, no. 4, pp. 290–302, 1999.

[5] J. C. Szepietowski and A. Reich, "Stigmatisation in onychomycosis patients: a population-based study," *Mycoses*, vol. 52, no. 4, pp. 343–349, 2009.

[6] J. C. Szepietowski, A. Reich, P. Pacan, E. Garlowska, and E. Baran, "Evaluation of quality of life in patients with toenail onychomycosis by Polish version of an international onychomycosis-specific questionnaire," *Journal of the European Academy of Dermatology and Venereology*, vol. 21, no. 4, pp. 491–496, 2007.

[7] Z. Manevitch, D. Lev, M. Hochberg, M. Palhan, A. Lewis, and C. D. Enk, "Direct antifungal effect of femtosecond laser on trichophyton rubrum Onychomycosis," *Photochemistry and Photobiology*, vol. 86, no. 2, pp. 476–479, 2010.

[8] E. M. Warshaw, "Evaluating costs for onychomycosis treatments: a practitioner's perspective," *Journal of the American Podiatric Medical Association*, vol. 96, no. 1, pp. 38–52, 2006.

[9] A. Tosti, B. M. Piraccini, C. Stinchi, and M. D. Colombo, "Relapses of onychomycosis alter successful treatment with systemic antifungals: a three-year follow-up," *Dermatology*, vol. 197, no. 2, pp. 162–166, 1998.

[10] B. Sigurgeirsson, J. H. Ólafsson, J. P. Steinsson, C. Paul, S. Billstein, and E. G. Evans, "Long-term effectiveness of treatment with terbinafine versus itraconazole in onychomycosis: a 5-year blinded prospective follow-up study," *Archives of Dermatology*, vol. 138, no. 3, pp. 353–357, 2002.

[11] H. Jelinkova, T. Dostalova, J. Duskova et al., "Er: YAG and alexandrite laser radiation propagation in root canal and its effect on bacteria," *Journal of Clinical Laser Medicine and Surgery*, vol. 17, no. 6, pp. 267–272, 1999.

[12] J. Frucht-Pery, M. Mor, R. Evron, A. Lewis, and H. Zauberman, "The effect of the ArF excimer laser on Candida albicans in vitro," *Graefe's Archive for Clinical and Experimental Ophthalmology*, vol. 231, no. 7, pp. 413–415, 1993.

[13] R. H. Keates, P. C. Drago, and E. J. Rothchild, "Effect of excimer laser on microbiological organisms," *Ophthalmic Surgery*, vol. 19, no. 10, pp. 715–718, 1988.

[14] E. Vural, H. L. Winfield, A. W. Shingleton, T. D. Horn, and G. Shafirstein, "The effects of laser irradiation on Trichophyton rubrum growth," *Lasers in Medical Science*, vol. 23, no. 4, pp. 349–353, 2008.

[15] R. K. Scher, A. Tavakkol, B. Sigurgeirsson et al., "Onychomycosis: diagnosis and definition of cure," *Journal of the American Academy of Dermatology*, vol. 56, no. 6, pp. 939–944, 2007.

[16] C. Grover and A. Khurana, "An update on treatment of onychomycosis," *Mycoses*, vol. 55, pp. 541–551, 2012.

[17] C. Carney, A. Tosti, R. Daniel et al., "A new classification system for grading the severity of onychomycosis: onychomycosis severity index," *Archives of Dermatology*, vol. 147, no. 11, pp. 1277–1282, 2011.

[18] N. Zaias, G. Rebell, M. N. Zaiac, and B. Glick, "Onychomycosis treated until the nail is replaced by normal growth or there is failure," *Archives of Dermatology*, vol. 136, no. 7, p. 940, 2000.

[19] M. Lecha, I. Effendy, M. F. de Chauvin, N. Di Chiacchio, and R. Baran, "Treatment options: development of consensus guidelines," *Journal of the European Academy of Dermatology and Venereology*, vol. 19, supplement 1, pp. 25–33, 2005.

[20] R. Baran and P. de Doncker, "Lateral edge nail involvement indicates poor prognosis for treating onychomycosis with the new systemic antifungals," *Acta Dermato-Venereologica*, vol. 76, no. 1, pp. 82–83, 1996.

[21] R. K. Scher and R. Baran, "Onychomycosis in clinical practice: factors contributing to recurrence," *British Journal of Dermatology, Supplement*, vol. 149, supplement 65, pp. 5–9, 2003.

[22] C. N. Burkhart, C. G. Burkhart, and A. K. Gupta, "Dermatophytoma: recalcitrance to treatment because of existence of fungal biofilm," *Journal of the American Academy of Dermatology*, vol. 47, no. 4, pp. 629–631, 2002.

[23] A. K. Gupta, C. Drummond-Main, E. A. Cooper, W. Brintnell, B. M. Piraccini, and A. Tosti, "Systematic review of non-dermatophyte mold onychomycosis: diagnosis, clinical types, epidemiology, and treatment," *Journal of the American Academy of Dermatology*, vol. 66, no. 3, pp. 494–502, 2012.

[24] E. Sarifakioglu, D. Seçkin, M. Demirbilek, and F. Can, "In vitro antifungal susceptibility patterns of dermatophyte strains causing tinea unguium," *Clinical and Experimental Dermatology*, vol. 32, no. 6, pp. 675–679, 2007.

[25] E. White, "Life, death, and the pursuit of apoptosis," *Genes and Development*, vol. 10, no. 1, pp. 1–15, 1996.

[26] E. P. Armour, D. McEachern, Z. Wang, P. M. Corry, and A. Martinez, "Sensitivity of human cells to mild hyperthermia," *Cancer Research*, vol. 53, no. 12, pp. 2740–2744, 1993.

[27] E. Cuende, J. E. Ales-Martinez, L. Ding, M. Gonzalez-Garcia, -A. C. Martinez, and G. Nunez, "Programmed cell death by bcl-2-dependent and independent mechanisms in B lymphoma cells," *The EMBO Journal*, vol. 12, no. 4, pp. 1555–1560, 1993.

[28] G. Deng and E. R. Podack, "Suppression of apoptosis in a cytotoxic T-cell line by interleukin 2- mediated gene transcription and deregulated expression of the protooncogene bcl-2," *Proceedings of the National Academy of Sciences of the United States of America*, vol. 90, no. 6, pp. 2189–2193, 1993.

[29] C. Carney, W. Cantrell, J. Warner, and B. Elewski, "Treatment of onychomycosis using a submillisecond 1064-nm neodymium: yttrium-aluminum-garnet laser," *Journal of the American Academy of Dermatology*, vol. 69, no. 4, pp. 578–582, 2013.

[30] H. Hees, C. Raulin, and W. Bäumler, "Laser treatment of onychomycosis: an in vitro pilot study," *Journal der Deutschen Dermatologischen Gesellschaft*, vol. 10, no. 12, pp. 913–918, 2012.

[31] J. A. Ledon, J. Savas, K. Franca, A. Chacon, and K. Nouri, "Laser and light therapy for onychomycosis: a systematic review," *Lasers in Medical Science*, vol. 69, no. 4, pp. 578–582, 2013.

[32] R. N. Zhang, D. K. Wang, F. L. Zhuo, X. H. Duan, X. Y. Zhang, and J. Y. Zhao, "Long-pulse Nd: YAG, 1064-nm laser treatment for onychomycosis," *Chinese Medical Journal*, vol. 125, no. 18, pp. 3288–3291, 2012.

[33] L. G. Hochman, "Laser treatment of onychomycosis using a novel 0.65-millisecond pulsed Nd:YAG 1064-nm laser," *Journal of Cosmetic and Laser Therapy*, vol. 13, no. 1, pp. 2–5, 2011.

[34] E. Bornstein, W. Hermans, S. Gridley, and J. Manni, "Near-infrared photoinactivation of bacteria and fungi at physiologic temperatures," *Photochemistry and Photobiology*, vol. 85, no. 6, pp. 1364–1374, 2009.

28

Leprosy Continues to Occur in Hilly Areas of North India

Deepak Dimri,[1] Arti Gupta,[2] and Amit Kumar Singh[2]

[1]*Department of Dermatology, Veer Chandra Singh Garhwali Government Medical Science and Research Institute, Uttarakhand 246174, India*
[2]*Department of Community Medicine, Veer Chandra Singh Garhwali Government Medical Science and Research Institute, Uttarakhand 246174, India*

Correspondence should be addressed to Deepak Dimri; drdeepakdimri19@gmail.com

Academic Editor: Giuseppe Stinco

Background. The aim of present study was to describe the profile of leprosy patients attending the outpatient department of dermatology in tertiary care hospital in Srinagar, Uttarakhand, North India. *Methodology.* This descriptive retrospective study. Patient data at the time of diagnosis were retrieved onto a predesigned proforma, which concerned the following variables at the time of registration: age, sex, and residence. Newly registered outpatients leprosy cases between 2009 and 2014 were included in the study. *Results.* It was found that 65 were multibacillary leprosy cases. Males constituted 62.8% of all leprosy cases. The majority (83.7%) belonged to the age group of 18–60 years. Of the total 48.8% of the new leprosy cases were from the Pauri district. The leprosy incidence rate in this population was 2.71 per 1000 patients. *Conclusion.* Leprosy still continues to be a communicable disease of concern. The lower incidence in women and children provokes the need to strengthen contact screening, early case detection, and referral activities in the population to sustain elimination.

1. Introduction

Hansen's disease, commonly known as leprosy, is a chronic, granulomatous, infectious disease that primarily affects the skin and the peripheral nerves [1]. Leprosy was eliminated as a public health problem from world in 2000 and from India in December 2005 with prevalence rate less than 1 per 10,000 population [2]. According to World Health Organization, the registered prevalence globally at the beginning of 2012 was 181 941 [3]. Leprosy, although quite rare, continues to occur. In India, a total of 1.27 Lakhs new cases were detected during the year 2013-14, which gives Annual New Case Detection Rate of 9.98 per 100,000 population. The prevalence rate of leprosy in India was 0.68 per 10,000 population with 0.86 Lakhs cases on record as on 1st April 2014 [4]. Also studies have reported discordance between NLEP figures and those reported by dermatologists [5].

The foundation for leprosy elimination was the introduction of antibacterial dapsone monotherapy. The World Health Organization (WHO) introduced multidrug therapy in 1981 due to dapsone resistance. Multidrug therapy since its introduction has not changed except for duration of treatment, which is 1 year in multibacillary cases and continues to be 6 months in paucibacillary cases of leprosy [2]. Adequate and timely treatment of leprosy is critical as it is an important cause of preventable disability [6]. There are gray areas in leprosy elimination as the new cases constantly occur across the country. With the above thought, the aim of this study was to describe the profile of leprosy patients attending the outpatient department in tertiary care hospital in Srinagar, Uttarakhand, North India.

2. Materials and Methods

This descriptive retrospective study was conducted at the Medical College Hospital, VCSG Government Medical Sciences and Research Institute, Uttarakhand, which is tertiary care teaching hospital in Northern India. Medical records of all leprosy cases registered by self-reporting between 2009

TABLE 1: Demographic profile of new cases of leprosy in a tertiary care hospital in Srinagar, Garhwal, North India (2009–2014).

Characteristic	Category	Number of cases (%)
Age group	0–18 years	9 (6.9)
	19–60 years	108 (83.7)
	>60 years	12 (9.4)
Sex	Female	48 (37.2)
	Male	81 (62.8)
District	Pauri	63 (48.8)
	Rudraprayag	16 (12.4)
	Chamoli	6 (4.6)
	Tehri	6 (4.6)
	Others	38 (29.6)
Total		129 (100)

TABLE 2: Observed incidence rates of leprosy per 1000 patient by sex and age in a tertiary care hospital in Srinagar, Garhwal, North India (2009–2014).

Age category (years)	Total new cases		New leprosy cases		Incidence rate per 1000 patient		
	Female	Male	Female	Male	Female	Male	Total
<18	4065	5002	5	4	1.23	0.79	0.99
18–60	17789	17569	41	67	2.30	3.8	3.05
>60	1199	1841	2	10	1.66	5.43	3.94

and March 2014 were retrospectively assessed. All cases registered received WHO recommended fixed duration multidrug therapy. The WHO classification of dividing leprosy into PB (≤5 lesions) and MB (>5 lesions) was used to make the diagnosis [7]. In the present the study the number of MB cases was estimated using the Uttarakhand state data of leprosy [4]. Patient data at the time of diagnosis were retrieved onto a predesigned proforma, which concerned the following variables at the time of registration: age, sex, and residence. Newly registered outpatients leprosy cases between 2009 and 2014 were included in the study. Data were entered in Microsoft excel spreadsheet and analysed with SPSS version 17.0 (Chicago, IL, USA). Descriptive analysis was done. Patients less than 18 years of age were considered as children, and proportions were given wherever necessary.

3. Results

A total of 47465 new patients were examined between 2009 and 2014 in outpatient department of dermatology in medical college hospital of VCSG Government Medical Sciences and Research Institute. Of the total 129 new cases of leprosy were detected during the year 2009–14. Of the total, 65 were multibacillary leprosy cases. Males constituted 62.8% of all leprosy cases. Of the total 129 new leprosy cases registered in the institute between 2009 and 2014, 9 were child cases up to 18 years of age. The average child proportion over a period of 5 years was 6.9%. The majority (83.7%) belonged to the age group of 18–60 years. The youngest diseased child was in 7–12 years of age. Nearly half (48.8%) of the new leprosy cases were from the Pauri district (Table 1). The leprosy incidence rate in this population was 2.71 per 1000 person years.

TABLE 3: Observed incidence rates of leprosy per 1000 patient by district in a tertiary care hospital in Srinagar, Garhwal, North India (2009–2014).

District	Total new case	New leprosy cases	Incidence rate per 1000 patient
Pauri	23527	63	2.67
Rudraprayag	2314	16	6.91
Chamoli	1119	6	5.36
Tehri	2453	6	2.44
Others	18052	38	2.11
Total	47465	129	2.71

The increase in incidence rate with age reflects the age structure of the population. In addition, the relative increase of incidence rate contributed to by young adults, in particular males, reflects their tendency to seek health care easily compared to women and children in hilly terrains. A total of 9 child cases were recorded in less than 18 years of age, indicating the incidence rate of leprosy among children as 0.99/1,000 patient (Table 2). The incidence rate of leprosy among patient by residence shows the increase in incidence rate with distance travelled (Table 3).

4. Discussion

The overall observed incidence rate of leprosy among patient attending outpatient department during the study period was 2.71 per 1000. The prevalence rate of leprosy in Uttarakhand as on March 2014 was 0.22 per 10,000 population. The annual new case detection rate in Uttarakhand as in March 2014

TABLE 4: Statistics of leprosy in Uttarakhand as in March 2014 [4] compared with present study.

S. no.	Variable	Uttarakhand (as in March 2014) [4]	Present study (2009–14)
1	Total population (n)	10663516	47465*
2	Total no. of districts (n)	13	5
3	Total cases of leprosy (n)	237	129
4	Proportion of multibacillary cases (%)	119	65
5	Annual new case detection rate per 10000 population	3.53	5.4

*Patients.

was 3.53 per 10,000 population. The present study reported higher incidence rate of leprosy compared to leprosy data of Uttarakhand. The major reason been the present study is a hospital based study (Table 4) [4].

A male preponderance was seen in our study. This was comparable to other studies. The primary reasons for males preponderance were their greater outdoor activity and increased opportunities for health care [1, 8, 9]. The proportion of new child cases of leprosy in present study was less than 10% of new caseload. Majority of pediatric cases of leprosy in our study belonged to the older age group that is above 12 years. Other studies from Delhi, Andhra Pradesh, Karnataka, and Maharashtra also reported a lesser occurrence in children less than 5 years [8–11]. Similar was the finding of a hospital based study conducted in Nepal [12].

The incidence rate by age, sex, and residence illustrates that each of these factors is an important determinant of leprosy risk. The incidence of leprosy was more prevalent among adults than among younger individuals in present study. The high incidence rates among older adults may be interpreted in various ways. It reflects stable incidence rate in the population for several years prior to this study. Moreover, it could be that individuals were infected late in life or incubation periods were very long. In addition, the incidence rates were higher among males than females over 18 years of age. This was contrary to a population-based study in Malawi where the children and females were found to have higher incidence of leprosy [13]. Alternatively, if incidence rates had been declining in the population for many years, the observed high incidence rates among older adults would be attributable to infections contracted many years previously when transmission of *M. leprae* was more intense than at the time of these surveys. There are no data from the past allowing us to discriminate between these explanations. In addition, the shift in new leprosy case detection towards older ages had occurred over time in Norway [14].

The present study found the increase in incidence rate with distance travelled. Primary reason for this increase of incidence rate can be due to lower number of all patients from distant areas. Other causes are due to low income, lack of knowledge, difficult terrains, and lack of proper transport; sick population of difficult terrain do not visit private health institutions for their medical treatment [15, 16].

The present study was conducted at one tertiary health care setting in North India and hence it cannot be generalised to whole of India. Though the profile was stratified by age and sex, it was not possible to classify on socioeconomic structure and clinical and microbiological features. A relatively long incubation period of leprosy and the chances of misdiagnosing indeterminate skin patches in the initial stages may lead to misclassification of cases.

5. Conclusion

Leprosy still continues to be a communicable disease of concern. Our study reports the epidemiology of leprosy in tertiary care hospital. The lower incidence in women and children provokes the need to strengthen contact screening, early case detection, and referral activities in the population to sustain elimination.

Abbreviations

NLEP: National Leprosy Elimination Programme
MB: Multibacillary
PB: Paucibacillary.

Conflict of Interests

The authors declare that there is no conflict of interests regarding the publication of this paper.

References

[1] S. Thakkar and S. Patel, "Clinical profile of leprosy patients: a prospective study," *Indian Journal of Dermatology*, vol. 59, no. 2, pp. 158–162, 2014.

[2] S. Dogra, T. Narang, and B. Kumar, "Leprosy—evolution of the path to eradication," *Indian Journal of Medical Research*, vol. 137, no. 1, pp. 15–35, 2013.

[3] World Health Organization, "Global leprosy situation, 2012," *Weekly Epidemiological Record*, vol. 87, no. 34, pp. 317–328, 2012.

[4] National Leprosy Eradication Programme (NLEP), *Progress Report for the Year 2013-14*, Central Leprosy Division, Directorate General of Health Services, New Delhi, India, 2015, http://nlep.nic.in/pdf/Progress%20report%2031st%20March%202013-14.pdf.

[5] S. Arora, S. Baveja, A. Sood, and G. Arora, "Containing leprosy: current epidemiological status, detection and management strategies, and experiences at a tertiary level center," *Astrocyte*, vol. 1, no. 1, pp. 23–27, 2014.

[6] I. S. Ukpe, "A Study of health workers' knowledge and practises regarding leprosy care and control at primary care clinics in Eerstehoek area of Gert Sibande district in Mpumalanga Province, South Africa," *South African Family Practice*, vol. 48, no. 5, p. 16, 2006.

[7] World Health Organization, "Chemotherapy of leprosy for control programmes," WHO Tech Rep Ser 675, WHO, Geneva, Switzerland, 1982.

[8] C. Grover, S. Nanda, V. K. Garg, and B. S. N. Reddy, "An epidemiologic study of childhood leprosy from Delhi," *Pediatric Dermatology*, vol. 22, no. 5, pp. 489–490, 2005.

[9] S. Jain, R. G. Reddy, S. N. Osmani, D. N. J. Lockwood, and S. Suneetha, "Childhood leprosy in an urban clinic, Hyderabad, India: clinical presentation and the role of household contacts," *Leprosy Review*, vol. 73, no. 3, pp. 248–253, 2002.

[10] V. P. Shetty, U. H. Thakar, E. D'Souza et al., "Detection of previously undetected leprosy cases in a defined rural and urban area of Maharashtra, Western India," *Leprosy Review*, vol. 80, no. 1, pp. 22–33, 2009.

[11] P. Chaitra and R. M. Bhat, "Postelimination status of childhood leprosy: report from a tertiary-care hospital in South India," *BioMed Research International*, vol. 2013, Article ID 328673, 4 pages, 2013.

[12] K. D. Burman, A. Rijal, S. Agrawal, A. Agarwalla, and K. K. Verma, "Childhood leprosy in Eastern Nepal: a hospital-based study," *Indian Journal of Leprosy*, vol. 75, no. 1, pp. 47–52, 2003.

[13] J. M. Ponnighaus, P. E. M. Fine, J. A. C. Sterne et al., "Incidence rates of leprosy in Karonga District, northern Malawi: patterns by age, sex, BCG status and classification," *International Journal of Leprosy and Other Mycobacterial Diseases*, vol. 62, no. 1, pp. 10–23, 1994.

[14] A. Meimaa, L. M. Irgensb, G. J. van Oortmarssen, J. H. Richardusa, and J. D. F. Habbemaa, "Disappearance of leprosy from Norway: an exploration of critical factors using an epidemiological modelling approach," *International Journal of Epidemiology*, vol. 31, no. 5, pp. 991–1000, 2002.

[15] D. B. Karki, H. Dixit, and A. Neopane, "Medical camps and their usefulness," *Kathmandu University Medical journal*, vol. 3, no. 12, pp. 449–450, 2005.

[16] B. Venkatashivareddy, A. Gupta, and A. K. Singh, "Health camp profile and its cost in Hilly terrains, North India," *Clinical Epidemiology and Global Health*, vol. 3, supplement 1, pp. S101–S106, 2015.

29

Macular Amyloidosis and Epstein-Barr Virus

Yalda Nahidi,[1] **Naser Tayyebi Meibodi,**[1] **Zahra Meshkat,**[2] **and Narges Nazeri**[3]

[1]*Skin Research Center, School of Medicine, Mashhad University of Medical Sciences, Mashhad 9176699199, Iran*
[2]*Virology Research Center, School of Medicine, Mashhad University of Medical Sciences, Mashhad 9176699199, Iran*
[3]*Pathology Department of Mashhad University of Medical Sciences, Mashhad 9176699199, Iran*

Correspondence should be addressed to Naser Tayyebi Meibodi; naser_tayyebi@yahoo.com

Academic Editor: Jag Bhawan

Background. Amyloidosis is extracellular precipitation of eosinophilic hyaline material of self-origin with special staining features and fibrillar ultrastructure. Macular amyloidosis is limited to the skin, and several factors have been proposed for its pathogenesis. Detection of Epstein-Barr virus (EBV) DNA in this lesion suggests that this virus can play a role in pathogenesis of this disease. *Objective.* EBV DNA detection was done on 30 skin samples with a diagnosis of macular amyloidosis and 31 healthy skin samples in the margin of removed melanocytic nevi by using PCR. *Results.* In patients positive for beta-globin gene in PCR, BLLF1 gene of EBV virus was positive in 23 patients (8 patients in case and 15 patients in the control group). There was no significant difference in presence of EBV DNA between macular amyloidosis (3.8%) and control (23.8%) groups ($P = 0.08$). *Conclusion.* The findings of this study showed that EBV is not involved in pathogenesis of macular amyloidosis.

1. Introduction

Amyloidosis is the extracellular deposition of a group of fibrous proteins. There is a variety of approaches for classification of amyloidosis, but the simplest method is division into systemic and organ-specific (localized) types. Skin is an involved tissue in both types. Cutaneous localized amyloidosis is of two types: (i) keratinic, which may be primary or secondary, and (ii) nodular. The secondary type is secondary to other skin lesions such as skin tumors, inflammatory skin disorders, and phototherapy. Two types of keratotic amyloidosis have been identified: macular and lichen amyloidosis, and the latter is more common. In keratotic amyloidosis, keratin depositions originating from basal keratinocyte are mainly CK5 positive. Keratotic type is mostly observed in South-East Asia, South America, and China. It has familial (10%) and sporadic forms, and the latter is more common in women [1]. The most common sites of involvement are upper back (interscapular area) and extremities (shins and arms), although they have also been described on face, trunk, and thighs [2]. Macular amyloidosis lesions usually appear in the form of hyperpigmented patches with indefinite margins composed of grayish brown macules, often with a reticulated or rippled appearance [3] (Figure 1). Itching is a common symptom before the onset of amyloidosis [1].

The pathogenesis of this disorder is not fully elucidated, except for the fact that the deposited keratin is derived from keratinocytes [1]. Two pathogenic mechanisms have been proposed including apoptotic (fibrillar) theory and secretory theory [4]. Based on apoptotic theory, degeneration of damaged keratinocytes in the basal layer is followed by the conversion of these colloid bodies by dermal histiocytes and fibroblasts into amyloid in the papillary dermis [5] (Figure 2). According to the secretory theory, deposits of amyloid derived from degenerated basal keratinocytes spread into papillary dermis through the damaged lamina densa [6]. There are several etiologic factors implicated in the pathogenesis of macular amyloidosis: racial factors [7], genetic predisposition, environmental factors [8], sex (female) [9, 10], female hormones [11], exposure to sunlight [12], friction (long term abrasion) [12–14], atopy [15], autoimmunity (based on association with systemic lupus erythematosus, dermatomyositis, systemic sclerosis, sarcoidosis, and IgA nephropathy) [16, 17], and infection with EBV [18, 19]. EBV,

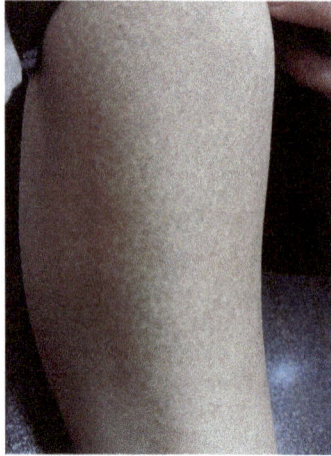

FIGURE 1: Hyperpigmented patch composed of small brown macules in a rippled or reticulated pattern on the arm.

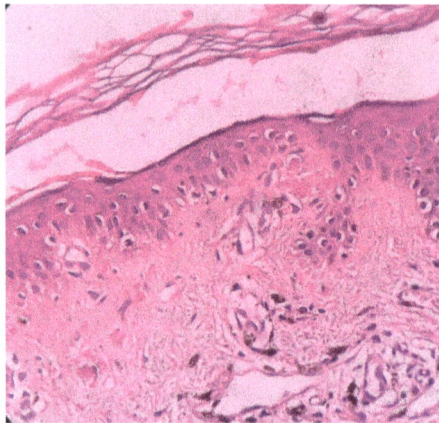

FIGURE 2: Small globular hyaline materials of amyloid in the papillary dermis.

the presence of which has been reported in epidermis of macular amyloidosis, is likely to act as a factor contributing to degeneration of keratinocytes [1].

The role of EBV in etiopathogenesis of primary cutaneous amyloidosis has been evaluated in only two prior studies including a single case report [18] and a case series of 27 patients from China [19]. Considering the shortage of studies on the association between EBV and macular amyloidosis, we set out to perform a study in this regard in Iran. Perhaps antiviral agents can be used in the future for treatment of this disease in case of association with EBV.

2. Materials and Methods

In this case-control study, 38 macular amyloidosis samples and 38 healthy skin samples around excised melanocytic nevi from age- and sex-matched patients without macular amyloidosis were enrolled in the clinical examination based on a nonrandom objective-oriented sampling. Inclusion criteria included paraffin blocks with sufficient tissue in archives of

Pathology Department of Imam Reza Hospital in Mashhad diagnosed with macular amyloidosis based on pathology report and clinical presentation. Exclusion criteria included blocks with imperfect data in records and insufficient samples for PCR.

In the case group, amyloid deposition was confirmed by optical microscopy and Congo red staining. In the next step, six 5 μm sections were prepared from each of the blocks in case and control groups in sterile conditions using sterile blade and were placed in sterile Eppendorf tubes.

2.1. Deparaffinization. Xylol/ethanol was used to deparaffinize the paraffinized tissues. One mL xylol was added to microtubes containing tissue sections and incubated in room temperature for half an hour with constant shaking. In the next step, microtubes were centrifuged in 13,000 rpm for 10 minutes, and their supernatant was discarded. These two steps were repeated once. Five hundred μL of 100% ethanol was added to the precipitate and centrifuged for 10 m in 13,000 rpm after several inversions of microtube, and the supernatant was then removed. This step was repeated again. Finally, the resulting precipitate was placed in room temperature to completely evaporate ethanol but not the precipitate.

2.2. DNA Extraction. DNA extraction was done using BIO BASIC INC (Canada) kit with lot number 8401-140116. Lysis buffer-T was used for extraction. In the next step, 100 μL extraction buffer and 10 μL proteinase K were added to each microtube and were mixed. Tissue samples were added to the mixture and incubated at room temperature for 10 minutes. Then, the samples were incubated at 95°C for 3 minutes to inactivate proteinase K. One hundred μL Universal Buffer NST was added to the tubes and inverted 10 times. The obtained mixture was used for PCR.

2.3. PCR. In this study, PCR was used to detect the presence of EBV genome in macular amyloidosis. After DNA extraction from paraffinized blocks, the quality of DNA extracted from paraffin-embedded tissues was determined using beta-globin gene primers. GH20 and PC04 beta-globin gene primers used in this study amplified a 260 bp fragment. The sequence of these primers was as follows:

GH20: 5′ GAA GAG CCA AGG ACA GGT AC 3′.

PC04: 5′ CAA CTT CAT CCA CGT TCA CC 3′.

The samples producing the 260 bp fragment using the desired primers were considered favorable for amplification of EBV virus BLLF1 gene.

Presence of EBV sequence in the extracted DNA samples was tested using Cinna Gen kit with lot number 935701 (Sina Clon, Iran). This kit has been designed to determine the quality of EBV DNA in infected samples using PCR. Optimized 1x PCR as a mixture of recombinant *Taq* DNA polymerase, PCR buffer, MgCl$_2$, dNTPs, and primers was the reagent used for mixing. The highly specific and repetitive region of BLLF1 gene encoding gp 350/220 is amplified by primers. They can detect at least 30 copies of EBV. The

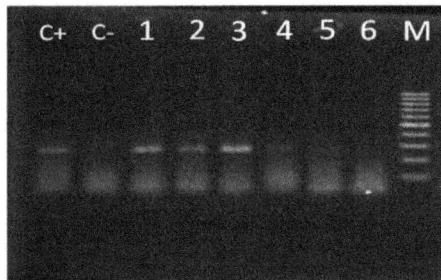

FIGURE 3: PCR results of beta-globin gene: in terms of amplification, samples 1, 2, and 3 are part of positive beta-globin gene (260 bp band) and samples 4, 5, and 6 are negative. C+ and C− indicate positive and negative controls, respectively, and M represents the DNA marker.

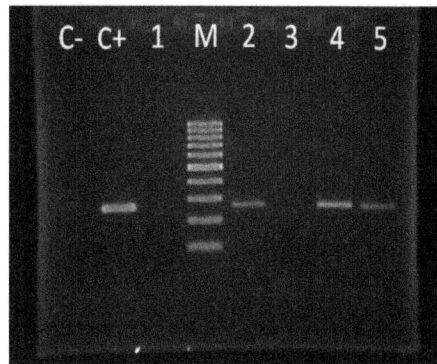

FIGURE 4: PCR results of BLLF1 gene of EBV: samples 2, 4, and 5 are positive (239 bp or 256 bp bands) and samples 1 and 3 are negative. C+ and C− indicate positive and negative controls, respectively, and M represents the DNA marker.

presence of 239 bp or 256 bp fragments indicates a positive test result.

Data analysis was performed using SPSS 11.5 software. Graphs and statistical tables were used to describe data and Chi-square and independent t-tests were used to compare EBV in healthy and patients' samples. In all tests, the significance level of 0.05 was considered.

3. Results

Fifty percent of the patients were male (19/38) and 50% were female (19/38). Three patients were in the age group under 20 years (7.9%), 5 patients 20–30 years (13.2%), 10 patients 30–40 years (26.3%), 13 patients 40–50 years (34.2%), 4 patients 50–60 years (10.5%), and 3 patients over 60 years (7.9%). The minimum and maximum ages were 19 and 76 years, respectively. There were 27 cases of infection in the trunk (71.1%) and 11 cases in the extremities (28.9%). The study and control group were matched for age ($P = 0.535$) and sex ($P = 0.646$).

PCR was conducted for beta-globin gene in 76 samples (38 cases and 38 controls), which was positive in 61 samples (30 samples in case group and 31 in the control group) and was negative in 15 samples (8 samples in case and 7 in control group) (Figure 3).

In 61 samples positive for beta-globin gene in PCR, BLLF1 gene from EBV was positive in 23 cases (8 cases in study group and 15 cases in control group) and was negative in 38 cases (22 cases in the study group and 16 cases in the control group) (Figure 4).

PCR of BLLF1 gene from EBV was 26.7% positive in study group and 48.4% positive in control group. Chi-square test results showed no correlation between EBV and macular amyloidosis ($P = 0.08$) (Table 1).

4. Discussion

Amyloidosis is known as extracellular deposition of eosinophilic hyaline material of self-origin with specific staining and ultrastructural characteristics. This disorder can occur in the background of systemic diseases or may be limited to the skin. Macular amyloidosis is limited to the skin

TABLE 1: Percentage distribution of PCR results from BLLF1 gene of EBV in 30 patients with macular amyloidosis and 31 melanocytic nevus samples among samples positive for beta-globin gene.

EBV DNA PCR	Study groups				Chi-square test results
	Cases		Controls		
	Number	Percent	Number	Percent	
Positive	8	26.7	15	48.4	$P = 0.08$
Negative	22	91.7	16	76.2	
Total	30		31		61

[1]. EBV may stimulate the secretion of amyloid material by keratinocytes or may be a stimulus for degeneration of keratinocytes and conversion of degenerated keratinocyte filaments into amyloid [1, 18]. Recent studies have indicated the role of epithelial cells in continued reproduction of EBV. EBV cell surface receptors found in less differentiated squamous epithelium suggest the direct infection of epidermal keratinocytes. Infection may occur in germinative layers; however, virus replication is only feasible through maturation and differentiation of cells. The expression of cytokeratin in human keratinocytes is changed in vitro after infection with EBV, resulting in their conversion to fibroblasts [18, 19]. Fibroblasts can phagocytize keratin aggregates and convert them to amyloid [18].

Drago et al. showed this correlation in Italy in 1996. Their patient was a 30-year-old female with a ten-year history of itchy brown papules and macules on the chest and back with symptoms of chronic fatigue syndrome. They could show EBV genome in epidermal lesions using in situ hybridization technique. EBV genome was principally shown in basal epidermal cells as well as higher layer cells, especially in the cytoplasm. Serological tests for EBV were also positive in the patient. Antiviral therapy with acyclovir and interferon alpha improved skin lesions and general symptoms in the patient [18]. Another study was conducted by Chang et al. on skin tissue of 27 patients with a diagnosis of lichen and macular amyloidosis in Taiwan in 1997. In situ hybridization method indicated EBV DNA in lesions of 11 patients (40.7%), while the control group (including three patients with secondary cutaneous amyloidosis, two patients with primary systemic amyloidosis, and four patients with chronic simplex lichen) lacked EBV DNA [19].

According to this study, there was no correlation between EBV and macular amyloidosis ($P = 0.08$). EBV DNA was present in 8 patients with macular amyloidosis and 15 controls in our study. The difference in rate of detection of EBV DNA between macular amyloidosis patients and controls in this study with the mentioned studies can be due to the following reasons:

(1) Lack of association between macular amyloidosis and EBV infection: there are a few studies presenting insufficient evidence for a definitive correlation between EBV and macular amyloidosis, so based on the results of our study we could make this conclusion.

(2) Methodology (PCR versus in situ hybridization): we used a sensitive method for detection of EBV DNA with positive and negative controls. Based on the previous studies, PCR is as sensitive as in situ hybridization [20, 21]. However, as we did not use in situ hybridization, we could not localize the exact infected cell with EBV in our controls which might be the circulating B cells of the skin instead of keratinocytes. As we used positive and negative controls in our PCR kit for EBV, the positive cases in our control group could not be false positive.

(3) Controls: the controls in our study were the healthy skin around melanocytic nevi, but the controls in Chang study were other cutaneous disorders.

(4) Type of cutaneous amyloidosis: in our study, all the patients had macular amyloidosis, but in both the previous studies [18, 19] most of the patients were of lichen amyloidosis.

5. Conclusion

According to the results of this study, there was no correlation between EBV and macular amyloidosis. We recommend the use of fresh tissue or quickly frozen biopsy punch as well as simultaneous serological study of patients for anti-EBV antibody to achieve more accurate results for comparative study of EBV DNA in macular amyloidosis. In situ PCR can also be used to localize the EBV DNA positive cells in the samples. Other genes can be used to detect EBV in the tissue since some EBV samples are mutated for BLLF1 gene used in this study [22].

Also, we recommend performing a comparative study on detection of EBV in both involved and uninvolved skin of the patients with macular amyloidosis.

Conflict of Interests

The authors declare no conflict of interests.

Acknowledgments

The authors express their profound gratitude for research deputy of MUMS for financial support and approval of the research proposal (no. 911283) related to thesis of Narges Nazeri. Financial support by research deputy of Mashhad University of Medical Sciences is acknowledged.

References

[1] A. Fernandez-Flores, "Cutaneous amyloidosis: a concept review," The American Journal of Dermatopathology, vol. 34, no. 1, pp. 1–14, 2012.

[2] J. T. Al-Ratrout and M. B. Satti, "Primary localized cutaneous amyloidosis: a clinicopathologic study from Saudi Arabia," International Journal of Dermatology, vol. 36, no. 6, pp. 428–434, 1997.

[3] A. Bandhlish, A. Aggarwal, and R. Koranne, "A clinico-epidemiological study of macular amyloidosis from North India," Indian Journal of Dermatology, vol. 57, no. 4, pp. 269–274, 2012.

[4] Y. Horiguchi, J.-D. Fine, I. M. Leigh, T. Yoshiki, M. Ueda, and S. Imamura, "Lamina densa malformation involved in histogenesis of primary localized cutaneous amyloidosis," Journal of Investigative Dermatology, vol. 99, no. 1, pp. 12–18, 1992.

[5] H. Kobayashi and K. Hashimoto, "Amyloidogenesis in organ-limited cutaneous amyloidosis: an antigenic identity between epidermal keratin and skin amyloid," Journal of Investigative Dermatology, vol. 80, no. 1, pp. 66–72, 1983.

[6] D. M. Touart and P. Sau, "Cutaneous deposition diseases: part I," Journal of the American Academy of Dermatology, vol. 39, no. 2, pp. 149–171, 1998.

[7] W.-J. Wang, C.-Y. Huang, Y.-T. Chang, and C.-K. Wong, "Anosacral cutaneous amyloidosis: a study of 10 Chinese cases," British Journal of Dermatology, vol. 143, no. 6, pp. 1266–1269, 2000.

[8] V. Eswaramoorthy, I. Kaur, A. Das, and B. Kumar, "Macular amyloidosis: etiological factors," The Journal of Dermatology, vol. 26, no. 5, pp. 305–310, 1999.

[9] A.-G. Kibbi, N. G. Rubeiz, S. T. Zaynoun, and A. K. Kurban, "Primary localized cutaneous amyloidosis," International Journal of Dermatology, vol. 31, no. 2, pp. 95–98, 1992.

[10] Y. T. Chang, C. K. Wong, K. C. Chow, and C. H. Tsai, "Apoptosis in primary cutaneous amyloidosis," British Journal of Dermatology, vol. 140, no. 2, pp. 210–215, 1999.

[11] A. Rasi, A. Khatami, and S. M. Javaheri, "Macular amyloidosis: an assessment of prevalence, sex, and age," International Journal of Dermatology, vol. 43, no. 12, pp. 898–899, 2004.

[12] V. K. Somani, H. Shailaja, V. N. V. L. Sita, and F. Razvi, "Nylon friction dermatitis: a distinct subset of macular amyloidosis," Indian Journal of Dermatology, Venereology and Leprology, vol. 61, no. 3, pp. 145–147, 1995.

[13] L. Onuma, M. Vega, R. Arenas, and L. Dominguez, "Friction amyloidosis," International Journal of Dermatology, vol. 33, no. 1, p. 74, 1994.

[14] M. Siragusa, R. Ferri, V. Cavallari, and C. Schepis, "Friction melanosis, friction amyloidosis, macular amyloidosis, towel melanosis: many names for the same clinical entity," European Journal of Dermatology, vol. 11, no. 6, pp. 545–548, 2001.

[15] D. D. Lee, C. K. Huang, P. C. Ko, Y. T. Chang, W. Z. Sun, and Y. J. Oyang, "Association of primary cutaneous amyloidosis with atopic dermatitis: a nationwide population-based study in Taiwan," *British Journal of Dermatology*, vol. 164, no. 1, pp. 148–153, 2011.

[16] A. Tanaka, K. Arita, J. E. Lai-Cheong, F. Palisson, M. Hide, and J. A. McGrath, "New insight into mechanisms of pruritus from molecular studies on familial primary localized cutaneous amyloidosis," *British Journal of Dermatology*, vol. 161, no. 6, pp. 1217–1224, 2009.

[17] M. J. Dahdah, M. Kurban, A.-G. Kibbi, and S. Ghosn, "Primary localized cutaneous amyloidosis: a sign of immune dysregulation?" *International Journal of Dermatology*, vol. 48, no. 4, pp. 419–421, 2009.

[18] F. Drago, E. Ranieri, A. Pasturino, S. Casazza, F. Crovato, and A. Rebora, "Epstein-Barr virus-related primary cutaneous amyloidosis. Successful treatment with acyclovir and interferon-alpha," *British Journal of Dermatology*, vol. 134, no. 1, pp. 170–174, 1996.

[19] Y. T. Chang, H. N. Liu, C. K. Wong, K. C. Chow, and K. Y. Chen, "Detection of Epstein-Barr virus in primary cutaneous amyloidosis," *British Journal of Dermatology*, vol. 136, no. 6, pp. 823–826, 1997.

[20] N. Suh, H. Liapis, J. Misdraji, E. M. Brunt, and H. L. Wang, "Epstein-Barr virus hepatitis: diagnostic value of in situ hybridization, polymerase chain reaction, and immunohisto-chemistry on liver biopsy from immunocompetent patients," *American Journal of Surgical Pathology*, vol. 31, no. 9, pp. 1403–1409, 2007.

[21] Z.-L. Qi, X.-Q. Han, J. Hu et al., "Comparison of three methods for the detection of Epstein-Barr virus in Hodgkin's lymphoma in paraffin-embedded tissues," *Molecular Medicine Reports*, vol. 7, no. 1, pp. 89–92, 2013.

[22] A. Janz, M. Oezel, C. Kurzeder et al., "Infectious Epstein-Barr virus lacking major glycoprotein BLLF1 (gp350/220) demonstrates the existence of additional viral ligands," *Journal of Virology*, vol. 74, no. 21, pp. 10142–10152, 2000.

30

Skin Protection Behaviors among Young Male Latino Day Laborers: An Exploratory Study Using a Social Cognitive Approach

Javier F. Boyas,[1] **Vinayak K. Nahar,**[2,3] **and Robert T. Brodell**[3,4,5]

[1]*School of Social Work, University of Alabama, Box 870314, Tuscaloosa, AL 35487, USA*
[2]*Department of Health, Exercise Science & Recreation Management, University of Mississippi, 215 Turner Center, P.O. Box 1848, University, MS 38677, USA*
[3]*Department of Dermatology, University of Mississippi Medical Center, 2500 N. State Street, Jackson, MS 39216, USA*
[4]*Department of Pathology, University of Mississippi Medical Center, 2500 N. State Street, Jackson, MS 39216, USA*
[5]*Department of Dermatology, University of Rochester School of Medicine and Dentistry, Rochester, NY 14642, USA*

Correspondence should be addressed to Javier F. Boyas; javierboyas@hotmail.com

Academic Editor: Herbert Honigsmann

Latino Day Laborers (LDLs) are employed in occupations where multiple work hazards exist. One such hazard is the overexposure to solar ultraviolet radiation for continuous periods of time. Regular sun exposure can put individuals at increased risk of developing skin cancers, especially without adequate protection. The purpose of this cross-sectional exploratory study was to use a social cognitive framework to assess skin protective behaviors among LDLs. A community-based nonrandom and purposive sample of LDLs was recruited in two states: Mississippi and Illinois. The study sample consisted of 137 male participants, of which the majority were of Mexican ancestry (72%). The average age was 35.40 (SD = 9.89) years. Results demonstrated that a substantial number of LDLs do not adequately practice sun protection behaviors on a regular basis. The skin cancer knowledge scores were very modest. The most frequently indicated barriers towards sun protection were "inconvenient," "forget to use," and "not being able to reapply sunscreen." Overall, LDLs had moderate confidence in their abilities to adopt successful sun protection strategies. This study underscores the need for intervention programs aimed at LDLs to reduce extended time in the sun and increase use of sun protective measures when working outdoors.

1. Introduction

The workplace is an overlooked determining factor of health and health disparities [1]. Work determines a person's income, health insurance benefits, and psychosocial functioning, all of which influence individual health [1–3]. However, it also relates to how much an individual is exposed to varying types of occupational hazards. It is well established that Latino Day Laborers (LDLs) are often employed in occupations that are highly hazardous, highly stressful, and low paying, are exposed to poor working conditions, and lack health insurance coverage [2–5]. Research on the risks associated with occupational exposures for LDLs continues to grow. Research suggests that LDLs are usually hired for jobs that involve a number of workplace threats, such as working with unsafe mechanized tools and equipment, environments with high noise levels, exposure to dangerous chemicals, work in risky heights, lack of personal protective equipment, and little to no safety oversight [2, 6]. However, the hazard of regular exposure to solar ultraviolet radiation (UVR) is one area that has remained completely unexplored. Continuous contact with UVR is commonplace for LDLs given that they are most frequently employed in job sectors such as landscaping, gardening, roofing, painting, and construction [5, 7]. These work activities commonly take place outdoors, which expose LDLs to considerable sun contact.

Overexposure to UVR for continuous periods of time, without proper protection, during peak periods of intense sun, can put individuals at risk of developing melanoma or other nonmelanoma forms of skin cancers [8]. Skin cancer is one of the top 10 new cancer diagnoses among adults in the USA [9, 10], and incidence rates in the USA have continued to soar in the past 35 years [11]. Among Latinos, incidence rates of melanoma are on the rise and they have risen at an annual rate of 2.9%, which is comparable to rates among non-Hispanic whites [12]. This is problematic given that only one in fourteen Latinos reports ever having a physician skin examination [13]; only 3.2% of Latinos have been told how to perform a skin self-examination [14]; and Latinos, relative to non-Hispanic whites, were less likely to wear sun protective clothing or sunscreen with a protection factor of 15 or higher [14]. These findings may partially explain why Latinos are often diagnosed at an earlier age and are diagnosed at advanced stages of melanoma and often have poorer cancer survival rates than non-Hispanic whites [9, 15]. Thus, research is needed that can assist this high risk and vulnerable population in the prevention of skin cancer.

Our research is important given that LDLs are typically employed in outdoor jobs, such as construction, landscaping, and framing, where UVR exposure is continuous. LDLs who are outdoor workers often experience regular exposure to solar UVR for extended periods of time, which can place this population at an increased risk of developing skin cancer [16–18]. Despite this recognition, to the best of our knowledge, no published studies have investigated the extent to which LDLs engage in skin protective behaviors. Thus, this is the first exploratory study that seeks to establish the sun protective perceptions and practices of LDLs. Our study utilized social cognitive theory (SCT) to help us understand cognitive and social factors that contribute to skin protective behaviors of LDLs [19]. The data collected as part of this study was based on social cognitive theory applied to health behavior [19, 20]. Social cognitive theory suggests that social and physical environments influence behavior. Moreover, there are incessant reciprocal exchanges among people and their environments and behaviors [19]. The purpose of this study was to use a social cognitive framework to identify psychosocial forms of self-efficacy in relation to employing sun protective strategies, intention to protect oneself from the sun, perceived workplace support, and perceived barriers and benefits associated with skin protective behaviors.

2. Methods

2.1. Sample and Procedures. The current study utilized cross-sectional data from the 2014 Mississippi Survey on Health Practices. To participate in this study, possible participants had to self-identify as either Hispanic or Latino, be at least 18 years of age, actively seek informal and short-term contingent employment, have no cognitive limitations, be not institutionalized, and reside in Mississippi or Illinois. In all, we surveyed a total of 138 participants: 77 of the participants were from Mississippi, whereas 61 were from Illinois. One of

the participants was a female day laborer. However, she was deleted from the analysis.

A community-based nonrandom and purposive sample of Latino participants was recruited in two states: Mississippi and Illinois. In Mississippi, the sample was recruited from multiple cities, including Hernando, Holly Springs, Oxford, and Southaven. The recruitment strategy varied in each state. In Mississippi, we relied on multiple strategies. The participants were recruited through advertisements (English and Spanish) and referrals from collaborating Latino/Hispanic serving social and health care providers. Recruitment flyers were posted at sites that day laborers frequently visit, such as Mexican *taquerias*, Laundromats, Catholic churches, and construction sites. In addition, face-to-face recruitment methods were also employed at various construction sites. A snowball technique was also used. We asked all participants if they could recommend someone else who was appropriate for the study. This strategy was beneficial given that day laborers are considered a hard-to-track population. This is especially true in some of the smaller southern towns where this population does not have a long history nor can they congregate on street corners or building supply store parking lots like they would in metropolitan areas. In Illinois, the sample was recruited from three common street corners where day laborers gather in the northwest side of Chicago. In Illinois, we approached LDLs seeking employment during the morning hours.

Data were collected from July 2014 to November 2014 from various urban, rural, and semirural communities in Mississippi and Illinois. This time frame allowed us to examine the summer sun protective behaviors in order to avoid a possible recall bias. In Mississippi, there are more extended periods of sunshine and warm temperatures that carry over well into the fall season. As such, data collection continued until November. However, in Illinois, data collection stopped in early October. That is because, in the Midwest, the number of sunny and warm days becomes less as the fall approaches. Informed consent authorizing participation in this study was provided to participants along with a self-report questionnaire. The questionnaire was available in English and Spanish. An option of an oral reading of the survey was offered to all participants. This measure was taken to ensure that potential respondents with literacy concerns did not have to disclose that they were illiterate and were not discouraged from participating in the survey. Study participants voluntarily completed a roughly 55-minute self-administered questionnaire developed primarily from established and validated instruments. Participants were given the opportunity to fill out the survey before or after work and received a $20.00 research honorarium. Members of the research team, which included the principal investigator and three bilingual/bicultural research assistants, administered data collection. Prior to the administration of the survey, all research assistants were trained for two hours on culturally sensitive data collection procedures. Institutional Review Board permission was obtained in order to ensure minimal risk to study participants.

2.2. Measures. A survey instrument was developed utilizing established scales and measures from prior research [21–29]. Some of these instruments were available in Spanish [26]. If a Spanish version was a not available, the research team, which consisted of two Mexican Americans, one Peruvian, and one Venezuelan, translated the instruments. All translations were first carried out independently. Then, the group discussed how to best structure the items, with the intention of making the language suitable to a population that is characterized by low levels of educational attainment.

A total of nine items were used to identify sun protection behaviors (e.g., wide-brimmed hat, long-sleeved shirt, shirt with collar, limiting midday sun, sunglasses, sunscreen, gloves, and covering head and face) [26]. These items were measured using a five-point scale (1 = "never"; 5 = "always"). For example, "During the summer months at work, how often do you wear sunscreen with sun protection factor (SPF) of 15 or higher when you are in the sun for more than 15 minutes?"; additionally, information on sunscreen use behavior (e.g., thorough application, SPF values, and reapplication) was assessed by three questions [26].

To assess perceived benefits of sun protection strategies, participants were asked to rate their level of agreement (1 = "strongly agree"; 5 = "strongly disagree") with three statements [21, 23]. The questions, for example, focused on "decrease the risk of skin cancer" and "decrease skin aging."

Twelve Likert-rated (1 = "strongly disagree"; 5 = "strongly agree") statements were used to assess perceived barriers among respondents for not engaging in sun protection behaviors [21, 23]. Three example statements are "I want to get a suntan," "sun protective clothing is too hot to wear," and "sunscreen is greasy."

Self-efficacy (i.e., the degree of confidence that an individual has in his/her ability to conduct a particular behavior) scale consisted of seven items that asked participants about their confidence level to use recommended sun protection measures (e.g., seeking shade, wide-brimmed hat, long-sleeved shirt, long pants, sunglasses, and sunscreen) [28–31]. Response categories ranged from 1 ("not at all confident") to 10 ("highly confident and certainly can do").

LDLs were asked about their sources of information (i.e., television, radio, newspaper, health care workers, family, friends, coworkers, and employer and supervisor) regarding protecting themselves from too much sun [21]. For each of the 9 items, responses were measured on a three-point scale (1 = "yes"; 0 = "no").

Knowledge regarding skin cancer (nonmelanoma skin cancer and melanoma) and risk factors was assessed by 24-item scale developed by Cottrell and colleagues (2005) (1 = "correct"; 0 = "incorrect") [25]. For example, "The most common form of skin cancer is - Basal cell carcinoma or Squamous cell carcinoma or Melanoma?" The total possible score for knowledge ranged from 0 to 24, with a higher score indicating higher skin cancer related knowledge.

Intentions to engage in sun protection practices (e.g., applying sunscreen, wearing protective clothing, long-sleeved shirt, seeking shade, and using sunglasses) were measured by five questions, using a five-point scale (1 = "strongly agree"; 5 = "strongly disagree"). Participants were asked if they would intend to use sun protection at work every time they go in the sun for more than 15 minutes during the summer months.

The authors developed the two workplace support items. We asked LDLs to state how much they think their supervisor(s) engage(s) in sun protective behaviors. They were also asked to assess how much they think their coworkers engage in sun protective behaviors. Both items were 5-point Likert-type coded as follows: 1 = never; 5 = always.

Skin screening was assessed by three questions [22]. The first question assessed if they ever had their skin checked for changes, which could be skin cancer (1 = "yes"; 0 = "no"). The second question assessed who checked their skin (1 = "I did," 2 = "skin doctor," 3 = "my partner did," 4 = "general practitioner," 5 = "a friend did," and 6 = "another family member did"). The third question assessed when they had their most recent skin exam (1 = "Within last year," 2 = "1 to 3 years ago," 3 = "Over 3 years ago," and 4 = "I do not know").

2.3. Analytic Strategy. Univariate statistics (i.e., frequencies and percentages) were used to describe all the variables collected in this study. Bivariate analyses were used to determine if statistical differences existed between data collected in Illinois and Mississippi. Additional bivariate analyses were conducted to determine if significant differences exist by legal status and education level in relation to major study constructs. The analyses were all conducted using Statistical Package for Social Sciences (SPSS) version 21 (Chicago, IL). Significance level was set at 0.05 *a priori*.

3. Results

The sample description is presented in Table 1. The men in our sample were mainly of Mexican ancestry (72%). The second largest group was from Central America (18%). The average age was 35.40 (SD = 9.89) years. In terms of legal status, the largest group was undocumented (35%). Our sample was not highly educated; 44% reported less than an 8th grade education. The majority of the sample who were foreign born reported receiving their education in their country of origin (88%). Those participants who were born in another country have been in the USA an average of 11.15 (SD = 9.48) years. The majority of participants were married ($n = 69$). The majority lived with roommates ($n = 53$). Of those that reported having roommates, the average number of roommates was 3.86. Sixty-nine percent reported earning less than \$20,000 a year in 2014. In terms of work types, the majority worked in multiple areas, such as construction, painting, roofing, and lawn mowing. However, the largest group reported working in the area of construction (42%). All of the LDLs worked for private employers. The majority of the respondents were outdoor workers who spent 4.66 (minimum 1; maximum 6) hours outside in the sun between 10 a.m. and 4 p.m. Only 7.3% of LDLs reported ever having their skin examined for changes, which could be skin cancer.

Data were examined to determine if statistical differences existed between the data collected in Mississippi and Illinois; however, no significant differences were found in any of the

TABLE 1: Sociodemographic characteristics of the Latino Day Laborers.

	n (%)
Ethnic background	
Colombian	1 (0.7%)
Cuban	1 (0.7%)
Ecuadorian	6 (4.5%)
Guatemalan	11 (8.2%)
Honduran	9 (6.7%)
Mexican	97 (72.4%)
Nicaraguan	1 (0.7%)
Peruvian	2 (1.5%)
Puerto Rican	3 (2.2%)
Salvadoran	3 (2.2%)
Racial background	
White/Caucasian	34 (24.8%)
African American	1 (0.7%)
Indigenous	50 (36.5%)
More than one race	48 (35%)
Legal status	
United States citizen	16 (11.9%)
Naturalized citizen	12 (8.9%)
Permanent legal resident	19 (14.1%)
Work permit	24 (17.8%)
Nonimmigrant visa	14 (10.4%)
Noncitizen and not permanent legal resident	50 (37%)
Level	
Less than elementary school	61 (44.5%)
Completed elementary school but not high school	27 (19.7%)
High school diploma	2 (1.5%)
Associate degree	41 (29.9%)
Bachelor's degree	5 (3.6%)
Graduate or professional degree	1 (7%)
Skin type	
Always burn, never tans	29 (21.5%)
Usually burn, tans with difficulty	5 (3.7%)
Sometimes mild burn, gradually tans to a light brown	24 (17.8%)
Rarely burn, tan with ease to a moderate brown	45 (33.3%)
Very rarely burns, tans very easily	17 (12.6%)
Never burns, tans very easily, deeply pigmented	15 (11.1%)
Educated in native country	
Yes	115 (83.9%)
No	22 (16.1%)
Marital status	
Single	45 (33.3%)
Married	69 (51.1%)
Separated	4 (3%)
Divorced	3 (2.2%)
Widowed	1 (7%)
Living with partner	13 (9.6%)
Living arrangements	
Roommates	53 (39.8%)
Spouse	15 (11.3%)
Spouse and children	23 (17.3%)
Relatives	21 (15.8%)
Live-in partner	11 (8.3%)
Alone	10 (7.5%)

TABLE 1: Continued.

	n (%)
Type of work	
Construction	57 (41.6%)
Roofing	4 (2.9%)
Landscaping	25 (18.2%)
Painting	15 (10.9%)
Cementing	2 (1.5%)
Lawn mowing	8 (5.8%)
Clean-up	1 (0.7%)
Welding	1 (0.7%)
Multiple	24 (17.5%)
Health insurance coverage	
Yes	21 (16.3%)
No	108 (83.7%)
Household income (yearly)	
Less than $20,000	95 (69.3%)
$21,000 to $30,000	41 (29.9%)
$31,000 to $40,000	1 (0.7%)

	Mean (SD)
Age (years)	35.40 (9.89)
Lived in USA (years)	11.15 (9.48)

sun protective perception or behavior variables. Two areas where they did differ were in the areas of legal status and acculturation levels. A higher number of LDLs reported being undocumented in Mississippi compared to Illinois (x^2 = 13.084, $p \leq 0.05$). We also found that acculturation levels of LDLs were significantly higher in Illinois (M = 6.65; SD = 3.13), compared to Mississippi (M = 5.65; SD = 2.71).

In terms of sun protective behaviors, the most frequently reported method was use of wearing something over their head, such as a hat, cap, or visor (see Table 2). The LDLs reported "always" or "often" wearing something on their head 26% of the time. The largest portion though, 41%, reported wearing something on their head only some of the time. The next two most reported sun protective practices were wearing sunglasses and wearing hats with a surrounding 2.5-inch brim. Twelve percent of respondents reported "always" or "often" wearing sunglasses, while 8% reported "always" or "often" wearing a hat with a surrounding brim of at least 2.5 inches. Some of the information on lack of practicing sun protective behaviors was concerning. For example, 59% of LDLs reported never using sunscreen, while 76% reported never wearing any protective gear over their face, such as a handkerchief or filter mask. More than half of the sample also reported never wearing a hat with a surrounding brim of at least 2.5 inches, gloves, a long-sleeved shirt, or a shirt with a collar.

In terms of protecting oneself from UVR by way of sunscreen with SPF 15, the majority of the sample did not report wide use. In all, only 6% reported wearing sunscreen "always" or "often." In terms of where they apply it, 35%

TABLE 2: Sun protection behaviors of Latino Day Laborers.

	Never	Sometimes	About half the time	Often	Always
	n (%)	n (%)	n (%)	n (%)	n (%)
Wear something on your head (any type of hat, cap, or visor)	8 (5.8%)	56 (40.9%)	37 (27%)	24 (17.5%)	12 (8%)
Wear hat with a surrounding brim of at least 2.5 inches	71 (51.8%)	40 (29.2%)	15 (10.9%)	6 (4.4%)	5 (3.6%)
Wear a long-sleeved shirt	76 (55.5%)	45 (32.8%)	14 (10.2%)	1 (0.7%)	1 (0.7%)
Wear shirt with a collar	70 (51.1%)	52 (38%)	10 (7.3%)	4 (2.9%)	1 (0.7%)
Limit the time you are exposed to the sun at midday	49 (35.8%)	59 (43.1%)	26 (19%)	3 (2.2%)	0 (0%)
Wear sunscreen with SPF of 15 or higher	81 (59.1%)	33 (24.1%)	15 (10.9%)	6 (4.4%)	2 (1.5%)
Wear sunglasses	43 (31.4%)	56 (40.9%)	21 (15.3%)	11 (8.0%)	6 (4.4%)
Wear gloves	73 (53.3%)	49 (35.8%)	11 (8%)	4 (2.9%)	0 (0%)
Wear any protective gear over your face (hankie, filter mask)	104 (75.9%)	27 (19.7%)	6 (4.4%)	0 (0%)	0 (0%)

TABLE 3: Sun protection self-efficacy of the Latino Day Laborers.

	Mean (SD)
Seek shade	4.98 (2.51)
Wear a wide-brimmed hat with a surrounding brim of at least 2.5 inches	5.35 (3.22)
Wear a long-sleeved shirt	5.51 (3.34)
Wear long pants	6.89 (2.83)
Wear sunglasses	6.13 (3.32)
Wear work gloves	5.60 (3.49)
Wear sunscreen with a sun protection factor (SPF) of 15 or higher	4.75 (2.69)

TABLE 4: Sun protection barriers of the Latino Day Laborers.

	Mean (SD)
Not concerned about sun exposure	3.74 (0.93)
Sun protection clothing is too hot to wear	3.99 (0.86)
Not always convenient to protect myself from the sun	4.17 (0.74)
Often forget to protect myself from the sun	4.16 (0.90)
Sun protection measures are expensive	3.60 (0.93)
Use of sun protection measures is time consuming	3.85 (0.60)
Use of sunscreen is too feminine	2.85 (1.00)
I don't like the smell of sunscreen	2.93 (0.87)
Sunscreen is greasy	3.45 (1.09)
Sunscreen attracts dirt	3.46 (1.06)
Sunscreen sweats off of me	4.04 (0.77)
I can't reapply sunscreen	4.12 (0.64)

reported applying sunscreen to their face. Another 28% applied sunscreen to their neck, 22% applied it to their ears, 27% applied it to their upper arms, 34% applied it to their lower arms, and 24% applied it to their hands. The highest area to be left unprotected by sunscreen was the legs; 88% reported not applying sunscreen to that part of their body. On the day of data collection, only 17% were wearing sunscreen. When asked how many times a day they applied sunscreen when they are at work, their average was low (M = 0.61; SD = 1.03).

Levels of self-efficacy in relation to using different practices to protect themselves from the sun varied among LDLs (see Table 3). Collectively, our indicators suggest that LDLs had moderate confidence in their abilities to use various strategies to protect themselves. The highest level of confidence was professed for wearing long pants (M = 6.89; SD = 2.83), wearing sunglasses (M = 6.13; SD = 3.32), and wearing work gloves (M = 5.60; SD = 3.49). The two areas that LDLs were least confident in using were using sunscreen (M = 4.75; SD = 2.69) and seeking shade (M = 4.98; SD = 2.51).

In terms of perceived barriers, LDLs reported having multiple barriers to protecting themselves from the sun between 10 a.m. and 4 p.m. (see Table 4). The top three barriers were as follows: not always being convenient to protect oneself from the sun (M = 4.17; SD = 0.74), often

forgetting to protect oneself from the sun (M = 4.16; SD = 0.90), and not being able to reapply sunscreen (M = 4.12; SD = 0.64). Other barriers included sunscreen sweating off of them, sun protective clothing being too hot to wear, sun protective measures were too time consuming, and being concerned about sun exposure. LDLs did not believe that sunscreen was too feminine (M = 2.85; SD = 1.00) or that sunscreen had a bad smell (M = 2.93; SD = 0.87). LDLs were neutral on sun protective measures being expensive, sunscreen being greasy, and sunscreen attracting dirt.

Turning to benefits of protecting themselves while out in the sun for more than 15 minutes between 10 a.m. and 4 p.m., LDLs were asked about doing so to decrease skin aging, decrease sunburn, and decrease the risk of developing skin cancer. In terms of aging, 64% either "strongly agreed" or "agreed" that this was a perceived benefit of protecting themselves from the sun. Sixty-one percent of LDLs either "strongly agreed" or "agreed" that a perceived benefit of protecting themselves from the sun was to decrease the likelihood of sunburn. Last, 73% of LDLs reported protecting themselves from the sun to decrease the risk of developing skin cancer.

LDLs were also surveyed about their future intent to engage in a series of sun protective behaviors. The strongest intention reported was to seek shade during the peak hours of the day (M = 3.55; SD = 1.24). They were least likely to report future intentions to engage in using sunscreen with SPF 15 or better (M = 2.80; SD = 1.22). They were more neutral about intending to wear protective clothing, such as hats, wear long-sleeved shirts, and wear sunglasses.

LDLs were also surveyed about their perception of whether their supervisors and coworkers engage in sun protective behaviors. Our results suggest that LDLs perceived that neither their supervisors (M = 2.50; SD = 1.02) nor coworkers (M = 2.66; SD = 1.13) often engage in sun protective behaviors.

With regard to receiving information about sun protection, television (88.2%) and radio (77.1%) were indicated most frequently by participants, followed by family (62%), friends (47.1%), newspapers (46.6%), coworkers (39.3%), health care workers (37.4%), and supervision (34.1%).

We sought to also establish how much LDLs knew about skin cancer and whether they could identify risk factors associated with melanoma. The knowledge scores were very modest. The overwhelming number of the participants reported not knowing answers to the questions. In terms of identifying risks associated with melanoma, we asked if they could identify them from 8 different risk factors. Collectively, LDLs were able to identify a modest number (M = 2.60; SD = 1.55). Given this lack of knowledge, we examined whether achieved education levels could partially explain this result. However, we found that education was only significantly associated with self-efficacy (t = 2.178; $p \leq 0.05$), but not SPBs (t = −1.020; $p \geq 0.05$); barriers (t = 1.170; $p \geq 0.05$); or being able to identify skin cancer risk factors (t = −0.402; $p \geq 0.05$). LDLs with some college level training beyond a high school diploma were able to express higher levels of self-efficacy (M = 44.72; SD = 17.24) in relation to using sun protective strategies, compared to LDLs with a high school diploma or less (M = 37.90; SD = 17.48).

Given that Mississippi included more persons who were not legal, we examined whether legal status shaped SPBs, barriers, self-efficacy, and being able to identify skin cancer risk factors. We collapsed the categories so that LDLs who reported being legal (citizen by birth, naturalized citizen, and permanent legal resident) were in one category and LDLs with a work permit and nonimmigrant visa and noncitizen nor permanent legal resident were grouped in another. Significant differences were found in the areas of SPBs (t = 5.709; $p \leq 0.001$) and being able to identify skin cancer risk factors (t = 5.252; $p \leq 0.001$). LDLs who held a legal status reported using more SPBs (M = 19.36; SD = 5.78), compared to LDLs who were not legal (M = 14.60; SD = 3.85). Legal LDLs were able to properly identify more skin cancer risk factors (M = 3.40; SD = 1.67), compared to LDLs who were not legal (M = 2.17; SD = 1.31). Legal status did not have a significant effect on reporting barriers or self-efficacy.

4. Discussion

We used a social cognitive approach to identify the practices and beliefs of sun protection behaviors among LDLs. Our results suggest that sun protection practices are necessary given the length of time LDLs are exposed to UVR. On average, LDLs spend 4.66 hours outdoors during peak periods of sun intensity. Further complicating matters, only 7.3% of the respondents had ever had their skin examined, despite continuous UVR contact. Thus, LDLs are exposed to dangerous levels of UVR, without any attention given to protection or having their skin examined. This finding is consistent with the broader literature that suggests that very few Latinos have ever had a physician skin exam [13]. These two findings call for health promotion professionals to assist LDLs in protecting themselves out in the field, by educating them about the harms and risks associated with continuous exposure to UVR during peak periods of intense sun. They could also assist in educating them about the benefits of having skin exams. Although encouraging LDLs to have physician skin exams is preferred, it is not likely given that so many of them do not have access to health care resources because they are uninsured. Thus, at the very least, LDLs should be trained on how to perform self-skin examinations. This might be one strategy that could help; however, it has to be a health message that has to be conveyed to this population continuously. In one study, Latinos in one southern state reported that they were not told by their physicians to get self-skin examinations, which is why they did not perform them [12]. Thus, getting reminders from health professionals may help LDLs adhere to having skin examinations on a continual basis.

In terms of sun protective behaviors, LDLs reported concerning levels of unsafe sun practices. They reported a low frequency of wearing protective clothing during summer. LDLs also indicated that they did not do much to limit the sun exposure at midday. Furthermore, many of the LDLs reported not using sunscreen with SPF 15. Our findings suggest that they were not currently applying sunscreen and it was unlikely that this practice would change in the future. A large portion reported never applying sunscreen and many also reported that their future intent to engage in a series of sun protective behaviors did not include applying sunscreen. The reported levels of sunscreen use and wearing a long sleeve shirt were much lower among LDLs compared to other reports of sun protective behaviors among US Latinos [32, 33], and other studies focused on outdoor workers [34]. LDLs reported higher levels of using hats compared to broader Latina/o samples [32]. This finding can be partially explained by the low levels of acculturation of our sample, which could point to a cultural contrast in norms among LDLs. It has been maintained that sunscreen is a US cultural norm [32] that may not be reflective of norms in other cultures or countries. Varying degrees of sun protective behaviors have been linked to differences in acculturation levels among Latinos. For example, Andreeva and colleagues (2009) found that Latinos with lower levels of acculturation were significantly less likely to use sunscreen compared to those who were more acculturated [32]. In that study, lower levels of acculturation had a negative effect on sun protective behaviors, such as applying sunscreen. However, other research suggests that lower levels of acculturation can have a protective effect as well. Coups and colleagues (2013) found that less acculturated Latinos were more likely to wear sun protective clothing and seek shade but were less likely to report sunbathing and indoor tanning [33]. These contradictory findings suggest that the relationship between acculturated Latinos and sun protective behaviors is complex.

Poor sun-safe practices reported by LDLs may be attributed to a lack of knowledge. In this study, LDLs demonstrated that they lacked knowledge about skin cancer and they were not able to identify risk factors associated with melanoma, which is consistent with findings of the broader Latino population in terms of skin cancer knowledge [35]. The knowledge scores that were obtained in this study were not usable data because the overwhelming majority of respondents stated that they did not know the answer or provided an incorrect answer. Our measure on identifying risk factors further corroborated this knowledge gap. This finding establishes that education and awareness about skin cancer and risk factors are necessary among LDLs. Despite this recognition, prevention interventions that target LDLs and the broader Latina/o population remain inadequate [35]. More interventions are needed that can target the Latina/o population as a whole but also that address the unique workplace risks faced by LDLs. Given that the majority of LDLs receive sun protection information from television and radio, it would be beneficial for skin cancer agencies to collaborate with media channels in order to develop effective sun safety programs.

The barriers reported by LDLs should be taken into account as interventions are being developed. Our findings suggest that LDLs may not have the option of seeking shade, stopping work to reapply sunscreen, or thinking about how to better protect oneself from the sun. These are barriers that should be addressed through interventions that target these areas. For example, what can be done to protect oneself when time and flexibility are an issue and there are not many ways to stop work to think about seeking shade? These barriers should likely be addressed structurally through public policies. It may be that the US Occupational and Safety Health Administration (OSHA) has to take a more proactive role in considering the harmful effects of UVR as a legitimate occupational risk hazard. This position is not very pronounced in their information on personal protective equipment [36]. Their informational document does not address specifically the type of gear and/or equipment needed to properly protect oneself from UVR.

The LDLs reported varying levels of self-efficacy in regard to sun protective practices when in the sun for more than 15 minutes during peak times. Most reported moderate levels of confidence in wearing sun protective clothing. However, they were less inclined to make compromises towards wearing sunscreen and seeking shade. Not wearing sunscreen was consistently reported across various measures used in this study. However, it is not known whether the reported levels of self-efficacy towards using sunscreen are low due to an outright unwillingness to apply it or because it is part of the descriptive norms in which they work. It has been maintained that descriptive norms have a powerful influence on behavior in ways that may lead individuals to adopt risky health behaviors [37]. In regard to lacking self-efficacy in seeking shade, it may be that LDLs lack self-efficacy because they are mainly outside workers and they have very little latitude in terms of stopping work merely to take a break from the sun. This may cause them to be dismissed and then face the challenge of securing another job. LDLs may be willing to work through continuous exposure to UVR and overlook this risk simply because of the need to keep their job. The economic pressures faced by LDLs can make them averse to leaving a job, even if it is hazardous [38]. These findings warrant additional research to look into identifying what strategies could be used to enhance the self-efficacy and motivation of LDLs to regularly apply sunscreen and seek shade whenever possible during work hours. It is recommended that interventions be designed using Motivational Interviewing (MI) as an intervention approach to help LDLs strengthen their level of self-efficacy in relation to sun protective behaviors in order to reduce the number of unsafe sun practices, such as not applying sunscreen and not seeking shade. MI-based prevention interventions have been successful in enhancing self-efficacy and motivating the readiness of participants to practice safer sex and ensuring positive behavior change [39].

The workplace environment appears to be another type of barrier. Supervisors and coworkers were not identified as a frequent source of information about protecting from too much sun. Moreover, LDLs reported not having high beliefs that their supervisors and coworkers engage in sun protective behaviors. This can influence them to potentially espouse the same blasé attitude towards sun-safe practices and behaviors. Other research has established that descriptive norms predict sun protection behaviors [40]. Supervisors and coworkers may socially reject the use of sun protective strategies. This behavior can be demonstrated indirectly by not using or discussing sun-safe practices. This may be especially true in the environment where LDLs work, where supervisors' and coworkers' norms regarding sun protective behaviors serve as group-level referent informational influences [40]. Health promotion professionals should consider whether conducting sun safety educational training sessions at worksites could be a viable path in modifying workplace descriptive and injunctive norms in support of greater use of sun protection practices. Mobile training, like clinics, may be a viable approach to promote better sun protective practices among LDLs. This training should not just target the workers but the supervisors as well. Supervisors can play an integral part in shaping the attitudes and behaviors workers exhibit in the workplace. They themselves can model the behaviors that promote more adherence to using sunscreen practices. In general, the Latino culture strongly supports respect for authority figures, such as supervisors [41]. This cultural trait can be used positively. The respect for authority figures may facilitate recommendations made by supervisors to increase use of sun-safe practices among LDLs [41].

5. Limitations

This research is subject to some limitations. Due to the small sample size and nonrandom sampling design, the generalizability of the findings to all LDLs may be limited. We believe participation in this research was impacted by recent anti-immigrant public policies in neighboring states, Alabama and Georgia. Latino immigrants experience a great deal of stress and fear in relation to being "discovered" and then deported [42]. Even LDLs who are legal may have opted out of participating because they may have feared being harassed or exploited. It is likely that the sociopolitical climate could have exacerbated their fear and discouraged LDLs from participating. Further, the majority of the participants in this study were males recruited from only two states; therefore, sample may not be entirely representative of all LDLs. Future studies should involve diverse LDL samples collected from larger geographic areas. Another limitation of our study is that findings are reliant on self-report responses, which might have introduced recall bias in the study. However, previous studies have validated self-report of sun protection using observational methods [43, 44]. Moreover, we tried to increase the sun protection recall accuracy by collecting data during summer months or a little after the end of summer months. Lastly, the majority of our sample reported low levels of acculturation. This issue could have influenced the overall results. Despite these limitations, this study provides firsthand information critically required to develop specific intervention programs to improve adoption of skin cancer prevention behaviors among this population group.

6. Conclusions

In summary, the findings of this study suggested that a substantial number of LDLs, in particular those who are not legal, do not adequately practice sun protection behaviors on a regular basis. Our results underscore the need for intervention programs aimed at LDLs to reduce extended time in the sun and increase use of sun protective measures when working outdoors. This is important given that LDLs continue to work in areas where the exposure to levels of UVR remains high. Moreover, since overall knowledge of skin cancer among this occupational group was considerably low, LDLs should be specifically educated on their vulnerability of future skin cancer risk and importance of comprehensive preventive strategies. Hence, future interventions should incorporate components to effectively minimize LDLs' barriers towards sun protection and improve their self-efficacy in wearing sunscreen and protective clothing, especially because SPBs are malleable behaviors. Doing so may provide a path for reducing the risk of developing skin cancer amongst such a susceptible group.

Ethical Approval

The approval for this research was obtained from University of Mississippi Institutional Review Board (IRB).

Conflict of Interests

Javier F. Boyas, Ph.D., and Vinayak K. Nahar, M.D., M.S., and Ph.D. Candidate, have no conflict of interests to report. Robert T. Brodell, M.D., discloses the following potential conflict of interests: honoraria have been received from presentations for Allergan, Galderma, and PharmaDerm, a division of Nycomed US Inc. Consultant fees have been received from Galderma Laboratories, L.P. Clinical trials have been performed for Genentech and Janssen Biotech, Inc. The material in this paper is not believed to be relevant to any of these reported conflicts.

Acknowledgments

The authors would like to thank all the participants who participated in this research study. They would also like to thank Zaksis Contractor for his help in data collection process.

References

[1] H. J. Lipscomb, D. Loomis, M. A. McDonald, R. A. Argue, and S. Wing, "A conceptual model of work and health disparities in the United States," *International Journal of Health Services*, vol. 36, no. 1, pp. 25–50, 2006.

[2] A. B. de Castro, J. G. Voss, A. Ruppin, C. F. Dominguez, and N. S. Seixas, "Stressors among Latino day laborers. A pilot study examining allostatic load," *American Association of Occupational Health Nurses*, vol. 58, no. 5, pp. 185–196, 2010.

[3] N. N. Menzel and A. P. Gutierrez, "Latino worker perceptions of construction risks," *American Journal of Industrial Medicine*, vol. 53, no. 2, pp. 179–187, 2010.

[4] Q. Williams Jr., M. Ochsner, E. Marshall, L. Kimmel, and C. Martino, "The impact of a peer-led participatory health and safety training program for Latino day laborers in construction," *Journal of Safety Research*, vol. 41, no. 3, pp. 253–261, 2010.

[5] O. A. Leclere and R. A. López, "The jornalero: perceptions of health care resources of immigrant day laborers," *Journal of Immigrant and Minority Health*, vol. 14, no. 4, pp. 691–697, 2012.

[6] S. J. Lowry, H. Blecker, J. Camp et al., "Possibilities and challenges in occupational injury surveillance of day laborers," *American Journal of Industrial Medicine*, vol. 53, no. 2, pp. 126–134, 2010.

[7] A. Valenzuela, N. Theodore, E. Melendez, and A. L. Gonzales, *On the Corner: Day Labor in the United States*, Center for the Study of Urban Poverty, University of California, Los Angeles, Calif, USA, 2006.

[8] V. K. Nahar, M. A. Ford, J. S. Hallam, M. A. Bass, and M. A. Vice, "Sociodemographic and psychological correlates of sun protection behaviors among outdoor workers: a review," *Journal of Skin Cancer*, vol. 2013, Article ID 453174, 10 pages, 2013.

[9] A. Jemal, R. Siegel, E. Ward et al., "Cancer statistics, 2008," *CA: A Cancer Journal for Clinicians*, vol. 58, no. 2, pp. 71–96, 2008.

[10] P. Rouhani, S. Hu, and R. S. Kirsner, "Melanoma in hispanic and black Americans," *Cancer Control*, vol. 15, no. 3, pp. 248–253, 2008.

[11] A. S. James, M. K. Tripp, G. S. Parcel, A. Sweeney, and E. R. Gritz, "Psychosocial correlates of sun-protective practices of preschool staff toward their students," *Health Education Research*, vol. 17, no. 3, pp. 305–314, 2002.

[12] C. Roman, A. Lugo-Somolinos, and N. Thomas, "Skin cancer knowledge and skin self-examinations in the Hispanic population of North Carolina: the patient's perspective," *JAMA Dermatology*, vol. 149, no. 1, pp. 103–104, 2013.

[13] E. J. Coups, J. L. Stapleton, S. V. Hudson, A. Medina-Forrester, J. S. Goydos, and A. Natale-Pereira, "Skin cancer screening among hispanic adults in the United States: results from the 2010 National Health Interview Survey," *Archives of Dermatology*, vol. 148, no. 7, pp. 861–863, 2012.

[14] F. Ma, F. Collado-Mesa, S. Hu, and R. S. Kirsner, "Skin cancer awareness and sun protection behaviors in white hispanic and white non-hispanic high school students in Miami, Florida," *Archives of Dermatology*, vol. 143, no. 8, pp. 983–988, 2007.

[15] J. N. Cormier, Y. Xing, M. Ding et al., "Ethnic differences among patients with cutaneous melanoma," *Archives of Internal Medicine*, vol. 166, no. 17, pp. 1907–1914, 2006.

[16] K. Glanz, D. B. Buller, and M. Saraiya, "Reducing ultraviolet radiation exposure among outdoor workers: state of the evidence and recommendations," *Environmental Health*, vol. 6, article 22, 2007.

[17] D. Reinau, M. Weiss, C. R. Meier, T. L. Diepgen, and C. Surber, "Outdoor workers' sun-related knowledge, attitudes and protective behaviours: a systematic review of cross-sectional and interventional studies," *British Journal of Dermatology*, vol. 168, no. 5, pp. 928–940, 2013.

[18] V. K. Nahar, M. A. Ford, J. F. Boyas et al., "Skin cancer preventative behaviors in state park workers: a pilot study," *Environmental Health and Preventive Medicine*, vol. 19, no. 6, pp. 467–474, 2014.

[19] A. Bandura, *Social Foundations of Thought and Action: A Social Cognitive Theory*, Prentice-Hall, Englewood Cliffs, NJ, USA, 1986.

[20] K. Glanz, R. A. Lew, V. Song, and V. A. Cook, "Factors associated with skin cancer prevention practices in a multiethnic population," *Health Education and Behavior*, vol. 26, no. 3, pp. 344–359, 1999.

[21] B. Marlenga, "The health beliefs and skin cancer prevention practices of Wisconsin dairy farmers," *Oncology Nursing Forum*, vol. 22, no. 4, pp. 681–686, 1995.

[22] K. D. Rosenman, J. Gardiner, G. M. Swanson, P. Mullan, and Z. Zhu, "Use of skin-cancer prevention strategies among farmers and their spouses," *American Journal of Preventive Medicine*, vol. 11, no. 5, pp. 342–347, 1995.

[23] K. M. Jackson and L. S. Aiken, "A psychosocial model of sun protection and sunbathing in young women: the impact of health beliefs, attitudes, norms, and self-efficacy for sun protection," *Health Psychology*, vol. 19, no. 5, pp. 469–478, 2000.

[24] J. A. Shoveller, C. Y. Lovato, L. Peters, and J. K. Rivers, "Canadian national survey on sun exposure and protective behaviors: outdoor workers," *Canadian Journal of Public Health*, vol. 91, no. 1, pp. 34–35, 2000.

[25] R. Cottrell, L. McClamroch, and A. L. Bernard, "Melanoma knowledge and sun protection attitudes and behaviors among college students by gender and skin type," *American Journal of Health Education*, vol. 36, no. 5, pp. 274–278, 2005.

[26] R. Salas, J. A. Mayer, and K. D. Hoerster, "Sun-protective behaviors of California farmworkers," *Journal of Occupational and Environmental Medicine*, vol. 47, no. 12, pp. 1244–1249, 2005.

[27] V. Hammond, A. I. Reeder, A. R. Gray, and M. L. Bell, "Are workers or their workplaces the key to occupational sun protection?" *Health Promotion Journal of Australia*, vol. 19, no. 2, pp. 97–101, 2008.

[28] D. Von Ah, S. Ebert, A. Ngamvitroj, N. Park, and D.-H. Kang, "Predictors of health behaviours in college students," *Journal of Advanced Nursing*, vol. 48, no. 5, pp. 463–474, 2004.

[29] D. Von Ah, S. Ebert, N. Park, A. Ngamvitroj, and D. H. Kang, "Factors related to cigarette smoking initiation and use among college students," *Tobacco Induced Diseases*, vol. 3, no. 1, pp. 27–40, 2005.

[30] A. Bandura, *Self-Efficacy: The Exercise of Control*, W.H. Freeman Publishers, New York, NY, USA, 1997.

[31] K. Glanz, B. K. Rimer, and F. M. Lewis, Eds., *Health Behavior and Health Education: Theory, Research and Practice*, Jossey Bass, San Francisco, Calif, USA, 4th edition, 2008.

[32] V. A. Andreeva, J. B. Unger, A. L. Yaroch, M. G. Cockburn, L. Baezconde-Garbanati, and K. D. Reynolds, "Acculturation and sun-safe behaviors among US Latinos: findings from the 2005 Health Information National Trends Survey," *American Journal of Public Health*, vol. 99, no. 4, pp. 734–741, 2009.

[33] E. J. Coups, J. L. Stapleton, S. V. Hudson et al., "Linguistic acculturation and skin cancer-related behaviors among Hispanics in the southern and western United States," *JAMA Dermatology*, vol. 149, no. 6, pp. 679–686, 2013.

[34] P. Madgwick, J. Houdmont, and R. Randall, "Sun safety measures among construction workers in Britain," *Occupational Medicine*, vol. 61, no. 6, pp. 430–433, 2011.

[35] C. Hernandez, S. Wang, I. Abraham et al., "Evaluation of educational videos to increase skin cancer risk awareness and sun-safe behaviors among adult hispanics," *Journal of Cancer Education*, vol. 29, no. 3, pp. 563–569, 2014.

[36] Occupational Safety and Health Administration, 2015, https://www.osha.gov/Publications/osha3151.pdf.

[37] A. E. Reid and L. S. Aiken, "Correcting injunctive norm misperceptions motivates behavior change: a randomized controlled sun protection intervention," *Health Psychology*, vol. 32, no. 5, pp. 551–560, 2013.

[38] N. Walter, P. Bourgois, H. M. Loinaz, and D. Schillinger, "Social context of work injury among undocumented day laborers in San Francisco," *Journal of General Internal Medicine*, vol. 17, no. 3, pp. 221–229, 2002.

[39] Z. Chariyeva, C. E. Golin, J. A. Earp, S. Maman, C. Suchindran, and C. Zimmer, "The role of self-efficacy and motivation to explain the effect of motivational interviewing time on changes in risky sexual behavior among people living with HIV: a mediation analysis," *AIDS and Behavior*, vol. 17, no. 2, pp. 813–823, 2013.

[40] H. Bodimeade, E. Anderson, S. La Macchia, J. R. Smith, D. J. Terry, and W. R. Louis, "Testing the direct, indirect, and interactive roles of referent group injunctive and descriptive norms for sun protection in relation to the theory of planned behavior," *Journal of Applied Social Psychology*, vol. 44, no. 11, pp. 739–750, 2015.

[41] M. C. Zea, T. Quezeda, and A. Z. Belgrave, "Latino cultural values: their role in adjustment in disability," *Journal of Social Behavior and Personality*, vol. 9, pp. 185–200, 1994.

[42] American Psychological Association, *Crossroads: The Psychology of Immigration in the New Century. The Report of the APA Presidential Task Force on Immigration. Working with Immigrant-Origin Clients, an Update for Mental Health Professionals*, American Psychological Association, 2002, http://www.apa.org/topics/immigration/executive-summary.pdf.

[43] S. S. Oh, J. A. Mayer, E. C. Lewis et al., "Validating outdoor workers' self-report of sun protection," *Preventive Medicine*, vol. 39, no. 4, pp. 798–803, 2004.

[44] K. Glanz, F. McCarty, E. J. Nehl et al., "Validity of self-reported sunscreen use by parents, children, and lifeguards," *American Journal of Preventive Medicine*, vol. 36, no. 1, pp. 63–69, 2009.

31

Clinicoepidemiological Observational Study of Acquired Alopecias in Females Correlating with Anemia and Thyroid Function

Kirti Deo, Yugal K. Sharma, Meenakshi Wadhokar, and Neha Tyagi

Department of Dermatology, Dr. D. Y. Patil Medical College and Hospital and Research Centre, Pimpri, Pune, Maharashtra 411018, India

Correspondence should be addressed to Meenakshi Wadhokar; meenakshiwadhokar@yahoo.co.in

Academic Editor: Elizabeth Helen Kemp

Alopecia can either be inherited or acquired; the latter, more common, can be diffuse, patterned, and focal, each having cicatricial and noncicatricial forms. This observational study of 135 cases in a semiurban Indian population aimed to detect the prevalence of various forms of acquired alopecia in females and correlate the same with levels of hemoglobin, serum ferritin, triiodothyronine, thyroxin, and thyroid stimulating hormone. The majority (84, 62.2%) of our cases of alopecia had telogen effluvium followed by female pattern alopecia (32, 23.7%). Stress (86, 63.7%), topical application of chemicals (72, 53.3%), systemic medications for concurrent illnesses (62, 5%), and pregnancy (14, 10.3%) were the common exacerbating factors. Neither low hemoglobin (<12 gm%, 73.4%) nor low serum ferritin (<12 μg/L, 6.7%) was found to be statistically significant. A majority (90, 90.9%) of 99 cases with anemia (hemoglobin levels of <12 gm%) had serum ferritin levels >12 μg/L. Though lack of vitamin B12 testing was a limitation of our study, its deficiency could be the probable cause of iron deficiency as the majority (58, 64.4%) of these cases, as indeed majority (89, 65.4%) of our study population, were vegetarians. Thyroid disorders (23, 17%, including 9 newly diagnosed) were not of significance statistically.

1. Introduction

The importance of human hair in social communication and sexual attraction is enormous, its loss (alopecia), shaft defects, or excess on the body are often accompanied by diminished sense of personal well-being, self-esteem, depressive moods, and withdrawal from society [1]. Alopecia, due to its multiple, virtually impossible to pinpoint, underlying causes and poor response to treatment, remains one of the most common entities that baffle dermatologists. Patient's anxiety compounds the scenario by causing increased hair loss on one hand and lack of response to treatment on the other. Lack of societal acceptance of hair loss in women, unlike in men, generates distress [2] leading not only to low self-esteem, poor body image, feeling of guilt, difficulty sleeping, and restriction in active social life [3] but also to overpresentation of women amongst those seeking treatment [4].

Alopecia can either be inherited or acquired; the latter, more common, is broadly classified into diffuse, patterned, and focal types, each further divided into scarring (cicatricial) and nonscarring (noncicatricial) forms [1]. The relatively rare inherited forms result either from improper development or nondevelopment of follicles or due to a defective hair shaft; the former has been divided again into focal (e.g., aplasia cutis congenita) or diffuse (e.g., ectodermal dysplasia) forms. The acquired hair shaft defects and increased hair breakage, commonly as a result of hair grooming practices, are reversible on cessation thereof and the inherited ones, though irreversible, also tend to improve with the advancing age [1]. Though the diagnosis of hair loss is mainly clinical, additional techniques like the hair pull test, video-dermoscopy, and histopathology are used to supplement history and examination.

The controversy regarding the association between nutritional factors and hair loss continues to persist. The supportive management with zinc and iron supplements is empirical rather than being based on unambiguous data regarding role of low serum zinc concentrations or deficient serum ferritin.

TABLE 1: Distribution of alopecia in the age groups.

Age in years	Telogen effluvium	Alopecia areata	Female pattern hair loss	Frontal fibrosing alopecia	Anagen effluvium	Total
15–20	3	2	1	0	0	6
21–30	47	11	10	0	0	68
31–40	29	3	11	1	1	45
41–50	5	1	8	0	0	14
51–60	0	0	2	0	0	2
Total	**84**	**17**	**32**	**1**	**1**	**135**

TABLE 2: Location of alopecia.

Location	Telogen effluvium	Alopecia areata	Female pattern hair loss	Frontal fibrosing alopecia	Anagen effluvium	Total
Diffuse	83	0	3	0	0	86
Parietal	1	7	0	0	0	8
Temporal	0	4	7	0	1	12
Vertex	0	5	22	1	0	28
Occipital	0	1	0	0	0	1
Total	**84**	**17**	**32**	**1**	**1**	**135**

As excessive intake of nutritional supplements may actually lead to increased hair loss, it appears logical to prescribe them in cases only with the proven deficiency [5].

This study aimed to detect the prevalence of various forms of acquired alopecia in females and their correlation with anemia and triiodothyronine (T3), thyroxin (T4), and thyroid stimulating hormone (TSH) levels.

2. Materials and Methods

This observational study comprised 135 consecutive female patients presenting to our department for the treatment of alopecia during the period of October 2014 to July 2015. Institutional ethical committee clearance and an informed consent of each patient were obtained and detailed history and examination undertaken to assess the type of alopecia, exacerbating factors, and associated systemic illnesses. Patients with diffuse hair loss, presence of one or more of the exacerbating factors, namely, stress, pregnancy, and application of chemicals, and positive hair pull test were considered to have telogen effluvium. Patients with reduction of number of hair, especially in biparietal, bitemporal, and vertex regions with preservation of anterior hair implantation line, were considered to have female pattern hair loss. However, overlapping of both of these diseases could occur in some cases. All patients were tested for hemoglobin (Hb), serum ferritin, and T3, T4, and TSH levels. The data obtained were analyzed statistically using SPSS version 22.0. Correlation between variables was calculated using Spearman's rank correlation coefficient and Chi-square test. A value of $p < 0.05$ was considered significant.

3. Results

The age of our study patients ranged from 15 to 60 (mean: 30.96 ± 8.489) years, with the majority (68, 50.4%) belonging to the third decade (Table 1). After onset of alopecia patients took one to 84 (mean: 15.64 ± 16.003) months to seek consultation, the largest segment (29, 21.5%) reporting after 12 months resulting in a significant, but mild positive, correlation (rho = 0.219; $p = 0.011$); OPD consultation gets increasingly delayed with the advancing age of the patients.

The first and second common types of alopecia in our study were telogen effluvium (TE) (84, 62.2%) and female pattern hair loss (FPHL) (32, 23.7%) (Table 1). The exacerbating factors found across the spectrum of alopecia were stress, in 86 (63.7%) patients; application of chemicals such as mehndi or dye, in 72 (53.3%); pregnancy and/or delivery six months preceding the presentation, in 14 (10.3%). Sixty-two (45.9%) patients were undergoing treatment for associated systemic illness(es): 21 (15.6%) for diabetes mellitus; 14 (10.4%) for polycystic ovarian disease; 11 (8.1%) for hypertension; 8 (5.9%) for hypothyroidism; 6 (4.4%) for hyperthyroidism; and 1 (0.7%) for tuberculosis and cancer each. Dandruff seen in 63 (46.7%) and oily scalp in 75 (55.6%) were not statistically significantly associated. The majority (86, 63.7%) of patients had diffuse hair loss followed by hair loss over the vertex (28, 20.7%) (Table 2). Family history of alopecia was given by only 6 (4.4%). FPHL, found in 8 (25%) postmenopausal cases in our study, revealed a statistically significant association ($p = 0.006$, strength of association, $\chi^2 = 21.36$). Characteristic nail pitting seen in 9 (52.9%) of 17 cases of alopecia areata was also associated significantly ($p = 0.001$, strength of association, $\chi^2 = 0.545$).

Hemoglobin levels ranged from 7.20 to 13.40 (mean: 10.97 ± 1.32) gm%; anemia (Hb < 12 gm%) was present in 99 (73.4%). Serum ferritin levels ranged from 5.10 to 200.70 (mean: 54.73 ± 41.5) µg/L. Iron deficiency was seen in 9 (6.7%) of our study population having serum ferritin < 12 µg/L; neither hemoglobin nor serum ferritin levels were statistically significant. Thyroid disorders present in 23 (17%) patients, including nine (6.7%) newly diagnosed ones, too, were not of statistical significance (Table 3).

TABLE 3: Thyroid disorders throughout the spectrum of alopecia (new + old cases).

	Telogen effluvium		Alopecia areata		Female pattern hair loss		Frontal fibrosing alopecia	Anagen effluvium	Total
	N	O	N	O	N	O			
Hypothyroidism	2	4	1	1	2	3	0	0	**13**
Hyperthyroidism	3	5	1	1	0	0	0	0	**10**
Euthyroid	70		13		27		1	1	**112**
Total	**84**		**17**		**32**		1	1	135

N: new; O: old.

TABLE 4: Comparison between prevalence of female pattern hair loss.

Age in years	Wang et al. [8] (%)	Paik et al. [9] (%)	Birch et al. [10] (%)	Gan and Sinclair [11] (%)	Present study (%)
15–20	—	—	—	—	0.7
21–30	1.30	0.2	12.3	12.00	7.4
31–40	2.30	2.3	17.00	—	8.1
41–50	5.40	3.8	25.40	25.00	5.9
51–60	7.50	7.4	27.90	—	1.4
61–70	10.30	11.7	41.10	41.00	—
71–80	11.80	24.7	53.60	50.00	—

4. Discussion

Despite its exact prevalence being difficult to estimate due to its subclinical nature [1], telogen effluvium is generally considered to be the most common type of alopecia in females followed by FPHL and alopecia areata [6]. Similar was the frequency of occurrence of these three types of alopecia in our study.

Telogen effluvium in women commonly occurs during the age of 30–60 years, usually commencing abruptly with or without a recognizable initiating factor [7]. Among the 84 patients of TE in our study, as also in a South Arabian one, its peak incidence (47, 56%) was during the third decade of life [7]. For unknown reasons, chronic TE seems to affect only women [7]. History of hair coming out along with the bulbs given by 74 (88.1%) of our 84 patients of TE was statistically significant ($p = 0.00$, strength of association, $\chi^2 = 24.180$); 10 (11.09%) of these developed it after pregnancy; 58 (69.1%) underwent a period of stress during the preceding six months and 53 (65.1%) were vegetarians. Positive hair pull test in all scalp areas indicative of associated TE was detected in 46 (54.8%) of these 84 cases; the Saudi Arabian study reported positive hair pull test in 61% of their cases of TE [7]. Sixty-three (75%) of our 84 patients of TE were anemic (Hb < 12 gm%) and 8 (9.5%) were iron deficient (serum ferritin < 12 μg/L).

Female pattern hair loss (FPHL) was observed in 32 (23.7%) patients in our study, 11 (34.4%) belonging to the third decade; unlike in most of the earlier studies, its prevalence was not seen to increase with age (Table 4) [8–11]. However, a comparison between prevalence studies is hampered by the lack of universally accepted criteria for diagnostic definition of this disease. Despite onset of FPHL during the reproductive years, there is a greater demand for its treatment among patients aged 25–40 years possibly explaining the preponderance of cases (21 of 32, 65%) aged 21–40 years in

our study [12]. Lesser prevalence with increasing age in our study could be due to only 2 (1.48%) cases belonging to the last decade of the age of our study population. Hair loss over the vertex was present in 22 (68.8%) patients followed by that on the temporal zone (7; 21.9%) and diffuse hair loss (3; 9.4%). In an Australian study, the majority (64.4%) of such patients exhibited bitemporal hair loss [11]. Twenty (62.5%) of our cases of FPHL gave history of application of mehndi/hair dye; 20 (62.5%) of irregular menses or menopause; and 15 (46.1%) of stress. Hypertension and diabetes mellitus were present in 8 (25%) and 7 (21.9%) cases, respectively. Hair pull test was positive in 15 (46.1%); 20 (62.5%) were anemic and 1 (3.1%) was iron deficient, reaffirming the lack of role of nutrition in causation of FPHL. Insignificant (1, 3.1%) incidence of positive family history in our FPHL patients, unlike that of 45.2% (Wang et al.) [8] and 19.2% (Paik et al.) [9], could probably be due to different, as yet unknown, underlying genetic factors in different ethnicities.

The prevalence (17, 12.6%) of alopecia areata (AA) in our study was almost half of that (25%) found in a the United States based study by McMichael et al. Unlike majority (11; 64.1%) of these patients in our study belonging to the third decade, majority of them in study by McMichael et al. belonged to 4th to 6th decades of life [13]. In a German study its highest prevalence was seen during 2nd to 4th decades of life, up to 66% of these patients being below 30 years of age and only 20% older than 40 years [14]. The onset below the age of 40 was reported in 70% of the patients of AA in a Greek study by Kyriakis et al., 48% having onset of AA before the age of 20 years [15]. The appearance of first patch before the age of 20 was seen in 60% of cases in a United States based study by Wasserman et al. Surprisingly, just 2 (12%) of our cases of AA developed first patch before the age of 20 [16]. AA was associated with stress during the six months preceding its onset in 11 (64.7%) of our study patients, similar to that of Taiwanese (50%) and Romanian (45.6%) studies [17, 18], corroborating the well-known role of psychological stress in precipitating AA [19, 20]. However, family history of AA in our study was rarely positive (1, 5.9%), as also remarked in previous studies: 9% (Sharma et al.) [21] and 4.6% (Tan et al.) [22].

Anagen effluvium and frontal fibrosing alopecia each occurred only in one case in our study.

Hemoglobin levels ranged from 7.20 to 13.40 (mean: 10.97 ± 1.32) gm% in our study. Ninety-nine (73.4%) patients were found to be anemic (Hb < 12 gm%); 68 (50.3%) were mild (Hb 10–11.99 gm%), 31 (23%) moderate (Hb 7–9.99 gm%), and none severe (Hb < 7 gm%). This classification of anemia was based on Indian (national family health survey 3, 2005-2006) Government survey in which 48.3% (3890 of 8053) of women in Maharashtra, the Indian state of our study population, were found to be anemic [mild (32.8%); moderate (13.8%); severe (1.7%)] [23] suggesting anemia to be a major factor underlying hair loss. The prevalence of anemia in a study of 4032 asymptomatic females in the Indian state of Andhra Pradesh was found to be 52% [24]. In our study population, serum ferritin levels ranged from 5.10 to 200.70 (mean: 54.73 ± 41.46) μg/L, nine (6.6%) being iron deficient (serum ferritin < 12 μg/L), as compared to that of 33.3% in studies conducted in Bangladesh and Iran [24, 25]. Out of 99 patients of anemia, 9 (9.1%) were found to have iron deficiency anemia. Among the 90 non-iron deficiency anemia patients, 58 (63.1%) were vegetarians who probably had underlying vitamin B12 deficiency. In a study by Sinclair no direct relationship between low serum ferritin and hair loss was established and determination of serum ferritin as a routine investigation in women with chronic diffuse telogen hair loss was not found useful, doubting the role of iron supplementation in management of hair loss [26].

Twenty-three patients (17%) were found to be suffering from thyroid disorders: 13 (9.63%) were suffering from hypothyroidism and 10 (7.4%) hyperthyroidism, similar to the overall prevalence (18.6%) of thyroid disorders in Maharashtra [23] and much more than 2.5% of hypothyroidism and hyperthyroidism each in a German study [27]. However, 9 (6.7%) patients, 5 (3.7%) with hypothyroidism and 4 (3%) with hyperthyroidism, were newly diagnosed during our study (Table 3).

5. Conclusion

Telogen effluvium was the most frequent type of alopecia found in our study. Exacerbating factors included stress, pregnancy, and application of chemicals. Anemia detected in approximately 3rd/4th of our study population would appear as the commonest cause of alopecia. While only a small minority were diagnosed as having iron deficiency anemia, a majority suffered probably from vitamin B12 deficiency, being vegetarians. According to our study serum ferritin levels did not have significant role in the pathogenesis of hair loss and may not need to be estimated routinely. Women suffering from recalcitrant hair loss should undergo thyroid function tests to reveal subclinical thyroid disorders. Appropriate counseling and treatment can then be specifically directed at the etiology of hair loss, thus improving the patient outcome.

Conflict of Interests

The authors declare that there is no conflict of interests regarding the publication of this paper.

Authors' Contribution

All authors contributed to concepts, design, definition of intellectual content, literature search, and clinical studies. Kirti Deo, Yugal K. Sharma, and Meenakshi Wadhokar contributed to paper preparation and editing. Kirti Deo and Yugal K. Sharma contributed to paper review.

References

[1] N. Otberg and J. Shapiro, "Hair growth disorders," in *Fitzpatrick's Dermatology in General Medicine*, L. A. Goldsmith, S. I. Katz, B. A. Gilcherst, A. S. Paller, D. J. Lefeell, and K. Wolff, Eds., pp. 979–1008, McGraw-Hill, New York, NY, USA, 8th edition, 2012.

[2] T. F. Cash, "The psychological effects of androgenetic alopecia in men," *Journal of the American Academy of Dermatology*, vol. 26, no. 6, pp. 926–931, 1992.

[3] T. F. Cash, V. H. Price, and R. C. Savin, "Psychological effects of androgenetic alopecia on women: comparisons with balding men and with female control subjects," *Journal of the American Academy of Dermatology*, vol. 29, no. 4, pp. 568–575, 1993.

[4] C. Grover and A. Khurana, "Telogen effluvium," *Indian Journal of Dermatology, Venereology and Leprology*, vol. 79, no. 5, pp. 591–603, 2013.

[5] D. H. Rushton, "Nutritional factors and hair loss," *Clinical and Experimental Dermatology*, vol. 27, no. 5, pp. 396–404, 2002.

[6] S. B. Shrivastava, "Diffuse hair loss in an adult female: approach to diagnosis and management," *Indian Journal of Dermatology, Venereology and Leprology*, vol. 75, no. 1, pp. 20–28, 2009.

[7] M. I. Fatani, A. M. Bin Mahfoz, A. H. Mahdi et al., "Prevalence and factors associated with telogen effluvium in adult females at Makkah region, Saudi Arabia: a retrospective study," *Journal of Dermatology & Dermatologic Surgery*, vol. 19, no. 1, pp. 27–30, 2015.

[8] T. L. Wang, C. Zhou, Y. W. Shen et al., "Prevalence of androgenetic alopecia in China: a community-based study in six cities," *British Journal of Dermatology*, vol. 162, no. 4, pp. 843–847, 2010.

[9] J.-H. Paik, J.-B. Yoon, W.-Y. Sim, B.-S. Kim, and N.-I. Kim, "The prevalence and types of androgenetic alopecia in Korean men and women," *British Journal of Dermatology*, vol. 145, no. 1, pp. 95–99, 2001.

[10] M. P. Birch, J. F. Messenger, and A. G. Messenger, "Hair density, hair diameter and the prevalence of female pattern hair loss," *British Journal of Dermatology*, vol. 144, no. 2, pp. 297–304, 2001.

[11] D. C. C. Gan and R. D. Sinclair, "Prevalence of male and female pattern hair loss in Maryborough," *The Journal of Investigative Dermatology*, vol. 10, no. 3, pp. 184–189, 2005.

[12] P. M. Ramos and H. A. Miot, "Female pattern hair loss: a clinical and pathophysiological review," *Anais Brasileiros de Dermatologia*, vol. 90, no. 4, pp. 529–543, 2015.

[13] A. J. McMichael, D. J. Pearce, D. Wasserman et al., "Alopecia in the United States: outpatient utilization and common prescribing patterns," *Journal of the American Academy of Dermatology*, vol. 57, no. 2, pp. S49–S51, 2007.

[14] A. M. Finner, "Alopecia areata: clinical presentation, diagnosis, and unusual cases," *Dermatologic Therapy*, vol. 24, no. 3, pp. 348–354, 2011.

[15] K. P. Kyriakis, K. Paltazidou, E. Kosma, E. Sofouri, A. Tadros, and E. Rachioli, "Alopecia areata preelnce by gender and age," *Journal of the European Academy of Dermatology and Venereology*, vol. 23, no. 5, pp. 572–573, 2009.

[16] D. Wasserman, D. A. Guzman-Sanchez, K. Scott, and A. Mcmichael, "Alopecia areata," *International Journal of Dermatology*, vol. 46, no. 2, pp. 121–131, 2007.

[17] S.-Y. Chu, Y.-J. Chen, W.-C. Tseng et al., "Psychiatric comorbidities in patients with alopecia areata in Taiwan: a case-control study," *British Journal of Dermatology*, vol. 166, no. 3, pp. 525–531, 2012.

[18] L. Manolache and V. Benea, "Stress in patients with alopecia areata and vitiligo," *Journal of the European Academy of Dermatology and Venereology*, vol. 21, no. 7, pp. 921–928, 2007.

[19] P. Sharma, A. Fernandes, A. Bharati et al., "Psychological aspects of Alopecia Areata," *Indian Journal of Mental Health*, vol. 2, no. 1, 2015.

[20] A. T. Güleç, N. Tanriverdi, Ç. Dürü, Y. Saray, and C. Akçali, "The role of psychological factors in alopecia areata and the impact of the disease on the quality of life," *International Journal of Dermatology*, vol. 43, no. 5, pp. 352–356, 2004.

[21] V. K. Sharma, G. Dawn, and B. Kumar, "Profile of alopecia areata in Northern India," *International Journal of Dermatology*, vol. 35, no. 1, pp. 22–27, 1996.

[22] E. Tan, Y.-K. Tay, C.-L. Goh, and Y. C. Giam, "The pattern and profile of alopecia areata in Singapore—a study of 219 Asians," *International Journal of Dermatology*, vol. 41, no. 11, pp. 748–753, 2002.

[23] International Institute for Population Sciences (IIPS) and Macro International, "National family health survey (NFHS-3)," Tech. Rep. 2005-06, IIPS, Mumbai, India, 2008.

[24] M. E. Bentley and P. L. Griffiths, "The burden of anemia among women in India," *European Journal of Clinical Nutrition*, vol. 57, no. 1, pp. 52–60, 2003.

[25] M. M. Karim, M. A. Wahab, L. Khondoker, and M. S. Khan, "Low iron level is related to telogen effluvium in women," *Bangladesh Journal of Medicine*, vol. 21, no. 2, pp. 84–89, 2013.

[26] R. Sinclair, "There is no clear association between low serum ferritin and chronic diffuse telogen hair loss," *British Journal of Dermatology*, vol. 147, no. 5, pp. 982–984, 2002.

[27] G. Lutz, "Hair loss and hyperprolactinemia in women," *Dermato-Endocrinology*, vol. 4, no. 1, pp. 65–71, 2012.

32

Epidermal Permeability Barrier in the Treatment of Keratosis Pilaris

Tanawatt Kootiratrakarn, Kowit Kampirapap, and Chakkrapong Chunhasewee

Institute of Dermatology, Bangkok 10400, Thailand

Correspondence should be addressed to Tanawatt Kootiratrakarn; tanawatt_k@hotmail.com

Academic Editor: Bruno A. Bernard

Objectives. To evaluate and compare the efficacy, safety, hydrating properties, and tolerability of 10% lactic acid (LA) and 5% salicylic acid (SA) in the therapy of keratosis pilaris (KP). *Material and Method.* Patients with KP were randomized for treatment with either 10% LA or 5% SA creams being applied twice daily for 3 months. The patients were clinically assessed at baseline and after 4, 8, and 12 weeks of treatment and 4 weeks after treatment. The functional properties of the stratum corneum (SC) were determined before treatment, 12 weeks, and follow-up phase by high-frequency conductance and transepidermal water loss (TEWL). *Results.* At the end of the trial, the mean reduction of the lesions from baseline was statistically significant for 10% LA (66%) and 5% SA (52%). During the treatment, higher conductance values were found on both group and this improvement was maintained until the follow up period. No significant differences in transepidermal water loss were observed after treatment. The adverse effects were limited to mild irritation localized on the skin without systemic side effect. *Conclusion.* The study demonstrated that 10% LA and 5% SA are beneficial to treat KP with the significantly clearance and marked improvement as by instrumental evaluation.

1. Introduction

Keratosis pilaris (KP) is a common benign disorder that presents an eruption of symmetrically distributed, keratotic follicular papules on the proximal extremities of young individuals. Although it is neither life-threatening nor physically debilitating, it can severely affect those individuals socially and psychologically. Furthermore, commonly employed treatments appear to show a lack of satisfactory efficacy. These medications have included an emollient cream and keratolytic agents containing lactic acid or salicylic acid [1]. In the present study, we evaluated the clinical outcome as well as the functions of the stratum corneum (SC) by employing a prospective split side-controlled trial of lactic acid and salicylic acid before and after topical treatment with representative keratolytic agents.

2. Material and Method

2.1. Patients and Procedures. A prospective, randomized, and clinical study comparing 10% lactic acid and 5% salicylic cream was carried out at the Institute of Dermatology,

Bangkok, Thailand. The protocol was approved by the Ethical Committee of the Institute of Dermatology and written informed consent was obtained from all participants.

The patients had a clinical diagnosis of keratosis pilaris, which showed the extensive keratotic follicular papules, almost entirely on the extensor and lateral aspect of proximal extremities, symmetrically. Fifty participants were enrolled in this clinical study. Patients were in good health and free of other skin disease or physical condition that would impair evaluation of treatment areas. Subjects were ineligible to participate if they (i) were sensitive to the ingredients in the formulations; (ii) were pregnant or lactating; (iii) had used topical therapy (emollients, moisturizers, corticosteroids) within 1 month prior to the study; (iv) were receiving concurrent systemic therapy with corticosteroids or retinoid. They were allowed to continue their usual daily activities throughout the trial.

2.2. Randomized Treatment Phase. The patients were enrolled in this study to evaluate the effect of 10% lactic acid versus 5% salicylic acid cream. The vehicle has been controlled by using base cream (8% stearyl alcohol, 4% cetyl alcohol, 18%

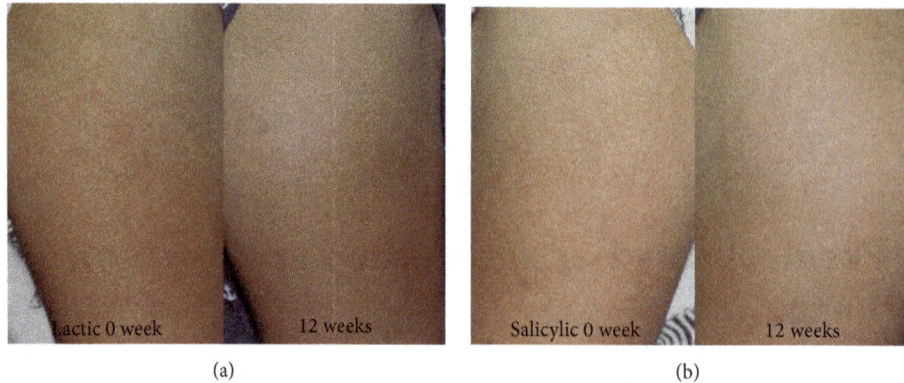

FIGURE 1: Clinical appearance of keratosis pilaris before and after 12 weeks of treatment with 10% lactic cream (a) and 5% salicylic cream (b). They show decreased hyperkeratotic papules at the end of trial.

liquid paraffin, 5.7% propylene glycol, 2% white beeswax, 5.5% sodium lauryl sulfate, and 1% paraben conc.) with active gradient 10% lactic acid or 5% salicylic acid, respectively. They were told to apply the one designated agents twice daily on each of their extensor upper arms by using one hand to apply one test medication to the opposite upper arm and vice versa. The information stored securely for each patient and examining dermatologists were blinded to this information. Patients were reexamined by the dermatologist at 4, 8, and 12 weeks after beginning the study and 4 weeks follow-up phase and any changes in number of lesions were documented in questionnaires designed for this purpose.

2.3. Subjective Self-Assessment. Self-assessments were solicited by questionnaire; study participants were interviewed and questioned regarding therapy benefits. An open-ended question asked patients if any treatment had been successful and, if so, to evaluate overall change in smoothness and dark spot of the affected area. The quantification of any amelioration in their KP was also done by marking the improved percentage from baseline.

2.4. Investigator Assessment. Investigators' evaluations were recorded via questionnaires by three independent dermatologists. At the end of treatment and follow-up phase, the change in the signs of papules and postinflammatory pigment alteration were evaluated in the overall disease severity by percent of improvement.

2.5. Biophysical Skin Parameters Obtained by Noninvasive Measurements. High-frequency conductance, which is a parameter for the hydration state of the skin surface, was measured with a skin surface hygrometer (Skicon 200, IBS Ltd., Hamamatsu, Japan) with a probe of 2 mm inner diameter and 4 mm outer diameter electrodes. Transepidermal water loss (TEWL), a parameter for the water barrier function of the stratum corneum SC, was measured with close-chamber evaporimeter (Vapometer, Delfin Technologies Ltd., Kuopio, Finland) [2]. All measurements were performed on the mid portion of the upper arm by a 30 min acclimatization time in a climate chamber, in which the room temperature and relative

humidity were adjusted to 25°C and the relative humidity was 65 to 70%, respectively. The conductance and TEWL were recorded at the baseline, week 12 of treatment and 4-week follow-up after complete treatment.

2.6. Statistical Analysis. Statistical analyses were performed with SPSS 16 for Windows software (SPSS Inc., Chicago, IL, USA). Scores of the clinical assessment were compared between each treated side using the Wilcoxon signed-ranks test. The values of the conductance, TEWL, were compared between each treatment with the paired t-test. P values of <0.05 were accepted as statistically significant.

3. Result

The age of onset of KP was as follows; during first decade in 57%, second decade 31%, and third decade 12%. Body sites affected included the arms (93%), legs (26%), face (6%), and buttocks (27%). Family history of KP was found in 67%. An associated atopic condition (allergic rhinitis, asthma, and eczema) was recorded in 42%. No seasonal variation was noted in our patients. Half of them felt that their skin was dry and considered that dry environment was a precipitating factor. Most of patients (65%) had previously sought and received treatments and felt dissatisfaction with the appearance, embarrassment, and lack of self-confidence. Social dysfunction has also been observed, including concerns about social appearances in public.

Fifty participants completed the monthly assessment for evaluation of treatment efficacy (Figure 1). Compared with baseline, both treatments showed a statistically significant reduction of lesions at the end of 4, 8, and 12 weeks of treatment ($P < 0.05$). The rate of decline was greater during the first 4 weeks and more gradually decreased during the next 4 weeks until the end of 12 weeks. The mean percentage of reduction from baseline up until the end of the trial was 66% in the lactic acid group and 52% with the salicylic acid group. The change from baseline until the end of the 12 weeks was statistically significant in both groups ($P < 0.05$). The mean difference between both groups from baseline until the end of 12 weeks was 14% which was statistically significant

TABLE 1: At the end of the 12-week treatment period, the obtained skin conductance values were significantly higher for each of the therapies, as compared with their respective baseline values. These obtained values were higher for the 10% lactic acid cream treated side than the 5% salicylic acid treated side. By contrast, TEWL showed no statistically significant changes in both lactic acid and salicylic acid-treated sites as compared with those values measured before treatment.

| | Conductance ($\pm$SD) | | TEWL ($\pm$SD) | |
	10% lactic	5% salicylic	10% lactic	5% salicylic
Base line	121.5 ± 60.0	124.5 ± 55.3	8.1 ± 1.6	7.9 ± 1.8
Week 12	$169.1 \pm 74.0^*$	$148.5 \pm 49.9^*$	7.7 ± 1.6	7.7 ± 1.4
4-week follow-up	$155.3 \pm 53.2^*$	$140.6 \pm 43.6^*$	7.5 ± 2.3	7.7 ± 1.2

$^*P < 0.05$.

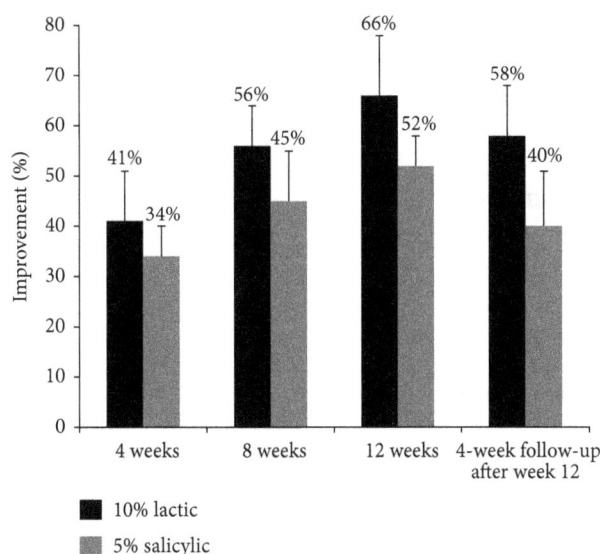

FIGURE 2: Compared with the baseline, both treatments showed a statistically significant reduction of the lesions at the end of 4, 8, and 12 weeks of treatment ($P < 0.05$). The observed rate of decline was greater during the first 4 weeks, becoming more gradual during the next 4 weeks until the end of 12 weeks. The mean percentage of reduction from the baseline up until the end of the trial was 66% for the lactic acid group in contrast to 52% for the salicylic acid group. These changes from the baseline until the end of the 12 weeks were all statistically significant in both groups ($P < 0.05$).

($P < 0.05$), the lactic acid group was more effective than the salicylic acid group (Figure 2).

The mean percentage change forming baseline to up until the 4 and 8 weeks was 41% and 56% in the lactic acid group and 34% and 45% in the salicylic acid group, respectively. Both treatment groups had a statistically significant reduction in the mean percentage improvement from baseline until the end of the 4 and 8 weeks ($P < 0.05$).

The patients in both groups assessed the aesthetic features of both creams. The greasiness of both creams was similar; however, the lactic acid group complained more about malodor and irritation when applying the cream. The adverse events reported during the present study showed only irritation, which was typically slightly burning or itching sensation with no visible reaction on the skin. These reactions were found more common in the lactic acid group than

the salicylic acid group but the difference was not statistically significant.

The instrumental assessments were summarized in Table 1. Although at the end of 12-week period showed no statistically significant changes in TEWL in either lactic acid or salicylic acid treated sites as compared with their data obtained before treatment, the skin conductance became significantly higher after treatment with both agents, as compared with their baseline values. These obtained data also showed the sustainable benefits even at 4-week follow-up phase.

4. Discussion

Keratosis pilaris is known to be a common disorder which affects 40% of population [3]. However, the disease has been poorly documented in the literature. The isolated form frequently appears in childhood with remission by adulthood in many patients. Most of our patients developed KP during the first decade of life, which agrees with the previous finding that KP commences in childhood and reaches its peak prevalence during adolescence. A family history of KP in 67% would support and agree with an autosomal dominant mode of inheritance. The families with incomplete penetrance had been postulated [4]. The increasing prevalence of KP in autosomal dominant ichthyosis had also been reported.

Patients' tolerance to the rough texture and cosmetic appearance of KP varies considerably and is frequently discordant with the clinical signs [5]. The interaction of KP and psychosocial issues is complex and, in adolescents, can be associated with developmental issues of body image, socialization, and sexuality [6, 7]. However, the study on the psychosocial impact of KP has not been documented. The impact of KP may have been underestimated. Our data showed that 40% of those with KP have significant effect on self-image and impacts in the quality of life; therefore, the effective treatment should result in the improvement of anxiety, depression, and body satisfaction.

The treatment usually begins with reassurance for the patient and a discussion of general skin care. Measures should be taken to prevent excessive skin dryness, such as decreasing the frequency of skin cleansing, brief water showers, and using mild soaps. The keratolytic agent such as one that contains lactic acid, salicylic acid, or urea may be beneficial. Lactic acid functions, primarily, as modulator of skin keratinization, although it also is referred to as humectant, pH adjuster, and mild irritation [8]. The application should show the reduction of corneocyte adhesion at the lowest levels of the stratum corneum, which results in desquamation of both normal and diseased skin, also resulting in normalization of retention hyperkeratosis. With continued treatment, the lactic acid 10% treatment site demonstrated a dramatic increase in turnover rate [9, 10]. Salicylic acid is a topical keratolytic agent which is believed at act by reducing cohesion between keratinocytes. Symptoms of toxicity form percutaneous absorption and contact sensitizer have been reported [11]. The urea cream usually produces keratolytic effect without the stimulatory response to basal cells, avoiding the production of excess or abnormal corneocytes [12]. We particularly like a cream preparation consisting of 10% lactic acid or salicylic acid. We hypothesize that, in the differences, mechanism of action may explain the differences seen in the two treatments. A follow-up study also may be desirable to study this important variable.

The present study confirmed the effectiveness of 10% lactic acid and 5% salicylic acid in the treatment of KP. Both medications showed greater statistically significant improvement of KP at the end of 4 weeks. However, the data indicated that clinical observation ratings by patients differed between the two treatments. Most measures showed that improvement was achieved in less time with 10% lactic acid cream than with 5% salicylic acid cream. Moreover, patients receiving 10% lactic acid showed rapid onset of improvement from baseline at the end of 4 weeks and sustained improvement afterwards until the end of 12 weeks. Furthermore, the investigators' overall assessment showed over 62.5% of patients treated with 10% lactic acid achieved marked improvement and clearance at the end of 12 weeks, which showed the high efficacy of this treatment. However, patients treated by 10% lactic acid showed mild local irritation as a side effect that was well tolerated.

The cutaneous bioengineering was also used to evaluate the mechanical and functional characteristics of the skin affected by KP. The most commonly used methods for evaluating moisturization are cutaneous electrical capacitance and TEWL. Cutaneous electrical capacitance involves the passage of low-frequency alternate current through the skin, whose electrical conductivity depends on the water contents of the SC and its integrity. TEWL determines the flow of evaporation of water through the SC, thus allowing evaluation of its barrier function. We found an increase in the hydration state of the SC when evaluated with the measurements of high-frequency conductance of the treated skin at the end of treatment. Conductance findings suggested that 10% lactic acid cream improves texture by the stimulation of cell growth upward towards the skin surface, which might produce outer skin hydration at a slower pace. Thus, it can be estimated that at end of treatment it showed greater hydration. Five percent salicylic acid cream showed improvement of hydration by directly removing the upper surface layer of dead cells, thereby softening the skin. This suggests that both may significantly decrease SC cohesion by only minimally disrupting skin barrier to water diffusion. Since corneodesmosomes are believed to be the major component providing SC cohesion

[12, 13], our results indicate that both treatments mainly affect their structure and seems not significantly to perturb the SC lipid composition and organization, which is mainly responsible for SC excellent barrier properties.

In conclusion, the clinical observation ratings by patients and investigators, as well as instrument measures, showed the effectiveness of the two treatments. The conclusion from the present study is that 10% lactic acid should be chosen as standard treatment for KP in preference to salicylic acid in the view of its higher efficacy. When this therapy was used for distressing or extensive keratosis pilaris, it has been observed to be effective, convenient, well-accepted, well-tolerated regimen.

Conflict of Interests

The authors declare that there is no conflict of interests regarding the publication of this paper.

References

[1] S. Hwang and R. A. Schwartz, "Keratosis pilaris: a common follicular hyperkeratosis," Cutis, vol. 82, no. 3, pp. 177–180, 2008.

[2] K. Kikuchi, H. Kobayashi, T. Hirao, A. Ito, H. Takahashi, and H. Tagami, "Improvement of mild inflammatory changes of the facial skin induced by winter environment with daily applications of a moisturizing cream: a half-side test of biophysical skin parameters, cytokine expression pattern and the formation of cornified envelope," Dermatology, vol. 207, no. 3, pp. 269–275, 2003.

[3] L. Poskitt and J. D. Wilkinson, "Natural history of keratosis pilaris," British Journal of Dermatology, vol. 130, no. 6, pp. 711–713, 1994.

[4] B. Mevorah, A. Krayenbuhl, E. H. Bovey, and G. D. van Melle, "Autosomal dominant ichthyosis and X-linked ichthyosis," Acta Dermato-Venereologica, vol. 71, no. 5, pp. 431–434, 1991.

[5] G. Yosipovitch, A. DeVore, and A. Dawn, "Obesity and the skin: skin physiology and skin manifestations of obesity," Journal of the American Academy of Dermatology, vol. 56, no. 6, pp. 901–916, 2007.

[6] M. Augustine and E. Jayaseelan, "Erythromelanosis follicularis faciei et colli: relationship with keratosis pilaris," Indian Journal of Dermatology, Venereology and Leprology, vol. 74, no. 1, pp. 47–49, 2008.

[7] S. M. Clark, C. M. Mills, and S. W. Lanigan, "Treatment of keratosis pilaris atrophicans with the pulsed tunable dye laser," Journal of Cutaneous Laser Therapy, vol. 2, no. 3, pp. 151–156, 2000.

[8] N. L. Novick, "Practical management of widespread, atypical kerotosis pilaris," Journal of the American Academy of Dermatology, vol. 11, no. 2 I, pp. 305–306, 1984.

[9] E. Berardesca, F. Distante, G. P. Vignoli, C. Oresajo, and B. Green, "Alpha hydroxyacids modulate stratum corneum barrier function," British Journal of Dermatology, vol. 137, no. 6, pp. 934–938, 1997.

[10] G. Grove and C. Zerweck, "An evaluation of the moisturizing and anti-itch effects of a lactic acid and pramoxine hydrochloride cream," Cutis, vol. 73, no. 2, pp. 135–139, 2004.

[11] S. J. Bashir, F. Dreher, A. L. Chew et al., "Cutaneous bioassay of salicylic acid as a keratolytic," International Journal of Pharmaceutics, vol. 292, no. 1-2, pp. 187–194, 2005.

[12] J. Ademola, C. Frazier, S. J. Kim, C. Theaux, and X. Saudez, "Clinical evaluation of 40% urea and 12% ammonium lactate in the treatment of xerosis," *The American Journal of Clinical Dermatology*, vol. 3, no. 3, pp. 217–222, 2002.

[13] S. J. Chapman, A. Walsh, S. M. Jackson, and P. S. Friedmann, "Lipids, proteins and corneocyte adhesion," *Archives of Dermatological Research*, vol. 283, no. 3, pp. 167–173, 1991.

33

Leprosy Reaction in Thai Population: A 20-Year Retrospective Study

Poonkiat Suchonwanit, Siripich Triamchaisri, Sanchawan Wittayakornrerk, and Ploysyne Rattanakaemakorn

Division of Dermatology, Department of Medicine, Faculty of Medicine, Ramathibodi Hospital, Mahidol University, Bangkok 10400, Thailand

Correspondence should be addressed to Poonkiat Suchonwanit; poonkiat@hotmail.com

Academic Editor: Craig G. Burkhart

Background. Leprosy is a chronic infectious disease that presents with varying dermatological and neurological symptoms. The leprosy reactions occur over the chronic course of the disease and lead to extensive disability and morbidity. *Objective.* To analyze and identify the risk factors which contribute to leprosy reactions. *Methods.* In a retrospective study, we reviewed the medical records of leprosy patients registered at the leprosy clinic, Ramathibodi Hospital, Thailand, between March 1995 and April 2015. One hundred and eight patients were included; descriptive analysis was used for baseline characteristics and a binary logistic regression model was applied for identifying risk factors correlated with leprosy reactions. *Results.* Of the 108 cases analyzed, 51 were male and 57 were female. The mean age of presentation was 45 years. The borderline tuberculoid type was the most common clinical form. Leprosy reactions were documented in 61 cases (56.5%). The average time to reaction was 8.9 months. From multivariate analysis, risk factors for leprosy reactions were being female, positive bacillary index status, and MB treatment regimen. *Conclusions.* Leprosy reactions are common complications in leprosy patients. Being female, positive bacillary index status, and multibacillary treatment regimen are significantly associated with the reactions. Early detection in cases with risk factors followed by appropriate treatment could prevent the morbidity of leprosy patients.

1. Introduction

Leprosy is a chronic disease caused by *Mycobacterium leprae*, which primarily affects the skin and nerves. Clinical characteristics are anesthetic skin lesions and peripheral nerve thickening. With the success of multidrug therapy (MDT) by the World Health Organization (WHO) in 1982, attention has changed to focus on the leprosy reactions, which are now the most significant problem in the management of patients.

Leprosy reactions are acute inflammatory processes occurring over the course of the disease. The reactions affect skin and nerves resulting in physical disability of the patients. There are two types of leprosy reaction. Type 1 reaction (reversal reaction, RR) is the development of acute erythema and the swelling of existing skin lesions due to the cell-mediate immunity. Type 2 reaction (erythema nodosum leprosum, ENL) is the appearance of skin nodules due to the

formation of immune complexes in the humoral immunity. Reaction episodes can take place at any time during the treatment course and can be aggravated by stress, infection, or pregnancy [1, 2].

Physical disabilities caused by leprosy reactions result from nerve damage during immunological processes. The high frequency of neuritis leads to significant morbidity. The most important strategies to prevent disability are early diagnosis and treatment of both leprosy and its reactions and the provision of education to the patients [3]. To be successful in this issue, it is important to discover the risks of developing leprosy reactions.

Despite a large number of leprosy cases, publication of data concerning leprosy reactions has been limited. The information about reactions in Thailand is incomplete and scant. The purpose of this study is to identify the risk factors of leprosy reactions and to provide the epidemiological data and clinical characteristics of the patients presenting to the leprosy clinic, Ramathibodi Hospital, Thailand, between March 1995 and April 2015.

2. Material and Methods

This was a retrospective study conducted at the Division of Dermatology, Ramathibodi Hospital, Mahidol University, Bangkok, Thailand. The study was approved by the Mahidol University Institutional Review Board for Ethics in Human Research and was conducted in accordance with the Declaration of Helsinki.

We reviewed the medical records of leprosy patients registered at the leprosy clinic of Ramathibodi Hospital between March 1995 and April 2015 and excluded those of incomplete medical records. Clinical and demographic data were collected from the records and evaluated by simple descriptive analysis.

In the present study, treatment regimens followed the modified WHO-recommended MDT. Paucibacillary (PB) patients received rifampicin and dapsone for 6 months, while multibacillary (MB) patients were treated with rifampicin, dapsone, and clofazimine for 24 months. Release from treatment (RFT) period was the follow-up period after completion of MDT up to 5 years. Late RR was defined as a development of RR after 6 months of MDT completion. Recurrent reaction was defined as recurrence of leprosy reaction (RR or ENL) more than 6 weeks after completing the treatment of previous reaction.

The statistical analysis was performed using IBM SPSS Statistics version 21.0. Descriptive analysis was used for the baseline characteristics. Univariate and multivariate analyses of factors correlated with leprosy reaction were performed using the binary logistic regression model. Variables with a p value less than or equal to 0.2 in the univariate analysis were included in the multivariate analysis. Correlations were expressed as an odds ratio (OR) and as a 95% confidence interval. A p value less than 0.05 was considered to be statistically significant.

3. Results

Of the 137 cases in the leprosy clinic, 29 patients were excluded because of incomplete medical records and loss of follow-up. One hundred and eight patients were eligible for this study.

The demographic and clinical characteristics of the patients were summarized in Table 1. The patients were 57 females (52.8%) and 51 males (47.2%). The range of ages was 21 to 71 years with a mean age of 45. Fifty-nine patients lived in Bangkok, the capital city, and 7 patients had a history of leprosy contact. Borderline tuberculoid (BT) was the most common clinical form of leprosy, followed by borderline lepromatous (BL), lepromatous (LL), tuberculoid (TT), indeterminate (I), and borderline borderline (BB) forms, respectively. The bacillary index (BI) value was positive in 59 patients with a mean BI value of 3.4. According to the types of MDT received, the MB cases were 53.7%, while the PB cases were 46.3%.

TABLE 1: Epidemiological characteristics and background clinical status.

	Number	Percentage
Age range	21–71 (mean = 45 years)	
Gender		
Male	51	47.2%
Female	57	52.8%
Residence		
Bangkok	59	54.6%
Other areas	49	45.4%
History of leprosy contact		
Yes	7	6.5%
No	101	94.5%
Clinical form of leprosy		
TT	19	17.6%
BT	35	32.4%
BB	2	1.9%
BL	28	25.9%
LL	20	18.5%
I	4	3.7%
BI status at diagnosis		
Negative	49	45.4%
Positive	59	54.6%
Treatment regimen		
PB	50	46.3%
MB	58	53.7%
Leprosy reaction		
No reaction	47	43.5%
Yes	61	56.5%
Reversal reaction	42	38.9%
ENL	19	17.6%
Total 108 patients		

The characteristics of leprosy reactions in our study were shown in Table 2. The reactions were documented in 61 cases (56.5%) and were predominant in the female patients. The average time to develop leprosy reaction was 8.9 months after starting treatment. Most reactions occurred in more than 6 to 12 months, during MDT treatment (34.4%). Type 1 reaction (RR) occurred more often than type 2 (ENL). BT leprosy was the form that most frequently developed leprosy reactions (Figure 1). Of the 42 patients with RR, 28 patients had evidence of skin reactions only, and the remaining 14 had both skin and nerve involvement, whereas in patients having ENL 11 had cutaneous involvement and the remaining 8 had skin and nerve involvement. Thirteen patients were diagnosed with reactions on the first visit, before the MDT treatment. Late reversal reactions were observed in 4 patients (6.6%). Nineteen patients (31.2%) experienced recurrent leprosy reactions which continued for up to 2 years.

For the univariate analysis, BI status and treatment regimen were significant risk factors for leprosy reactions (both had p value = 0.01). The following variables were included in the multivariate analysis (Table 3): female gender, history of

TABLE 2: Characteristics of leprosy reactions.

	Number	Percentage
Average time to develop reaction	8.9 months	
Onset of reaction		
At first diagnosis	13	21.3%
During MDT	44	72.1%
0–6 months	12	19.7%
>6–12 months	21	34.4%
>12 months	11	18%
After release from treatment	4	6.6%
0–6 months	—	
>6–12 months	3	5%
>12 months	1	1.6%
Gender		
Female	37	60.6%
Male	24	39.4%
Leprosy reaction		
Reversal reaction	42	68.8%
ENL	19	31.2%
Organ involvement in reaction		
Cutaneous	39	63.9%
Reversal reaction	28	45.9%
ENL	11	18%
Cutaneous and neuritis	22	36.1%
Reversal reaction	14	22.9%
ENL	8	13.2%
Recurrent reaction		
Yes	19	31.2%
No	42	68.8%
Total 61 patients		

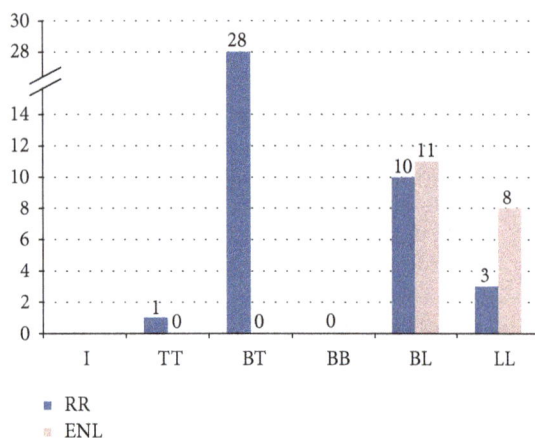

FIGURE 1: Distribution of the patients with leprosy reactions according to the clinical form.

leprosy contact, clinical presentation of BL and LL, positive BI status, and MB treatment regimen. When using multivariate analysis, female gender, positive BI status at diagnosis, and MB treatment regimen were risk factors for development of leprosy reactions (p value = 0.014, 0.004, and 0.012, resp.) (Table 4).

4. Discussion

Leprosy reactions are serious complications among leprosy patients. The reactions cause permanent nerve damage, resulting in disability and deformities. To prevent this morbidity, it is important to discover the risk of developing leprosy reactions. This study reported the epidemiological data, clinical characteristics, and risk factors to develop leprosy reactions in the patients registered at the leprosy clinic, Ramathibodi Hospital, Thailand, between March 1995 and April 2015.

The transmission of leprosy is person to person and depends on individual immunological conditions [4, 5]. Interestingly, our study reported that only six patients had a history of leprosy contact. The possible explanation could be disease transmission from patients with subclinical or unrecognized disease. For the type of leprosy, BT was the most common clinical form found in our study. This was consistent with the previous study in Thailand [6]. Our study reported that BB had the lowest prevalence. It is due to the fact that BB is the most unstable form of leprosy [7].

The frequency of leprosy reactions has been studied by several authors. In the present study, leprosy reactions occurred in 61 patients (56.5%). Most of the patients developed the reactions during the treatment and reactions were more prevalent in the patients treated with the MB regimen. The reactions in our study were predominantly in the RR category (68.8%). This is in contrast to the study from Thailand in 1994, when Scollard et al. reported that ENL was more prevalent than RR [8, 9]. ENL reactions were reported to occur in more than 50% of leprosy cases in the pre-MDT era [10]. The incidence of ENL reactions appears to have fallen with the use of the MDT regimen because of the combination of the bactericidal effect and the anti-inflammatory effect in MDT [11]. The varied frequencies of ENL could be due to the subjects in the studies, patients in the field, and patients reporting to the hospitals. Due to the use of widely different case definitions, it is difficult to compare the frequencies of leprosy reactions from different centers. Other factors contributing to the variation could be the duration of MDT, duration of the steroid regimen, and quality of the local leprosy control program.

Leprosy reactions were commonly found during the MDT and sometimes after release from treatment. Our study revealed that the reactions frequently developed in more than 6 to 12 months, during MDT. The average time to reaction was 8.9 months. The finding is in agreement with previous studies that leprosy reactions occur most frequently within 6 to 12 months after starting treatment [12]. The mechanism of leprosy reaction developing after treatment could be the intense release of microbial antigens due to the antibacterial action of MDT. However, most previous studies, including the present study, did not report a long term follow-up period. Because the leprosy reactions can also be observed at

TABLE 3: Univariate analysis.

Variables	Reaction			Odds ratio	95% CI	p value
	Yes	No	n			
Age range						
0–35	34	24	58	1.21	0.56–2.58	0.62
>35	27	23	50			
Gender						
Female	37	20	57	2.08	0.96–4.51	0.06*
Male	24	27	51			
Residence						
Bangkok	31	28	59	0.7	0.32–1.51	0.36
Other areas	30	19	49			
History of leprosy contact						
Yes	6	1	7	5.02	0.58–43.21	0.10*
No	55	46	101			
Clinical form of leprosy						
Tuberculoid (TT and BT)	29	25	54			
Lepromatous (BL and LL)	32	16	48	1.72	0.77–3.85	0.20*
I and BB	0	6	6			
BI status at diagnosis						
Negative	28	21	49			
Positive	33	26	59	2.65	1.24–5.65	0.01*
Treatment regimen						
PB	22	28	50			
MB	39	19	58	2.61	1.19–5.71	0.01*

*Including multivariate analysis.

TABLE 4: Multivariate analysis.

Variables	Odds ratio	95% CI	p value
Female gender	1.87	1.05–3.31	0.014*
History of leprosy contact	3.69	0.67–14.21	1.00
Lepromatous (BL and LL)	1.2	0.84–1.35	0.84
Positive BI status	1.75	1.19–2.56	0.004*
MB treatment regimen	1.45	1.06–4.21	0.012*

*Statistically significant.

the first diagnostic visit, this shows that the reactions are not necessarily only the result of the treatment. In our study, 13 patients were diagnosed with reactions at the time of the first visit. These findings are in agreement with previous studies from India [13]. This may be explained by the genetic susceptibility regarding the previous reports [14, 15].

Regarding the clinical form of leprosy, our study reported greater prevalence in the group classified as lepromatous end (BL and LL). This association could be explained by the fact that there were more cases in the study, and it related immunological response to the infection due to bacterial load and higher exposure to organisms.

In leprosy reactions, the involvement of the skin and nerves occurred either singly or together. Our study found that cutaneous involvement developed more often than involvement of both skin and nerves. The observations emphasize that neuritis can occur along with inflammatory skin lesions or independently. Examination of nerves should be performed on each visit to detect early signs of nerve inflammation, regardless of the presence or absence of any skin reaction.

Late reversal reaction occurs mostly within the first 3 to 4 years after completing the treatment [16, 17]. In our study, late RR developed in 4 patients (6.6%) and the time taken to develop that ranged between 8 months and 3 years after treatment. In the absence of a clear definition for late RR and because of the different MDT regimens used in various studies, an exact comparison of the frequencies is not possible.

Recurrent episodes of leprosy reactions are an important clinical phenomenon, which may result in continuing nerve damage and add to the degree of impairment. Our study reported that 31.2% of patients had recurrent episodes which continued for up to 2 years. To prevent the consequences, patients must be informed of the possibility and be educated to return for follow-up assessment. In addition, physicians should be aware of the need to diagnose even late reactions in the long term follow-up period.

From the multivariate analysis, risk factors for leprosy reactions identified to be significant in this study were sex, BI status, and treatment regimens. Females were at greater risk of developing leprosy reactions than males. Positive BI status patients and MB treated patients showed a higher tendency towards leprosy reactions. These results were similar to those of the study by Kumar et al. [13].

The most important limitation in this study is the small number of patients, which may therefore not allow correlation to be established with confidence. Another limitation is incomplete data due to the retrospective design of the study. Because our hospital is a tertiary referral center, the population in our study may not represent the general population. Some patients were referred with atypical symptoms or were susceptible to leprosy reactions. Finally, the follow-up time in our study was too short to evaluate the long term outcomes. To minimize the impact of these limitations, prospective long term studies using a large number of patients should be performed in the future.

In conclusion, this is the study of leprosy patients from the leprosy clinic, Ramathibodi Hospital, Thailand. Reversal reaction and erythema nodosum leprosum are common complications in leprosy patients. Female gender, a positive bacteriological index, and an MB treatment regimen were found to be the main risk factors for the occurrence of leprosy reactions. Although leprosy was expected to be eliminated by 2005, those patients who have successfully completed treatment still continue to develop late or recurrent leprosy reactions. Early detection in cases where risk factors exist and prompt treatment could prevent the disabilities that cause suffering to leprosy patients and their families.

Conflict of Interests

The authors declare that there is no conflict of interests regarding the publication of this paper.

References

[1] J. Cuevas, J. L. Rodríguez-Peralto, R. Carrillo, and F. Contreras, "Erythema nodosum leprosum: reactional leprosy," *Seminars in Cutaneous Medicine and Surgery*, vol. 26, no. 2, pp. 126–130, 2007.

[2] A. P. Ustianowski, S. D. Lawn, and D. N. Lockwood, "Interactions between HIV infection and leprosy: a paradox," *The Lancet Infectious Diseases*, vol. 6, no. 6, pp. 350–360, 2006.

[3] D. N. J. Lockwood and B. Kumar, "Treatment of leprosy," *British Medical Journal*, vol. 328, no. 7454, pp. 1447–1448, 2004.

[4] L. R. S. Kerr-Pontes, M. L. Barreto, C. M. N. Evangelista, L. C. Rodrigues, J. Heukelbach, and H. Feldmeier, "Socioeconomic, environmental, and behavioural risk factors for leprosy in North-east Brazil: results of a case-control study," *International Journal of Epidemiology*, vol. 35, no. 4, pp. 994–1000, 2006.

[5] D. N. J. Lockwood and S. Suneetha, "Leprosy: too complex a disease for a simple elimination paradigm," *Bulletin of the World Health Organization*, vol. 83, no. 3, pp. 230–235, 2005.

[6] S. Kananurak, "Positive of slit skin smear on new case detecton of leprosy patients at Raj Pracha Samasai Institute, 2002–2006," *Journal of Raj Pracha Samasai Institute*, vol. 3, pp. 167–175, 2006.

[7] G. O. Penna, A. M. Pinheiro, L. S. C. Nogueira, L. R. de Carvalho, M. B. B. De Oliveira, and V. P. Carreiro, "Clinical and epidemiological study of leprosy cases in the university Hospital of Brasília: 20 years—1985 to 2005," *Revista da Sociedade Brasileira de Medicina Tropical*, vol. 41, no. 6, pp. 575–580, 2008.

[8] D. M. Scollard, T. Smith, L. Bhoopat, C. Theetranont, S. Rangdaeng, and D. M. Morens, "Epidemiologic characteristics of leprosy reactions," *International Journal of Leprosy and Other Mycobacterial Diseases*, vol. 62, no. 4, pp. 559–567, 1994.

[9] D. M. Scollard, C. M. T. Martelli, M. M. A. Stefani et al., "Risk factors for leprosy reactions in three endemic countries," *The American Journal of Tropical Medicine and Hygiene*, vol. 92, no. 1, pp. 108–114, 2015.

[10] D. N. J. Lockwood, "The management of erythema nodosum leprosum: current and future options," *Leprosy Review*, vol. 67, no. 4, pp. 253–259, 1996.

[11] D. N. J. Lockwood and H. H. Sinha, "Pregnancy and leprosy: a comprehensive literature review," *International Journal of Leprosy and Other Mycobacterial Diseases*, vol. 67, no. 1, pp. 6–12, 1999.

[12] B. Naafs, J. M. H. Pearson, and H. W. Wheate, "Reversal reaction: the prevention of permanent nerve damage. Comparison of short and long-term steroid treatment," *International Journal of Leprosy*, vol. 47, no. 1, pp. 7–12, 1979.

[13] B. Kumar, S. Dogra, and I. Kaur, "Epidemiological characteristics of leprosy reactions: 15 years experience from North India," *International Journal of Leprosy and Other Mycobacterial Diseases*, vol. 72, no. 2, pp. 125–133, 2004.

[14] A. L. M. Sousa, V. M. Fava, L. H. Sampaio et al., "Genetic and immunological evidence implicates interleukin 6 as a susceptibility gene for leprosy type 2 reaction," *The Journal of Infectious Diseases*, vol. 205, no. 9, pp. 1417–1424, 2012.

[15] B. R. Sapkota, M. Macdonald, W. R. Berrington et al., "Association of TNF, MBL, and VDR polymorphisms with leprosy phenotypes," *Human Immunology*, vol. 71, no. 10, pp. 992–998, 2010.

[16] M. Becx-Bleumink and D. Berhe, "Occurrence of reactions, their diagnosis and management in leprosy patients treated with multidrug therapy; Experience in the leprosy control program of the All Africa Leprosy and Rehabilitation Training Center (ALERT) in Ethiopia," *International Journal of Leprosy and Other Mycobacterial Diseases*, vol. 60, no. 2, pp. 173–184, 1992.

[17] P. A. M. Schreuder, "The occurrence of reactions and impairments in leprosy: experience in the leprosy control program of three provinces in northeastern Thailand, 1987—1995 [correction of 1978-1995]. I. Overview of the study," *International Journal of Leprosy and Other Mycobacterial Diseases*, vol. 66, no. 2, pp. 159–169, 1998.

34

Five-Year Retrospective Review of Acute Generalized Exanthematous Pustulosis

Chitprapassorn Thienvibul, Vasanop Vachiramon, and Kumutnart Chanprapaph

Division of Dermatology, Faculty of Medicine, Ramathibodi Hospital, Mahidol University, Bangkok 10400, Thailand

Correspondence should be addressed to Kumutnart Chanprapaph; kumutnartp@hotmail.com

Academic Editor: Jean Kanitakis

Background. Acute generalized exanthematous pustulosis (AGEP) is an acute pustular eruption characterized by widespread nonfollicular sterile pustules. The aim of this study is to characterize the etiology, clinical features, laboratory findings, management, and outcome of patients with AGEP in Asians. *Patient/Methods.* A retrospective analysis was performed on patient who presented with AGEP between August 2008 and November 2012 in a tertiary center in Thailand. *Results.* Nineteen patients with AGEP were included. AGEP was generally distributed in seventeen patients (89.5%) and localized in two (10.5%). Fever and neutrophilia occurred in 52.6% and 68.4%, respectively. Hepatitis was found up to 26.3%. The most common etiology was drugs (94.7%), comprising of antibiotics (73.6%), proton pump inhibitors (10.5%), nonsteroidal anti-inflammatory drugs (5.3%), and herbal medicine (5.3%). Beta-lactams were the most common causal drug, particularly carbapenems and cephalosporins. This is the first report of *Andrographis paniculata* as an offending agent for AGEP. We found no differences between various treatment regimens (topical corticosteroid, systemic corticosteroid, and supportive treatment) regarding the time from drug cessation to pustules resolution ($P = 0.171$). *Conclusions.* We have highlighted the presentation of AGEP among Asians. We found high association with systemic drugs. Carbapenems were one of the leading culprit drugs. Finally, a localized variant was observed.

1. Introduction

Acute generalized exanthematous pustulosis (AGEP) is a pustular reaction characterized by an abrupt onset of numerous nonfollicular sterile pustules, arising within an erythematous and edematous background. It is rare with the reported incidence of one to five cases per million people per year [1]. The etiology includes systemic drugs (>90% of cases reported) especially antibiotics such as penicillin and macrolides, hypersensitivity to mercury, virus, contact dermatitis, and spider bite [2]. In this study, we described the demographic data, the etiologies, clinical features, laboratory findings, and management of patients with AGEP diagnosed in a tertiary hospital in Thailand.

2. Methods

2.1. Study Population.
The medical records of 19 patients diagnosed with AGEP treated at Ramathibodi Hospital,

Mahidol University, Bangkok, Thailand, from August 2008 and November 2012 were retrospectively reviewed. Patients 18 years of age and above who had definite or probable diagnosis of AGEP (final score ≥ 5) according to the grading system proposed by the study group of the European study of Severe Cutaneous Adverse Reactions (EuroSCAR) (Table 1) and with available histological data at the time of diagnosis were included in the study [1]. Patients who had psoriasis or pustular psoriasis confirmed histologically were excluded from the study.

2.2. Statistical Analysis.
Statistical analyses were performed using computer software (SPSS version 18; SPSS Inc., Chicago, IL). Categorical variables (e.g., gender, prior drug allergy, distribution, culprit drug, clinical findings, and laboratory abnormalities) are expressed in percentage. Continuous variables (e.g., drug-AGEP latent period and resolution time) are reported as median. To compare various treatment regimens

TABLE 1: Acute generalized exanthematous pustulosis validation score of the EuroSCAR study group [1].

Morphology	Score
Pustules	
Typical	2
Compatible	1
Insufficient	0
Erythema	
Typical	2
Compatible	1
Insufficient	0
Distribution/pattern	
Typical	2
Compatible	1
Insufficient	0
Pustular desquamation	
Yes	1
No/insufficient	0
Course	
Mucosal involvement	
Yes	−2
No	0
Acute onset (<10 d)	
Yes	0
No	−2
Resolution (<15 d)	
Yes	0
No	−4
Fever > 38°C	
Yes	1
No	0
Neutrophils > 7,000/mm	
Yes	1
No	0
Histology	
Other diseases	−10
Not representative/no histopathology	0
Exocytosis of neutrophils	1
Subcorneal and/or intraepidermal nonspongiform or unspecified pustule(s) with papillary edema or subcorneal and/or intraepidermal spongiform or unspecified pustules(s) without papillary edema	2
Spongiform subcorneal and/or intraepidermal pustule(s) with papillary edema	3

Interpretation: <0: no AGEP, 1–4: possible, 5–7: probable, and 8–12: definite.

in correlation to the time of disease regression, ANOVA test was used. A *P* value of <0.05 was considered statistically significant.

3. Results

From August 2008 and November 2012, 25 patients of AGEP were identified. Nineteen patients had definite or probable diagnosis of AGEP according to the EuroSCAR AGEP validation score (final score ≥ 5). Fourteen patients had scores consistent with definite diagnosis and 5 patients were classified as probable cases of AGEP. Six cases classified as possible AGEP were excluded. The details of all patients and their reported comorbidities are summarized in Table 2. Of the 19 cases, ten (52.6%) were female and nine (47.4%) were male. The age ranged from 19 to 84 years, mean age of 52 years. None of the patients had personal or family history of psoriasis.

Systemic drugs were the most common etiology. The criteria proposed by Naranjo et al. were used to identify the culprit drug [3]. The most frequent culprit was antibiotics in 14 patients (73.7%). Omeprazole was the offending drug in two patients (10.5%). Celecoxib and herbal drug, namely, the *Andrographis paniculata*, were the implicated medication in one patient. Among the culprit antibiotics, beta-lactams were the most common causal drug, particularly carbapenems and cephalosporins (3 patients each). One patient did not have history of drug exposure and had symptoms and signs suggesting viral infection such as fever, rhinorrhea, nasal congestion, cervical lymphadenopathy, myalgia, and arthralgia prior to skin eruption. The etiologies of AGEP in this study are shown in Figure 1. The latent period of drug administration before the onset of symptoms ranged from 1 hour to 25 days (median 3 days).

All patients presented with nonfollicular, pinpoint, and superficial pustules on erythematous background (Figure 2), which were generally distributed in 17 of the patients (Figure 3(a)). The remaining 2 patients had localized lesions on the face (Figure 4) and the upper back, respectively. Fever was presented in 10 patients (52.6%). Facial edema was observed in 6 patients (31.6%). Three patients (15.8%) had at least one area (oral, ocular) of mucosal involvement. Pustules which coalesced to form pus-filled bullae resulted in cutaneous erosion in one patient. Resolution of pustules with desquamation (Figure 3(b)) was seen in 17 patients (89.5%). Cervical lymphadenopathy was observed in 2 patients.

Thirteen patients (68.4%) had associated leukocytosis (normal 4,000–10,000/μL) and neutrophilia. Two patients (10.5%) had eosinophilia (eosinophil count ≥ 500/μL or above 10% if the leukocyte count was lower than 4,000/μL). Five patients (26.3%) had hepatocellular involvement (the highest level of serum aspartate aminotransferase and/or alanine aminotransferase exceeded two times the upper normal limit) which resolved later upon drug discontinuation and pustules resolution. None of the patients had other systemic involvement such as renal and pulmonary. Pus gram stain was performed in 12 patients and revealed numerous neutrophils without organism. Skin biopsy was carried out in every patient. All showed subcorneal pustules or intraepidermal pustules filled with neutrophils and some showed papillary dermal edema. Clinical characteristics and laboratory findings are summarized in Table 3.

TABLE 2: Patient data (demographics, underlying disease, drug exposure, onset of symptoms, EuroSCAR AGEP validation, and therapy).

Patient	Age (years)/ sex	Drug allergy history	Comorbidities	Possible etiology and duration between drug initiation and AGEP	EuroSCAR score	Therapy
1	28/F	No	Cervical carcinoma stage IIIb	Omeprazole (15 days)	8	Topical steroid
2	84/M	No	Pulmonary tuberculosis, diverticular bleeding	Isoniazid, rifampicin, pyrazinamide, and ethambutol (16 days)	10	Supportive
3	73/M	No	COPD, pulmonary tuberculosis	Amoxicillin (3 days)	8	Topical steroid
4	38/F	Yes	Submucous myoma, hyperthyroidism	Clindamycin (1 day)	9	Supportive
5	74/F	No	Subarachnoid hemorrhage	Meropenem (4 days)	8	Oral prednisolone
6	48/F	No	Cervical carcinoma stage IIIb	Celecoxib (11 days)	7	Topical steroid
7	38/F	No	Ruptured appendicitis, Graves' disease	Ceftriaxone (2 days)	8	Topical steroid
8	65/M	No	Congestive heart failure	Piperacillin/tazobactam Levofloxacin (4 days)	7	Oral prednisolone
9	45/M	No	Accidental fingers amputation	Cefazolin (2 days)	8	Oral prednisolone
10	71/F	Yes	Rheumatoid arthritis, subacute lupus erythematosus, and lymph node tuberculosis	Clindamycin (2 days)	9	Topical steroid
11	53/M	No	Atypical mycobacterial infection	Amikacin, clarithromycin, levofloxacin, and imipenem (25 days)	9	Oral prednisolone
12	33/F	Yes	Morbid obesity post-Roux-en-Y gastrojejunostomy, carcinoma of the ovary	Omeprazole (3 days)	9	Topical steroid
13	68/F	No	Renal failure, old stroke, and sepsis with pancytopenia	Meropenem (1 hour)	8	Topical steroid
14	38/M	Yes	No	Amoxicillin (2 days)	9	Oral prednisolone
15	31/M	No	Upper respiratory tract infection	Herbal medicine (1 day)	6	Topical steroid
16	73/M	No	Chronic kidney disease with infected arteriovenous fistula	Vancomycin (21 days)	7	Topical steroid
17	76/M	No	Double-vessel disease admitting for coronary artery bypass graft	Imipenem (4 days)	6	Topical steroid
18	19/F	No	Donor for liver transplantation	Cefoxitin (3 days)	8	Topical steroid
19	36/M	No	No	Viral infection	9	Oral prednisolone

COPD, chronic obstructive pulmonary disease.

Four patients had history of cutaneous adverse drug reaction. Three patients had recurrent AGEP and one had prior exanthematous drug eruption. Two patients had past history of beta-lactam-induced AGEP. The first patient previously had AGEP from penicillin and developed AGEP the second time from clindamycin. The other had the first and second episodes of AGEP from ampicillin and amoxicillin, respectively. One patient had multiple recurrent AGEP from numerous medications (amoxicillin, dicloxacillin, piroxicam, diclofenac, and omeprazole) and this time developed AGEP from omeprazole. Given that the same medication (omeprazole) was commenced in several events, proton pump inhibitor is believed to be the culprit drug on these occasions. One patient had maculopapular rash due to cinnarizine, acetazolamide, isoniazid, and rifampicin and developed AGEP this time from clindamycin.

Sixteen cases were hospitalized and 3 patients were seen at an outpatient department. Most cases (11 patients) were treated with topical corticosteroid. Six patients were given oral prednisolone, which were patients with extensive cutaneous diseases and/or systemic involvement such as hepatitis. The remaining 2 patients received supportive care. The median duration of drug cessation to resolution of pustules was 3 days (2–12 days). There was one patient

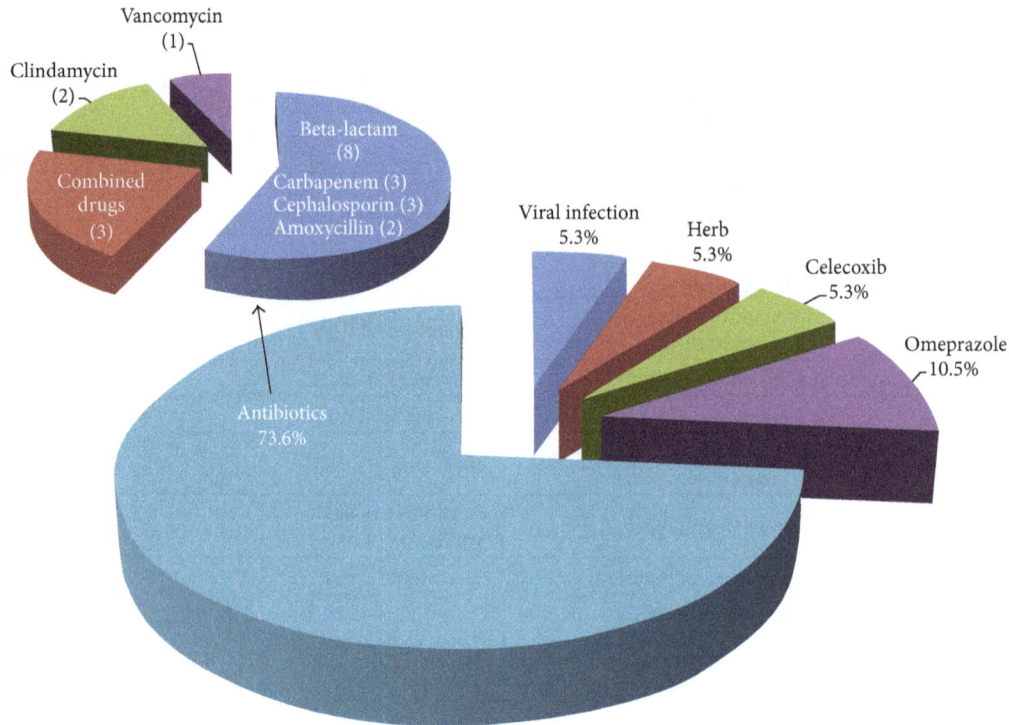

FIGURE 1: The etiology of acute generalized exanthematous pustulosis (AGEP) in this study.

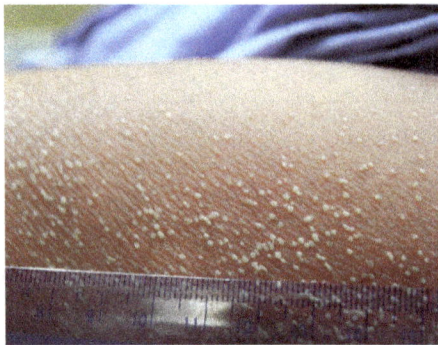

FIGURE 2: Nonfollicular, pinpoint, and superficial pustules on an erythematous background.

who had vancomycin-induced AGEP with exceptionally long resolution time of 12 days. This patient has chronic kidney disease stage 4 which leads to longer drug clearance time.

There were no differences between various treatment regimens regarding the median duration of medication cessation to resolution of pustules which were 2 days for topical corticosteroid, 3 days for oral prednisolone, and 2.5 days for supportive care (P = 0.171). One patient had protected clinical course and developed generalized erythema and desquamation necessitating gradual tapering of systemic steroids. Another patient had erosions on the back which turned into ulcers and required further wound care.

4. Discussion

We present here the first case series of AGEP in Thailand. The most common etiology for AGEP was beta-lactams antibiotics. Among these, carbapenems has emerged as one of the leading causes of AGEP, reflecting the increasing use of broad-spectrum antibiotics. We also present the first report of a herbal drug, namely, *Andrographis paniculata*, to be the offending agent for AGEP.

Our study revealed no sexual predominance, in agreement with the previous two large series [4, 5]. A high association with systemic drugs was found in this study (94.7%), similar to a large report by Roujeau et al. (87%) [4]. However, this is in contrast to two series done in Korea and Taiwan which found lower association with systemic drugs, 63.8% and 62.5%, respectively [6].

Antibiotics were the leading cause of AGEP (73.7%), followed by omeprazole (10.5%), celecoxib (5.3%), and herbal drug (5.3%). Interestingly, a more recent antibiotic implicated for drug resistant nosocomial infection in the carbapenem group, such as imipenem and meropenem, was found to be the cause of AGEP in 3 patients (15.8%). This may reflect drugs commonly given in a tertiary care setting.

Herbal drug was the cause of AGEP in one patient. *Andrographis paniculata*, in the family Acanthaceae, or Fa-thalai-chon in the Thai language, is one of the most popular medicinal plants used in traditional medicine in various Asian countries. Its aerial parts, roots, and whole plant have been used for centuries for the treatment of various ailments such as fever, sore throat, cough, and stomachache and as

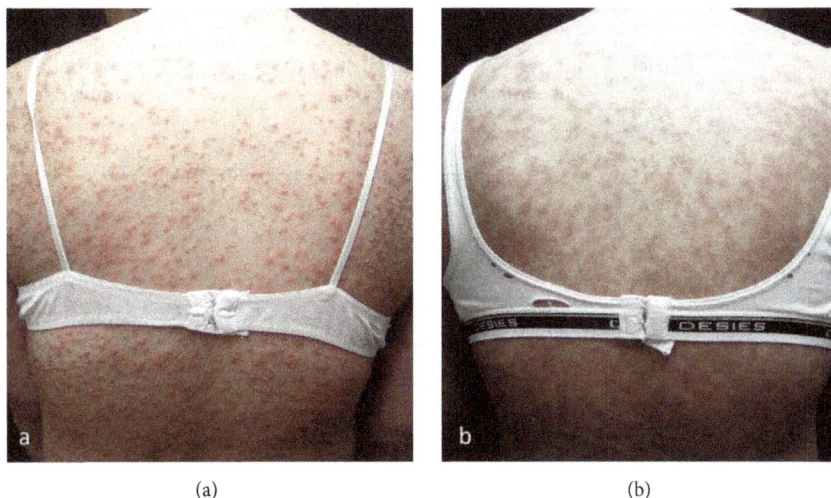

(a)   (b)

FIGURE 3: (a) Numerous small superficial pustules on erythematous base in a patient with AGEP. (b) Erythema and desquamation 3 days after discontinuation of culprit drug, and administration of systemic corticosteroid.

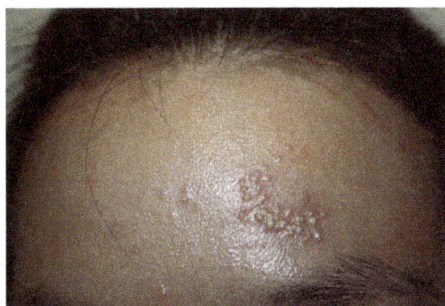

FIGURE 4: A 31-year-old female presented with ALEP on the face 1 day after taking herbal medicine.

antidiabetic and antioxidant agents [7, 8]. To the best of our knowledge, AGEP due to this herb has never been reported before. However, because it is commonly used in Asia, especially Thailand, and AGEP is a self-limiting disease, this particular side-effect might have been underestimated.

Viral infection was the suspected cause of AGEP in one patient based on the clinical presentation and peripheral blood picture profile; however, viral serology was not performed. Reports have shown that enterovirus, adenovirus, parvovirus B19, Epstein-Barr virus, cytomegalovirus, and hepatitis B virus were related to AGEP [9].

The pathophysiology of AGEP appears to be delayed type hypersensitivity to a specific drug. After exposure to the causative agent, activation of specific CD4 and CD8 occurs. These T cells then migrate to the skin and the drug-specific CD8 T cells use perforin/granzyme B and Fas ligand to cause keratinocytes apoptosis resulting in epidermal vesicle formation. Drug-specific T cells (mainly) and keratinocytes (to a lesser extent) produce CXCL8 (IL-8), a potent neutrophil-attracting chemokine, which leads to neutrophil accumulation within the vesicles. Moreover, interferon gamma

and granulocyte/macrophage colony-stimulating factor are enhanced which help increase the survival of neutrophils and augment the formation of neutrophil accumulation [10, 11]. Peripheral blood of AGEP patients shows increase in circulating Th (T helper) 17, as Th17 produces IL-17 and IL-22, which have synergistic effect on the production of CXCL8 by keratinocytes and further direct neutrophil aggregation [11, 12]. In addition, systemic involvement in AGEP such as hepatitis may be due to circulating IL-17 and IL-22 [13]. IL-22 is detected in many inflammatory diseases [13]. However, the exact mechanism of AGEP remains uncertain. Patch test and lymphocytic transformation test are promising diagnostic tests for this type of drug hypersensitivity. Although not a part of the EuroSCAR validation score, it has been well known that patch testing could induce dermatologic reaction with corresponding drug and could be one of the features of AGEP [14, 15].

In this study, the median latent period between drug initiation and skin eruption was 3 days (1 hour–25 days). However, the interval of more than 10 days was found in 5 patients. Two of these patients received omeprazole and celecoxib, which were nonantibiotics. This supports data from a previous study that drugs other than antibiotics had longer time between the administration of suspected drug and the onset of skin eruption [4]. In general, the short interval between drug administration and the development of rash in AGEP is probably from prior sensitization and/or an immune recall phenomenon induced by T cell reactivation. Therefore, patients are more likely to have had a lifetime exposure to antibiotics or to drugs of similar structures than from nonantibiotics. In another patient where omeprazole was the suspected culprit, the drug was commenced 3 days before the development of AGEP; however, this patient had previous recurrent AGEP from many kinds of drugs including omeprazole. The pattern with a short interval again is probably due to previous sensitization. The remaining 3

TABLE 3: Clinical characteristics and laboratory findings.

Pt.	Distribution	Fever	Facial edema	Oral involvement	Conjunctival involvement	Desquamation	Neutrophil count (/mL)	Eo	Hepatitis
1	Abdomen, arms, and ankles	−	−	−	−	+	4,602	−	−
2	Face, back, and upper chest	+	−	−	−	+	7,106	−	−
3	Face, axillae, and trunk	−	+	−	−	+	9,516	−	−
4	Face, trunk, arms, and legs	+	+	−	−	+	14,490	−	−
5	Abdomen, back	−	−	−	−	+	15,486	−	+
6	Face, trunk, arms, and legs	−	+	−	−	+	6,295	−	−
7	Trunk, hands, and feet	−	−	−	−	+	10,030	−	−
8	Neck, upper chest, and back	−	−	−	−	+	3,552	−	−
9	Axillae, groins, lateral trunk, inner thighs, and volar surfaces of arms	+	−	−	−	+	3,472	10% (WBC 5,260)	+
10	Proximal extremities	+	−	−	−	+	18,620	−	−
11	Chest, back, and intertriginous areas	+	−	−	−	+	13,975	−	+
12	Inframammary areas, lateral trunk, lower abdomen, and upper thighs	+	−	−	−	+	9,672	−	−
13	Inframammary areas, groins, and axillae	+	−	+	−	+	814	33% (WBC 1,480)	−
14	Face, trunk, and extremities (about 90% BSA)	+	+	−	+	+	11,025	−	+
15	Face	−	−	−	−	−	4,838	−	−
16	Face, neck, trunk, and proximal extremities	+	+	−	−	+	7,241	−	−
17	Upper back	−	−	−	−	−	9,316	−	−
18	Back, groins	−	−	−	−	+	11,398	−	−
19	Trunk, extremities	+	+	+	+	+	11,808	−	+

Remark: +, present; −, absent; Pt., patient; BSA, body surface area; WBC, white blood cells; Eo, eosinophils.

patients that had long incubation period from the start of drug to the development of skin symptoms could result from primary sensitization.

Localized lesions of AGEP were found in two patients, one on the face and one on the upper back. Prange and colleagues first defined acute localized exanthematous pustulosis (ALEP) in 2005 [16]. They suggested that ALEP was a variant of AGEP both clinically and histopathologically, localized to the flexural areas, face, neck, or chest.

Other less common features such as facial edema, mucosal involvement, blister, and erosion, which were found in our series, have been described previously [2, 4, 9, 17, 18]. Resolution of pustules with desquamation was found in all patients except for patients with localized lesions.

Fever (52.6%) and neutrophilia (68.4%) were detected lower than previous studies [4, 9, 17]. Eosinophilia was found in 10.5% corresponding to a previous report [9]. Hepatitis was found in 26.3% which was higher than prior reports [4, 6, 13]. Therefore, systemic involvement especially hepatitis should not be overlooked in patients with AGEP and withdrawal of the implicated drug is essential to avoid further hepatic injury.

History of prior cutaneous adverse drug reaction was detected in 4 patients (21.1%), comprising AGEP in 3 and maculopapular rash in 1. Recurrent AGEP is rarely reported in the literature. The major culprit drugs to cause recurrence are beta-lactam antibiotics, which is in consistence with an early report [19]. Herein, we also report another case with recurrent AGEP possibly from omeprazole.

The diagnosis of AGEP is determined on morphology, clinical presentation, laboratory data, and histopathology. Several diagnostic criteria have been proposed and a well-recognized scoring system elaborated by EuroSCAR project has been used in this study [1].

The differential diagnoses include generalized pustular psoriasis of Von Zumbusch, pustular vasculitis, pustular Sweet's syndrome, autoimmune blistering disease, and pustular eruption from infections such as bacterial folliculitis, dermatophyte, candida infection, herpes, and varicella infection. Although most can be excluded without difficulty, some may be a diagnostic challenge especially differentiating between AGEP and generalized pustular psoriasis [20].

Due to the self-limited and benign nature of this disease, treatment is usually not necessary except for symptomatic therapy and discontinuation of the offending drugs. However, in certain patients, the clinical course may be extensive and protracted necessitating systemic corticosteroids [17]. In this study, we found no differences between various treatment regimens (topical corticosteroid, systemic corticosteroid, and supportive treatment) regarding the duration of medication cessation to the resolution of pustules (P = 0.171). The clinical outcome was good in almost all patients. Only one patient had generalized erythema and desquamation requiring gradual tapering of systemic corticosteroid. Another patient with morbid-obesity had erosions on the back which ulcerated and required further wound care.

The limitations of this study are its retrospective nature and small number of subjects. Nevertheless, given the rarity of AGEP, large-scale studies are limited. Patch testing was not done as a part of the workup of AGEP.

Ethical Approval

This study received approval from the Mahidol University Institution Review Board (IRB) for human subject research (Protocol number 035645).

Consent

Informed consent was exempted by the Mahidol University Institution Review Board (IRB).

Conflict of Interests

The authors declare that there is no conflict of interests regarding the publication of this paper.

References

[1] A. Sidoroff, S. Halevy, J. N. B. Bavinck, L. Vaillant, and J.-C. Roujeau, "Acute generalized exanthematous pustulosis (AGEP)—a clinical reaction pattern," *Journal of Cutaneous Pathology*, vol. 28, no. 3, pp. 113–119, 2001.

[2] M. M. Speeckaert, R. Speeckaert, J. Lambert, and L. Brochez, "Acute generalized exanthematous pustulosis: an overview of the clinical, immunological and diagnostic concepts," *European Journal of Dermatology*, vol. 20, no. 4, pp. 425–433, 2010.

[3] C. A. Naranjo, U. Busto, E. M. Sellers et al., "A method for estimating the probability of adverse drug reactions," *Clinical Pharmacology and Therapeutics*, vol. 30, no. 2, pp. 239–245, 1981.

[4] J.-C. Roujeau, P. Bioulac-Sage, C. Bourseau et al., "Acute generalized exanthematous pustulosis. Analysis of 63 cases," *Archives of Dermatology*, vol. 127, no. 9, pp. 1333–1338, 1991.

[5] M. J. Choi, H. S. Kim, H. J. Park et al., "Clinicopathologic manifestations of 36 Korean patients with acute generalized exanthematous pustulosis: a case series and review of the literature," *Annals of Dermatology*, vol. 22, no. 2, pp. 163–169, 2010.

[6] S.-L. Chang, Y.-H. Huang, C.-H. Yang, S. Hu, and H.-S. Hong, "Clinical manifestations and characteristics of patients with acute generalized exanthematous pustulosis in Asia," *Acta Dermato-Venereologica*, vol. 88, no. 4, pp. 363–365, 2008.

[7] A. Okhuarobo, J. Ehizogie Falodun, O. Erharuyi, V. Imieje, A. Falodun, and P. Langer, "Harnessing the medicinal properties of *Andrographis paniculata* for diseases and beyond: a review of its phytochemistry and pharmacology," *Asian Pacific Journal of Tropical Disease*, vol. 4, no. 3, pp. 213–222, 2014.

[8] S. Chotchoungchatchai, P. Saralamp, T. Jenjittikul, S. Pornsiripongse, and S. Prathanturarug, "Medicinal plants used with Thai traditional medicine in modern healthcare services: a case study in Kabchoeng Hospital, Surin Province, Thailand," *Journal of Ethnopharmacology*, vol. 141, no. 1, pp. 193–205, 2012.

[9] E. Guevara-Gutierrez, E. Uribe-jimenez, M. Diaz-Canchola, and A. Tlacuilo-Parra, "Acute generalized exanthematous pustulosis: report of 12 cases and literature review," *International Journal of Dermatology*, vol. 48, no. 3, pp. 253–258, 2009.

[10] M. Britschgi and W. J. Pichler, "Acute generalized exanthematous pustulosis, a clue to neutrophil-mediated inflammatory processes orchestrated by T cells," *Current Opinion in Allergy and Clinical Immunology*, vol. 2, no. 4, pp. 325–331, 2002.

[11] J. Szatkowski and R. A. Schwartz, "Acute generalized exanthematous pustulosis (AGEP): a review and update," *Journal of the American Academy of Dermatology*, vol. 73, no. 5, pp. 843–848, 2015.

[12] R. Kabashima, K. Sugita, Y. Sawada, R. Hino, M. Nakamura, and Y. Tokura, "Increased circulating Th17 frequencies and serum IL-22 levels in patients with acute generalized exanthematous pustulosis," *Journal of the European Academy of Dermatology and Venereology*, vol. 25, no. 4, pp. 485–488, 2011.

[13] C. Hotz, L. Valeyrie-Allanore, C. Haddad et al., "Systemic involvement of acute generalized exanthematous pustulosis: a retrospective study on 58 patients," *British Journal of Dermatology*, vol. 169, no. 6, pp. 1223–1232, 2013.

[14] A. Barbaud, E. Collet, B. Milpied et al., "A multicentre study to determine the value and safety of drug patch tests for the three main classes of severe cutaneous adverse drug reactions," *British Journal of Dermatology*, vol. 168, no. 3, pp. 555–562, 2013.

[15] V. Jan, L. Machet, N. Gironet et al., "Acute generalized exanthematous pustulosis induced by diltiazem: value of patch testing," *Dermatology*, vol. 197, no. 3, pp. 274–275, 1998.

[16] B. Prange, A. Marini, A. Kalke, N. Hodzic-Avdagic, T. Ruzicka, and U. R. Hengge, "Acute localized exanthematous pustulosis (ALEP)," *Journal of the German Society of Dermatology*, vol. 3, no. 3, pp. 210–212, 2005.

[17] H. Y. Lee, D. Chou, S. M. Pang, and T. Thirumoorthy, "Acute generalized exanthematous pustulosis: analysis of cases managed in a tertiary hospital in Singapore," *International Journal of Dermatology*, vol. 49, no. 5, pp. 507–512, 2010.

[18] A. Sidoroff, A. Dunant, C. Viboud et al., "Risk factors for acute generalized exanthematous pustulosis (AGEP)—results of a multinational case-control study (EuroSCAR)," *British Journal of Dermatology*, vol. 157, no. 5, pp. 989–996, 2007.

[19] V. Mysore and A. Ghuloom, "A case of recurrent acute generalized exanthematous pustulosis due to beta-lactam antibiotics: a case report," *Journal of Dermatological Treatment*, vol. 14, no. 1, pp. 54–56, 2003.

[20] L. Duckworth, M. B. Maheshwari, and M. A. Thomson, "A diagnostic challenge: acute generalized exanthematous pustulosis or pustular psoriasis due to terbinafine," *Clinical and Experimental Dermatology*, vol. 37, no. 1, pp. 24–27, 2012.

Permissions

List of Contributors

Adilson Costa
Service of Dermatology of the Pontifical Catholic University of Campinas, Campinas, SP, Brazil
KOLderma Clinical Trials Institute, Campinas, SP, Brazil

Aline Siqueira Talarico, Carla de Oliveira Parra Duarte, Caroline Silva Pereira, Ellem Tatiani de Souza Weimann, Lissa Sabino de Matos, Livia Carolina Della Coletta, Maria Carolina Fidelis and Thaísa Saddi Tannous
Service of Dermatology of the Pontifical Catholic University of Campinas, Campinas, SP, Brazil

Cidia Vasconcellos
Department of Dermatology of the University of Sao Paulo, Sao Paulo, SP, Brazil

Doaa Salah Hegab
Faculty of Medicine, Dermatology and Venereology Department, Tanta University Hospitals, El Geish Street, Tanta, Gharbia Governorate 31111, Egypt

Mohammed Abd El Rahman Sweilam
Faculty of Medicine, Clinical Pathology Department, Tanta University Hospitals, El Geish Street, Tanta, Gharbia Governorate 31111, Egypt

Angeline Bhalerao
General Practice, Ipswich, Suffolk IP4 5PD, UK

Gurdeep S. Mannu
Oxford University Hospitals, Oxford OX3 9DU, UK

Asmaa M. Ele-Refaei and Fatma M. El-Esawy
Dermatology & Andrology Department, Faculty of Medicine, Benha University, Benha, Egypt

Hussein Mohamed Hassab-El-Naby, Yasser Fathy Mohamed, Hamed Mohamed Abdo, Mohamed Ismail Kamel and Osama Khalil Mohamed
Al-Hussein University Hospital, Gawhar Al Qaed Street, El Darrasa, Cairo 11633, Egypt
Dermatology, Venereology and Andrology, Faculty of Medicine, Al-Azhar University, Cairo 11823, Egypt

Wael Refaat Hablas
Al-Hussein University Hospital, Gawhar Al Qaed Street, El Darrasa, Cairo 11633, Egypt
Clinical and Chemical Pathology, Faculty of Medicine, Al-Azhar University, Cairo 11823, Egypt

Rafaela Koehler Zanella
Mãe de Deus Health System, Rua Soledade 569, 90470-340 Porto Alegre, RS, Brazil

Denis Souto Valente and Alexandre Vontobel Padoin
Graduate Program in Medicine and Health Sciences, School of Medicine, PUCRS (FAMED), Avenida Ipiranga 6681, 90619-900 Porto Alegre, RS, Brazil

Leo Francisco Doncatto
ULBRA School of Medicine, Lutheran University of Brazil (ULBRA), Avenida Farroupilha 8001, 92425-900 Canoas, RS, Brazil

Daniele Dos Santos Rossi and Aline Grimaldi Lerias
School of Medicine, PUCRS (FAMED), Avenida Ipiranga 6681, 90619-900 Porto Alegre, RS, Brazil

W. Nie and A. M. Deters
Westfalian Wilhelms University of Muenster, Institute for Pharmaceutical Biology and Phytochemistry, Hittorfstraße 56, 48149 Muenster, Germany

Mark Gorman and Andrew Hart
Canniesburn Plastic Surgery Unit, Glasgow Royal Infirmary, UK

Bipin Mathew
Hull Royal Infirmary, Hull, UK

Akiko Kamimura and Jennifer Tabler
Department of Sociology, University of Utah, Salt Lake City, UT 84112, USA

Maziar M. Nourian
School of Medicine, University of Utah, Salt Lake City, UT 84132, USA

Jeanie Ashby
Maliheh Free Clinic, Salt Lake City, UT 84107, USA

Ha Ngoc Trinh
Department of Sociology, Vietnam National University, Hanoi, Vietnam
Department of Sociology, University of Utah, Salt Lake City, UT 84112, USA

Nushean Assasnik
Health Society and Policy, University of Utah, Salt Lake City, UT 84112, USA

Bethany K. H. Lewis
Department of Dermatology, University of Utah, Salt Lake City, UT 84132, USA

Naveen Kumar, Satheesha Nayak Badagabettu and Sudarshan Surendran
Department of Anatomy, Melaka Manipal Medical College, Manipal University, Manipal Campus, Manipal 576104, India

Pramod Kumar
King Abdul Aziz Hospital, Al Jouf 42421, Saudi Arabia

Ranjini Kudva
Department of Pathology, Kasturba Medical College, Manipal, Manipal University, Manipal 576104, India

Murali Adiga
Department of Physiology, Kasturba Medical College, Manipal, Manipal University, Manipal 576104, India

M. R. Yaghoobi-Ershadi, N. Marvi-Moghadam, A. A. Akhavan and A. R. Zahrai-Ramazani
Department of Medical Entomology and Vector Control, School of Public Health, Tehran University of Medical Sciences, Tehran, Iran

R. Jafari and M. H. Arandian
Isfahan Research Station, National Institute of Health Research, Isfahan, Iran

H. Solimani
Yazd Health Research Station, National Institute of Health Research, Yazd, Iran

A. R. Dehghan-Dehnavi
School of Public Health, Yazd University of Medical Sciences, Yazd, Iran

Ana Filipa Pedrosa and Filomena Azevedo
Department of Dermatology and Venereology, Centro Hospitalar São João EPE Porto, Alameda Prof. Hernani Monteiro, 4200-319 Porto, Portugal

Paulo Morais and Carmen Lisboa
Faculty of Medicine, University of Porto, Alameda Prof. Hernani Monteiro, 4200-319 Porto, Portugal

Seyran Ozbas Gok and Emine Dervis
Department of Dermatology, Haseki Training and Research Hospital, 34080 Istanbul, Turkey

Asli Akin Belli
Department of Dermatology, Mugla Sitki Kocman University Training and Research Hospital, 48000 Mugla, Turkey

Christine Sävervall and Freja Lærke Sand
Department of Dermatology, Bispebjerg Hospital, 2400 Copenhagen NV, Denmark

Simon Francis Thomsen
Department of Dermatology, Bispebjerg Hospital, 2400 Copenhagen NV, Denmark
Center for Medical Research Methodology, Department of Biomedical Sciences, University of Copenhagen, 2200 Copenhagen N, Denmark

Jawaher Masmoudi, Rim Sellami, Uta Ouali, Leila Mnif, Ines Feki and Abdellaziz Jaoua
Department of Psychiatry A, Hédi Chaker University Hospital, Sfax, Tunisia

Mariam Amouri and Hamida Turki
Department of Dermatology, Hédi Chaker University Hospital, Sfax, Tunisia

Doaa Salah Hegab
Faculty of Medicine, Dermatology and Venereology Department, Tanta University Hospitals, El Geish Street, Tanta 31111, Egypt

Mohamed Attia Saad Attia
Faculty of Medicine, Clinical Pathology Department, Tanta University Hospitals, El Geish Street, Tanta 31111, Egypt

Abbas Darjani, Kiarash Mohammad Amini, Javad Golchai, Shahryar Sadre-Eshkevari and Narges Alizade
Department of Dermatology, Medical Faculty of Guilan University, Rasht, Iran

Zahra Mohtasham-Amiri
Department of Preventive and Community Medicine, Medical Faculty of Guilan University, 4163545851 Rasht, Iran

Hossein Kavoussi and Ali Ebrahimi
Dermatology Department, Imam Reza Hospital, Kermanshah University of Medical Sciences (KUMS), Kermanshah 6714415333, Iran

Mansour Rezaei
Health School, Family Health Research Center of Kermanshah University of Medical Sciences (KUMS), Kermanshah 6714415333, Iran

Katayoun Derakhshandeh and Alireza Moradi
Department of Pharmaceutics, School of Pharmacy, Hamadan University of Medical Sciences, Hamadan, Iran

Harif Rashidian and Reza Kavoussi
Kermanshah University of Medical Sciences (KUMS), Kermanshah 6714415333, Iran

Cody J. Connor
Department of Family Medicine, Broadlawns Medical Center, Des Moines, IA 50314, USA
Carver College of Medicine, University of Iowa, Iowa City, IA 52242, USA

Vincent Liu
Department of Dermatology, University of Iowa, Iowa City, IA 52242, USA
Department of Pathology, University of Iowa, Iowa City, IA 52242, USA

Jess G. Fiedorowicz
Department of Psychiatry, University of Iowa, Iowa City, IA 52242, USA
Department of Internal Medicine, University of Iowa, Iowa City, IA 52242, USA
Department of Epidemiology, College of Public Health, University of Iowa, Iowa City, IA 52242, USA

Alejandra García-Hernández, Rodrigo Roldán-Marín, Pablo Iglesias-Garcia and Josep Malvehy
Melanoma Unit, Dermatology Department, Hospital Clínic, C/Villaroel 170, 08036 Barcelona, Spain

Glynis Ablon
Ablon Skin Institute Research Center, Manhattan Beach, CA 90266, USA

Mamadou Kaloga, Ildevert Patrice Gbéry, Yao Isidore Kouassi, Elidjé Joseph Ecra, Sarah Kourouma, Kouadio Celestin Ahogo, Kouassi Alexandre Kouamé, Komenan Kassi, Kanga Kouame and Abdoulaye Sangaré
Department of Dermatology and Venereology, Teaching Hospital of Treichville, Abidjan, Côte d'Ivoire

Vagamon Bamba and Almamy Diabate
Department of Dermatology and Venereology, Teaching Hospital of Bouaké, Côte d'Ivoire

Joslyn S. Kirby, Elizabeth V. Seiverling and Sara Ferguson
Department of Dermatology, Penn State Milton S. Hershey Medical Center, Hershey, PA 17033, USA

Thomas Scharnitz
Penn State College of Medicine, Hershey, PA 17033, USA

Hadjh Ahrns
Department of Family and Community Medicine, Penn State Milton S. Hershey Medical Center, Hershey, PA 17033, USA

G. L. Morley and J. H. Matthews
College of Medical and Dental Sciences, University of Birmingham, Edgbaston, Birmingham B15 2TT, UK

I. Verpetinske
Russells Hall Hospital, Pensnett Road, Dudley, West Midlands DY1 2HQ, UK

G. A. Thom
Royal Perth Hospital, 197Wellington Street, Perth, WA 6000, Australia

R. M. Robati and F. Abdollahimajd
Skin Research Center, Shahid Beheshti University of Medical Sciences, Shohada-e Tajrish Hospital, Shahrdari Sreet, Tehran 1989934148, Iran

A.M. Robati
Department of Surgery, Bam University of Medical Sciences, Bam, Iran

Jillian W. Millsop
University of Utah, School of Medicine, 30 N 1900 E, Salt Lake City, UT 84132, USA

Raja K. Sivamani and Nasim Fazel
University of California, Davis, Department of Dermatology, 3301 C Street, Sacramento, CA 95816, USA

Kostas Kalokasidis
Dermatology and Laser Clinic, 88 Tsimiski Street, 54622 Thessaloniki, Greece

Meltem Onder
Dermatology and Laser Center, Reduitstrare 13, 76829 Landau, Germany
Gazi University Medical Faculty, Department of Dermatology, 06510 Ankara, Turkey

Myrto-Georgia Trakatelli
Aristotle University School of Medicine, Second Department of Dermatology and Venereology, 54622 Thessaloniki, Greece

Bertrand Richert
Université Libre de Bruxelles, Department CHU Brugmann-Saint Pierre, 1050 Brussels, Belgium

Klaus Fritz
Dermatology and Laser Center, Reduitstrare 13, 76829 Landau, Germany
Carol Davila University of Medicine, Dionisie Lupu Street, 020021 Bucharest, Romania
Osnabrueck University, Sedanstraße 115, 49090 Osnabrueck, Germany
Bern University, Department of Dermatology, 117 Inselspital, 3010 Bern, Switzerland

Deepak Dimri
Department of Dermatology, Veer Chandra Singh Garhwali Government Medical Science and Research Institute, Uttarakhand 246174, India

Arti Gupta and Amit Kumar Singh
Department of Community Medicine, Veer Chandra Singh Garhwali Government Medical Science and Research Institute, Uttarakhand 246174, India

Yalda Nahidi and Naser Tayyebi Meibodi
Skin Research Center, School of Medicine, Mashhad University of Medical Sciences, Mashhad 9176699199, Iran

Zahra Meshkat
Virology Research Center, School of Medicine, Mashhad University of Medical Sciences, Mashhad 9176699199, Iran

Narges Nazeri
Pathology Department of Mashhad University of Medical Sciences, Mashhad 9176699199, Iran

Javier F. Boyas
School of Social Work, University of Alabama, Box 870314, Tuscaloosa, AL 35487,USA

Vinayak K. Nahar
Department of Health, Exercise Science & Recreation Management, University of Mississippi, 215 Turner Center, P.O. Box 1848, University, MS 38677, USA
Department of Dermatology, University of Mississippi Medical Center, 2500 N. State Street, Jackson, MS 39216, USA

Robert T. Brodell
Department of Dermatology, University of Mississippi Medical Center, 2500 N. State Street, Jackson, MS 39216, USA
Department of Pathology, University of Mississippi Medical Center, 2500 N. State Street, Jackson, MS 39216, USA
Department of Dermatology, University of Rochester School of Medicine and Dentistry, Rochester, NY 14642, USA

Kirti Deo, Yugal K. Sharma, Meenakshi Wadhokar and Neha Tyagi
Department of Dermatology, Dr. D. Y. Patil Medical College and Hospital and Research Centre, Pimpri, Pune, Maharashtra 411018, India

Tanawatt Kootiratrakarn, Kowit Kampirapap and Chakkrapong Chunhasewee
Institute of Dermatology, Bangkok 10400, Thailand

Poonkiat Suchonwanit, Siripich Triamchaisri, Sanchawan Wittayakornrerk and Ploysyne Rattanakaemakorn
Division of Dermatology, Department of Medicine, Faculty of Medicine, Ramathibodi Hospital, Mahidol University, Bangkok 10400,Thailand

Chitprapassorn Thienvibul, Vasanop Vachiramon and Kumutnart Chanprapaph
Division of Dermatology, Faculty of Medicine, Ramathibodi Hospital, Mahidol University, Bangkok 10400, Thailand

www.ingramcontent.com/pod-product-compliance
Lightning Source LLC
Chambersburg PA
CBHW080524200326
41458CB00012B/4321